GENERAL TOXICOLOGY

Dr. Chebli Akli Islam

ALLIED HEALTH PRESS

General Toxicology

Author: **Dr. Chebli Akli Islam**

Allied Health Press
4164 Lakeshore Road
Burlington ON L7L 1A4
Canada
www.alliedhealthpress.com
Email: orders@arclereducation.com

ISBN: 978-1-77956-247-0

ABOUT THE AUTHOR

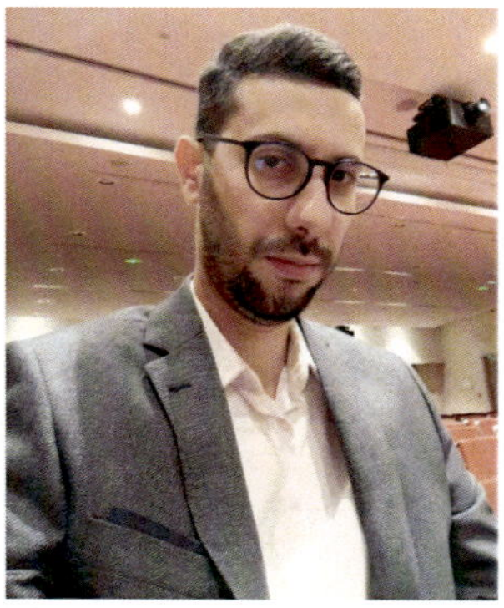

Dr. Chebli Akli Islam, PharmD, and holder of a PhD in Toxicology, epitomizes excellence in the field of hospital-university research. As a researcher at the University of Constantine, Faculty of Medicine, he passionately dedicates himself to studying various aspects of toxicology, including medicolegal, clinical, kinetic, food, and environmental toxicology. With over 10 years of experience, Dr. Chebli Akli Islam has cultivated expertise in a multitude of toxicological domains. His academic and professional career showcases an unwavering commitment to advancing knowledge in the field of toxicology. Dr. Chebli Akli Islam not only earned a pharmacy degree but also deepened his skills by pursuing a PhD in Toxicology, demonstrating his dedication to academic and scientific excellence. As a hospital-university researcher, Dr. Chebli Akli Islam tackles critical issues related to toxicology, such as toxic risk assessment in various contexts, identification of harmful substances in food and environmental products, and innovative solutions to mitigate the adverse effects of toxins on human health. His multidisciplinary expertise enables him to address the complex challenges of toxicology from different angles, ranging from clinical data analysis to the search for practical solutions to prevent poisonings and improve treatment protocols. Within the academic and scientific community, Dr. Chebli Akli Islam is recognized for his dedication to teaching and mentoring students, thereby inspiring future generations of researchers and healthcare professionals to pursue excellence in the field of toxicology. With his ambitious vision and unwavering commitment to scientific research, Dr. Chebli Akli Islam has become a prominent figure in the field of toxicology, making significant contributions to the safety and well-being of society.

Word Roots, Prefixes, and Suffixes by Chapter

Chapter 1 Introduction to Toxicology

Tox-: Poison or toxic substance (e.g., toxin, toxic).

Chem-: Chemical (e.g., chemical, chemotaxis).

Path-: Disease or suffering (e.g., pathology, pathogen).

Pharm-: Drug or medicine (e.g., pharmacology, pharmaceutical).

Anti-: Against (e.g., antidote, antitoxin).

Hyper-: Excessive or above normal (e.g., hypertoxic, hypersensitivity).

Hypo-: Below normal or deficient (e.g., hypotoxic, hypoglycemia).

-ology: Study of (e.g., toxicology, pharmacology).

-toxicity: The quality or state of being toxic (e.g., cytotoxicity, hepatotoxicity).

-gen: Producing or causing (e.g., carcinogen, mutagen).

-path: Disease or disorder (e.g., neuropath, pathogen).

Chapter 2 Different Classes of Toxicants and Their Characteristics: An Overview

Tox-: Poison, toxin

Pharmaco-: Drug or medicine

Chem-: Chemical

Carcin-: Cancer

Gen-: To produce or generate

Anti-: Against

Hyper-: Over, excessive

Sub-: Under, below

Pre-: Before

Chapter 3 Reproductive Toxicology

Tox - Poison or harmful substance

Repro - Related to reproduction

Gen - Origin or creation

Mut - Change

Terat - Monster or malformation

Embry - Embryo

Anti- - Against or opposing

Hyper- - Excessive or above normal

Hypo- - Under or below normal

Post- - After

-genesis - Formation or origin

-toxicity - The quality of being toxic

Chapter 4 Properties and Effects of Toxicity of Pesticides

Chem: Refers to chemistry or chemicals.

Pest: Refers to pests or harmful organisms.

Path: Refers to disease or suffering

Pharm: Refers to drugs or medicine.

Anti-: Against or opposing.

De-: Down, away, or reverse.

Hypo-: Under or below normal.

Hyper-: Over or excessive.

Pre-: Before or in advance.

-icide: Refers to killing.

-tox: Refers to poison or harmful effects.

Chapter 5 Exploring Environmental Toxicology: Understanding the Impact of Pollutants on Ecosystem and Human Health

Tox- (Greek: "poison")

Chem- (Greek: "chemistry")

Bio- (Greek: "life")

Ec- (Greek: "house, environment")

Path- (Greek: "disease")

Pollut- (Latin: "to make dirty")

Hyper- (Greek: "over, excessive")

Pre- (Latin: "before")

-ity (Latin: "quality of")

-logy (Greek: "study of")

-ation (Latin: "action or process")

-al (Latin: "pertaining to")

-ous (Latin: "full of")

Chapter 6 Toxicity and Mechanisms of Occupational Pollutants

Path (from Greek "pathos" meaning suffering or disease)

Expos (from Latin "expositus" meaning exposed)

Rad (from Latin "radius" meaning ray)

Carcin (from Greek "karkinos" meaning cancer)

Hyper- (over, above)

Inter- (between)

Over- (excessive)

-osis (condition or process)

-itis (inflammation)

-emia (blood condition)

Chapter 7 Properties and Effects of Natural Toxins and Venoms

Tox: From Greek "toxikon" meaning poison.

Ven: From Latin "venenum" meaning poison.

Nox: From Latin "noxa" meaning harm or injury.

Anti-: Against.

De-: Down, away, reverse.

Neo-: New.

-ic: Pertaining to.

-ous: Full of.

-ide: Used in chemistry to denote a compound.

Chapter 8 Toxicology and Their Impact on Human Health

Tox- (Toxic, Toxicity)

Bio- (Biotoxic)

Pharmaco- (Pharmacology, Pharmaceutics)

Anti- (Antidote, Antitoxin)

Hyper- (Hypertoxicity)

Sub- (Sublethal)

-ic (Toxicic)

-osis (Nephrosis)

-gen (Carcinogen)

Chapter 9 Prevention and Mitigation of Toxic Effects

Tox- / Toxic-: Poison

Therap-: Treatment

Protect-: To shield or guard

Prevent-: To stop something from happening

Mitig-: To make less severe

Anti-: Against, opposing

De-: Down, away, reverse

Pre-: Before, prior to

Pro-: For, in favor of

Non-: Not

-ic: Pertaining to

-al: Relating to

-ation: The action or process of

-ize: To make or become

-ate: To cause or perform an action

Table of Contents

6 Toxicity and Mechanisms of Occupational Pollutants 167

7 Properties and Effects of Natural Toxins and Venoms 185

LIST OF FIGURES

LIST OF TABLES

PREFACE

Toxicology, often described as the "Science of Safety," is an expansive field that not only delves into the adverse effects of chemicals on living organisms and the environment but also aims to mitigate these effects through predictive science and public health initiatives. It has evolved significantly from its origins in studying poisons, now focusing on understanding and preventing potential hazards posed by chemical exposures.

The discipline uses a variety of scientific methods to assess the risks associated with chemical substances. For instance, it is estimated that the global chemical industry exceeds $5 trillion in annual sales, and it introduces 1,000 to 2,000 new chemicals each year, underscoring the critical role of toxicologists in evaluating the safety of these substances. In the United States alone, the Environmental Protection Agency (EPA) oversees the regulation of chemicals under the Toxic Substances Control Act (TSCA), which affects thousands of new and existing chemicals. One of the key achievements in toxicology is the development of methodologies like dose-response assessment, which helps determine the level at which a substance causes harm. For example, the lethal dose (LD50) is a commonly used statistic to measure a substance's toxicity, indicating the dose required to kill half the members of a tested population. Toxicology also plays a crucial role in identifying carcinogens. According to the International Agency for Research on Cancer (IARC), there are more than 120 substances that have been identified as known human carcinogens. This knowledge helps in forming regulatory strategies to limit exposure to such dangerous substances.

The field has greatly benefited from advancements in technology such as bioinformatics and high-throughput screening, which allow for faster and more accurate toxicity testing. These technologies help predict adverse effects more efficiently, reducing the need for animal testing and accelerating the safety assessment process.

General Toxicology provides a comprehensive and foundational understanding of the principles, mechanisms, and effects of toxic substances on living organisms, particularly humans. This textbook is designed to cater to a wide audience, ranging from undergraduate and graduate students in toxicology, pharmacology, and environmental sciences to healthcare professionals and researchers who seek to deepen their understanding of the impact of toxins on health and the environment.

The book aims to equip its readers with the necessary tools to critically analyze the sources, pathways, and biological interactions of various toxins. Covering a broad spectrum of topics, including chemical properties of toxins, exposure routes, risk assessment, and the cellular and molecular basis of toxicity, the textbook serves as a crucial resource for students as they explore the complex interactions between toxic agents and biological systems.

This textbook also provides detailed insights into the latest methodologies and technologies used in the detection and analysis of toxic substances, offering practical skills that are applicable in both academic and professional settings. It is not only to impart theoretical knowledge but also to stimulate critical thinking and encourage a problem-solving approach towards contemporary toxicological challenges. It prepares readers to contribute effectively to the field of toxicology, enhancing their capability to manage and mitigate the effects of toxins in various contexts. This textbook is an invaluable resource for anyone committed to advancing their expertise in toxicology or related fields and for those involved in the development of safer chemicals and environmental practices.

Chapter

INTRODUCTION TO TOXICOLOGY

1

Contents

Introduction

The term "toxicology" has its etymological roots in the Greek words "Toxicon," which refers to "poison," and "logos," which signifies the act of studying or discourse. When combined, these terms evolve into the modern English word "toxicology," which is literally interpreted as the scientific discipline focused on the study of poisons. This field of study extends beyond merely understanding the fundamental chemical and physical properties of toxic substances; it also includes their detection, identification, and the profound impact they have on biological systems. Furthermore, toxicology investigates the treatment and prevention of illness states that arise from exposure to these poisons.

Moreover, the scope of toxicology is broad, encompassing the study of specific adverse effects associated with toxic substances, such as teratogenicity (the ability to cause developmental malformations), carcinogenicity (the capacity to cause cancer), immunotoxicity (the potential to impair immune system function), developmental toxicity (effects on developmental processes), mutagenesis (induction of genetic mutations), neurotoxicity (toxic effects on the nervous system), and endocrine disruption (interference with hormonal systems). These areas of research highlight the diverse and significant impact that toxic substances can have on health and the environment, underscoring the importance of the field in public health and safety (Timbrell & Barile, 2023).

Orientation and Directional Terms

Term	Definition	Illustration
Toxicology	The scientific study of the adverse effects of chemicals or physical agents on living organisms. It encompasses the identification, understanding, and management of toxic substances.	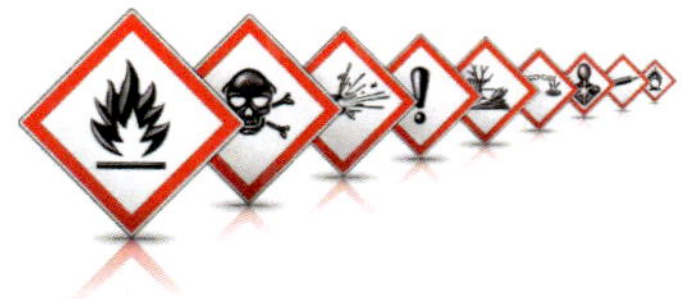
Antiquity	The ancient past, especially the period of classical and early civilizations such as those of Greece and Rome. It generally refers to historical periods prior to the Middle Ages.	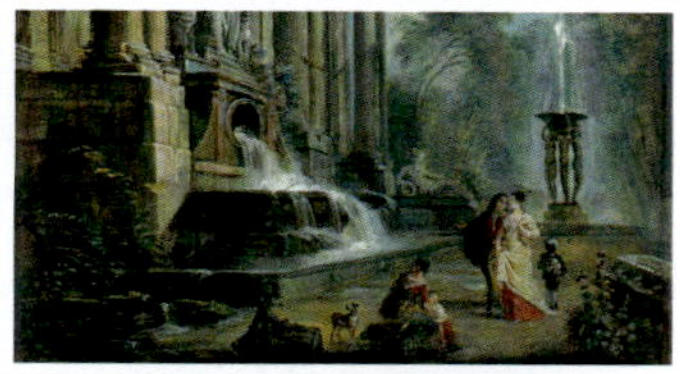
Organ Toxicant	A chemical or substance that specifically targets and causes damage to a particular organ in the body.	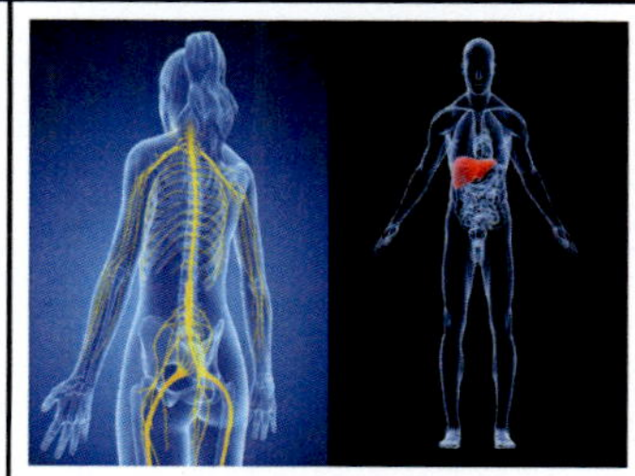
Xenobiotic	A chemical substance that is foreign to a biological system, including drugs, pollutants, and industrial chemicals. These substances can affect the organism in various ways.	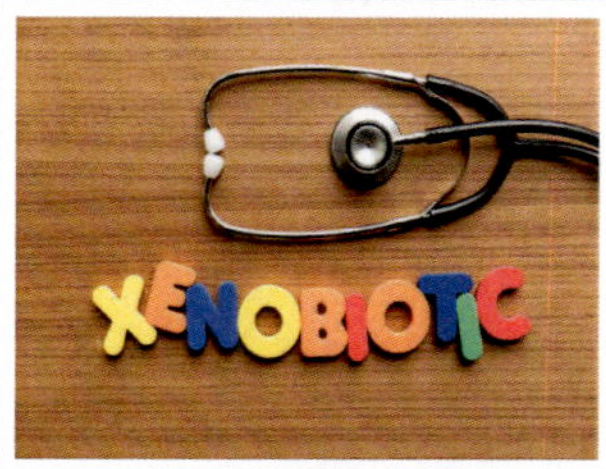
Systemic Toxicant	A toxicant that causes harm throughout the entire body or in multiple organ systems, rather than being localized to a specific area.	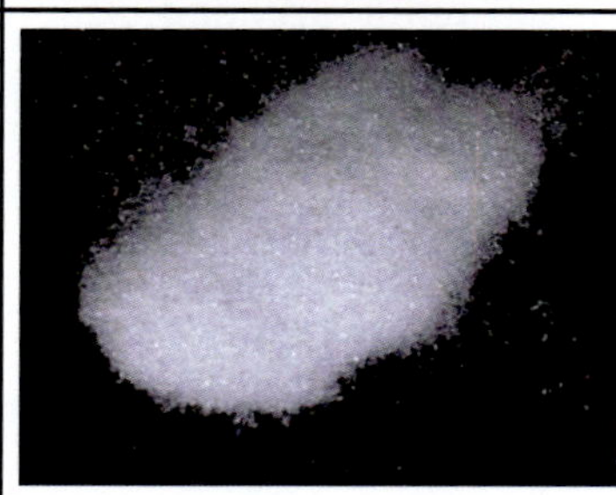

1.1. Historical Background

1.1.1. Antiquity

The understanding of poisons dates to the beginning of human civilization or even further. Toxins that were naturally occurring in plants and animals, along with a few minerals, were the only sources of the first poisons. Hunting was the primary intent behind their use. As "ordeal poisons," some of these substances were utilized, such as amygdalin derived from peach pits and physostigmine derived from *Physostigma venenosum* (also known as Calabar bean). Hunting animals (and sometimes even other people!) was a common practice that involved the use of poisons for arrows and darts. According to Wexler (2018), strophanthin, aconitine, extracts from hellebores, which are a cardiotoxic plant, and torte-nelmi venoms were among the most common types of arrow poisons. Ever since the beginning of time, people have had the knowledge that it is necessary to protect themselves against the potentially harmful effects of both plants and animals. Furthermore, they acquired the knowledge necessary to defeat their adversaries by poisoning them (Borzelleca, 2000).

Some of the earliest sources of information include historical texts, archaeology literature, and ancient publications on myths and legends. It is possible that the Ebers Papyrus, which was used in Egyptian medicine in the past and dates to 1550 BC, is the first medical record that includes such a wide variety of illnesses and treatments. Well-known poisons such as aconite, an old arrow poison, and opium (both as an antidote and as a poison) are among the many of these. According to Ramoutsaki, Ramoutsakis, Tsikritzis, & Tsatsakis (2000), Hippocrates is the "Father of Rational Medicine" (460–375 BC). To provide an ethical framework for the practice of therapies by individuals who are aware of copper, mercury, antimony, lead, and other substances that are poisonous and are at least somewhat familiar with their qualities, a group of medical professionals established the Hippocrates School. When it came to treating poisoning, they suggested using heated oil as a remedy and inducing vomiting to prevent the poisons from being absorbed. Hemlock, which contains the alkaloid coniine, was one of the poisons that was effective during that time period. According to Wexler (2014), the execution of Socrates was carried out with the use of hemlock in the year 470,390 BC. During the year 371 BC, Theophrastus, who was Aristotle's most devoted student, penned an early treatise on the poisons that plants contain. 204,135 BC, Nicander may have been the first person to conduct an experiment in the field of toxicology. In a similar vein, the history of poisonings committed in the name of murder is quite extensive. In 81 BC, Rome passed a law known as the Lex Cornelia, which was one of the earliest laws that prohibited the use of poisons for the purpose of killing (Wexler, 2017).

In the year 4080 AD, the Greek army physician Pedanius Dioscorides classified poisons according to the source from which they originated. Those that are mineral, vegetable, or animal. It is still important to distinguish between the therapeutic properties of natural chemicals and the hazardous properties of natural chemicals. Dioscorides' De Materia Medica, which is one of the most significant herbal publications in history, is a five-volume work that served as the model for all modern pharmacopeias (Clarkson & Magos, 2006).

1.1.2. Middle Ages

Between the fall of the Roman Empire and the publication of Maimonides' (Moses ben Maimon) (11351204) work Treatise on Poisons and Their Antidotes in 1198, a well-known Swiss philosopher, there was a pause in the development of toxicology. In this work, he discussed the treatment of poisonings caused by dogs, insects, and snakes. Poisoning art reached its pinnacle during the early Renaissance period, when Italians, in their customary practicality, brought it to its pinnacle. In addition, the poisoner emerged as a significant figure in the political arena (Walker-Meikle, 2014). Records kept by the city councils of Florence, particularly those kept by the notorious Council of Ten of Venice, contain a wealth of information regarding the political use of poisons. Once the act was carried out, the money was made. The names of the victims, the prices that were going to be charged, and the contracts that were going to be signed were all previously decided upon. According to Marquardt, Schafer, McClellan, & Welsch (1999), during that time period, a woman named Toffana was notorious for selling cosmetics that contained arsenic and consisted of specially formulated ingredients.

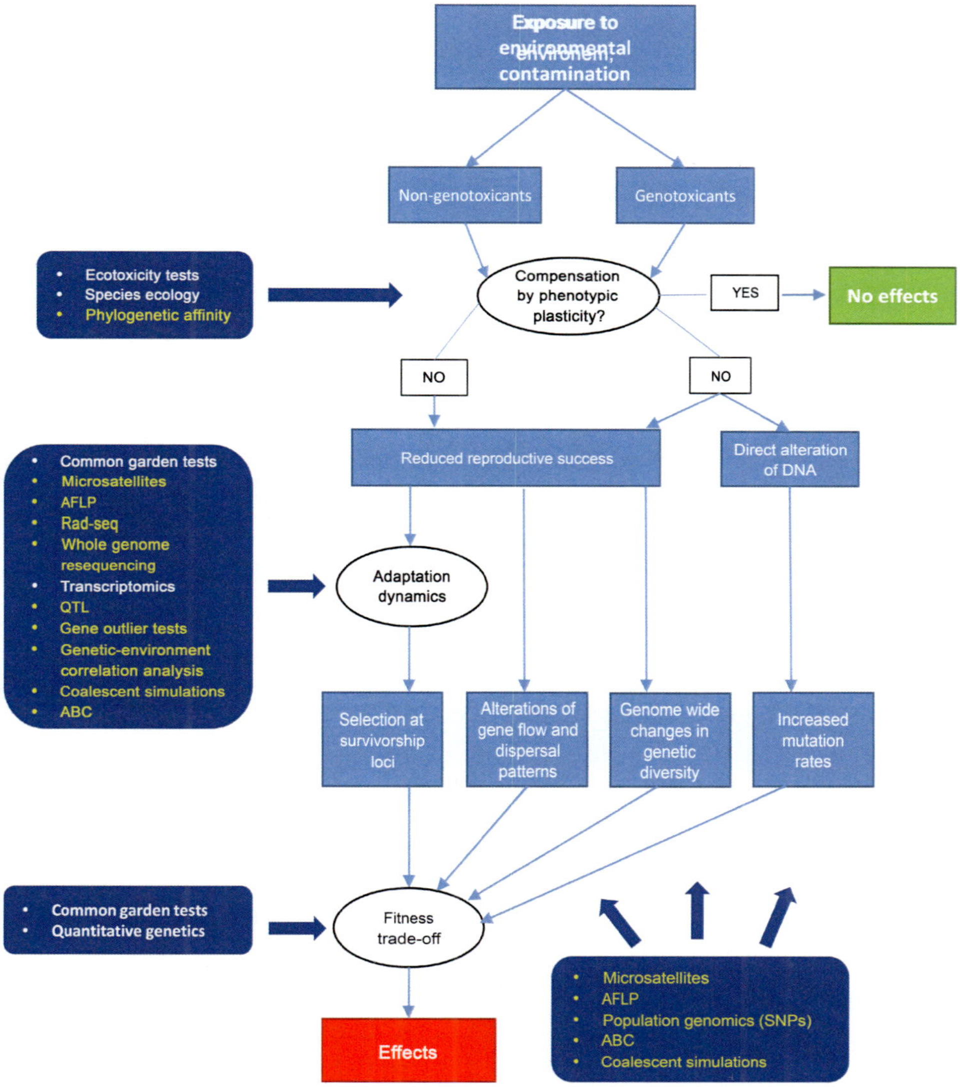

Figure 1.1. *Schematic of evolutionary of toxicology.*

Source: Rusconi, M., Bettinetti, R., Polesello, S., & Stefani, F., (2018). Evolutionary toxicology as a tool to assess the ecotoxicological risk in freshwater ecosystems. Water, 10(4), 490. https://doi.org/10.3390/w10040490.

Regrettably, during this time, the practice of employing poison as a method of murder spread across Europe, particularly in France and Italy, where schools were established to instruct students in the art of poisoning. More than 600 people lost their lives because of Madame Guilia Toffana's use of aqua Toffana, a white arsenic solution. She is one of the most notorious poisoners in history. It was possible to purchase this solution in Italy as a cosmetic. According to Pappas, Massoll, & Cannon (1999), the wave began to spread toward the end of the 16th century.

A wide range of social strata, from Italy to France, made extensive use of poisons as a means of eliminating opponents or individuals deemed undesirable. Throughout the 18th and 19th centuries, there was a persistent problem of criminal poisoning in various parts of the world (Radenkova-Saeva, 2008) (Figure 1.1). This problem took place in several different locations.

1.1.3. Age of Enlightenment

Philippus Aureolus Theophrastus Bombastus von Hohenheim-Paracelsus, a Renaissance man who called himself Paracelsus because he believed that his work went beyond that of Celsus, a Roman physician who lived in the first century and may have been the first to emphasize Toxicon, a toxic agent, as a chemical entity, was a significant figure in the field of science and medicine during the late Middle Ages (Magowska, 2007). The dose-response relationship was something he was familiar with, and he stated in his writings that "there is nothing that is not a poison." To differentiate between remedy and poison, the appropriate dose is required. During his lifetime, Paracelsus put forward several ideas that were considered groundbreaking at the time. These ideas are now considered fundamental concepts in the field of toxicology. He concentrated on Toxicon as a specific primary toxic chemical entity, as opposed to his earlier concentration on mixtures (Houston, 1994). Paracelsus progressed three fundamental ideas:

- To investigate chemical responses, it is necessary to conduct experiments.
- It is important to differentiate between the medicinal and harmful properties of substances.
- The toxic and therapeutic properties are intertwined and differentiated when the dose is taken into consideration.

According to Blaise (1998), it is possible to determine the degree of specificity for substances as well as the harmful and therapeutic effects of those substances.

A relatively new field of study, toxicology, was established through the scientific investigation of many dedicated individuals. Experimentation, rational thought, the relationship between dose and therapies (as opposed to harmful), and chemical responses are the factors that contribute to its development. Recent developments in all of the relevant fields have assisted us in gaining a more in-depth understanding of how harmful substances may influence both people and animals (Barker, 2017). In the year 1783, a German chemist named Friedrich Serturner (17831841) was the first person to successfully isolate a distinct narcotic molecule from opium. He named this molecule morphine, after Morpheus, the Roman god of sleep. After that, Mattie Josesph Benaventura Orfila, a Spanish physician who is frequently referred to as the "Father of Toxicology," established toxicology as a distinct profession and defined toxicology as the study of poisons. According to McCarty (2013), he believed autopsies should be carried out, along with a chemical examination of the viscera, to establish that poisoning was the causal factor in the death. It was his treatise Traite des Poisons, published in 1814, that laid the foundation for forensic toxicology. Between the years 1797 and 1882, one of his students, Robert Christison, published a condensed version of the English text under the title A Treatise on Poisons in the year 1829. In 1848, O. Costill published A Practical Treatise on Poisons, which is the first published treatise on clinical toxicology (Ware & Whitacre, 1994).

The pioneering French physiologist and toxicologist Francois Magendie (1783–1855) discovered the mechanisms of action of quinine, morphine, strychnine, emetine, and other alkaloids. He is known as the "Father of Experimental Pharmacology." Magendie lived from 1783 until 1855. By taking up man's investigation of arrow poisons and using them as a tool to get a deeper understanding of the workings of the body's many systems, Claude Bernard, a student of Magendie's went on to become an eminent scientist in his own right, took up the investigation of arrow poisons (Trestrail III, 2001). It was the responsibility of the German scientist Louis Lewin (1854–1929) to classify plants and medicines according to the psychological effects that they had on people. Additionally, he authored and published many books and papers about the toxicology of various substances, including methyl alcohol, chloroform, and opium.

His works that are among his most notable include Toxicologist's Perspective on Global History and A Textbook of Toxicology. These two discoveries—Paul Hermann Muller's discovery of the insecticidal capabilities of DDT in 1939 and the creation of dimercaprol (BAL) as an antidote for arsenic—contributed to the rapid advancement that occurred during the 20th century (Golberg, 1978). He was awarded the Nobel Prize in 1948 for his discovery of the remarkable effectiveness of DDT as a contact toxin against a variety of arthropods. Gerhard Schrader was a German scientist who lived from 1903 until 1990. He was working on the development of new insecticides when he made an unintended discovery that led to the creation of the highly lethal nerve agents soman, serin, tabun, and cyclosarin. Schrader and his team were able to determine the structural requirements for the insecticidal activity of anticholinesterase (anti-ChE) compounds, which ultimately resulted in the development of a new category of synthetic insecticides known as organophosphorus insecticides (OP). The phrase "Father of Nerve Agents" was coined to describe him (Marquardt et al., 1999).

1.2. Modern Toxicology

Toxicology has made significant strides since the 1900s. According to Langman & Kapur (2006), the production of pharmaceuticals, insecticides, synthetic textiles, and industrial chemicals all experienced significant increases during World War II. This was also the time when the field began to flourish exponentially within the industry.

Additionally, it was the beginning of a comprehensive understanding of the nature and mechanism of the effects that poisons have, as well as the development of specific antidotes for each of these poisons. Toxicology, in conjunction with other scientific disciplines, contributes to the development of safer chemicals suitable for use in pharmaceuticals, food additives, insecticides, industrial chemicals, and a wide range of substances that are necessary for day-to-day life (Langman & Kapur, 2006) (Figure 1.2).

As a result of the necessity for a prosperous society to protect itself from deleterious effects brought about by the introduction of physical agents, new chemicals, and a variety of industrial and consumer products, the various aspects of toxicology have expanded. As a result of this, the application of toxicology to the evaluation of safety and risk is of the utmost importance in the contemporary society that we are currently a part of (Krebs & McKeague, 2020).

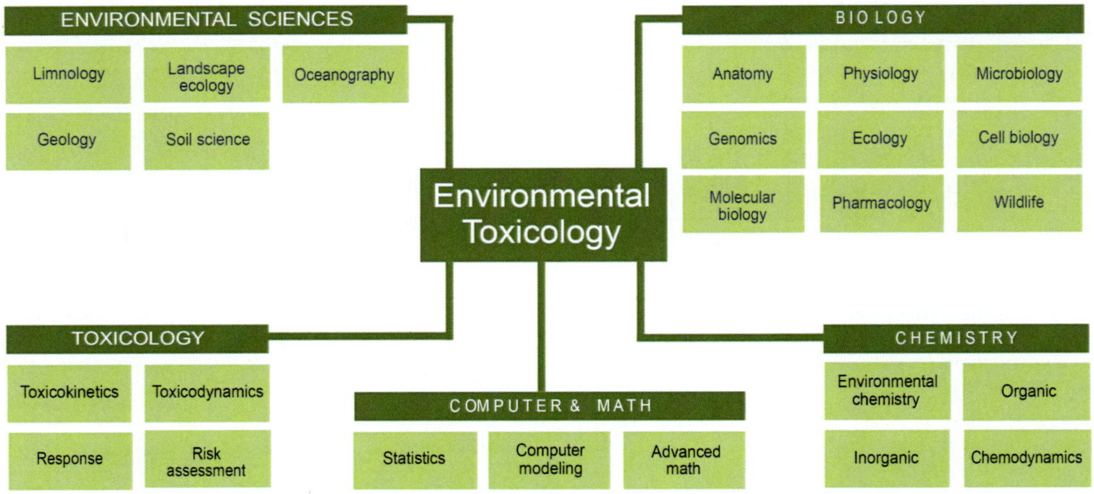

Figure 1.2. *Illustration of green toxicology.*

Source: https://en.wikipedia.org/wiki/File:Branches_of_Environmental_Toxicology_-_Entox-fields_lrg.png.

Beginning in the middle of the 1950s, the Food and Drug Administration of the United States Administration increased its commitment to toxicology. Arnold Lehman was the individual in charge of this endeavor. In 1955, Lehman, Fitzhugh, and their fellow employees formally established an experimental program to evaluate the safety of cosmetics, pharmaceuticals, and foods. In 1982, the Food and Drug Administration (FDA) of the United States made modifications to a program (Luch, 2012). The Delaney clause, which was included in these amendments in 1958, stated, in a broad sense, that any chemical that has been shown to be carcinogenic in laboratory animals or in people could not be added to the food supply in the United States. Regardless of how one feels about Delaney, it has proven to be an extremely helpful starting point for the construction of risk assessment models as well as the comprehension of the complexities of the biological phenomenon known as carcinogenicity (Langman & Kapur, 2006).

At the tail end of the 1960s, it was discovered that a contaminant known as 2,3,7,8-Tetrachlorodibenzo-p-dioxin (TCDD) was present in a herbicide known as Agent Orange. This discovery was the first discovery of its potentially harmful effects, and it was published in 1957 under the title "Chick Edema Factor."

This trend did not show any signs of slowing down by the time the 1970s and 1980s rolled around (Hodgson, 2004). During this time period, there was an exponential increase in the number of pieces of legislation, journals, and new societies that were engaged with toxicology. In the present day, the United States of America is home to a multitude of governmental, professional, and other scientific organizations, each of which serves a large number of members, numbering in the hundreds of thousands. Additionally, there are over 120 periodicals that are especially devoted to toxicology and other topics that are associated with it. Examples of this diversification include the undergraduate toxicology program, the engineering program, the public health program, the pharmacy program, the graduate program in toxicology in medical schools, and the public health program in public pharmacies. In recent years, there has been a growing trend among undergraduate liberal arts universities to incorporate toxicology courses into their biology and chemistry curricula (Massaro, 1997). Several definitions of toxicology include the following:

1.2.1. Toxicology

To a layperson, the term "toxicology" refers to the study of the ways in which chemicals can cause harm to living organisms. Toxicology, on the other hand, is now acknowledged as both a scientific field and an art that is practiced, much like medicine. The field of toxicology is concerned with the study of poisons and everything that is associated with them, including how they are discovered and identified, how they have an effect on living things, how they are treated, and how they are prevented from causing harm (Hodgson, 2012).

1.2.2. Xenobiotic

The term "xenobiotics" comes from the Greek word "xeno," which means "strange." Xenobiotics are foreign compounds that have biological activity. It is not possible to use them in a biosynthetic pathway or to break them down to generate energy. Pesticides, secondary plant metabolites, alkaloids, drugs, industrial chemicals, toxins from molds, plants, animals, and environmental pollutants are all examples of this all-encompassing category of structurally unfavorable substances (Rieger et al., 2002). Other examples include alkaloids, drugs, and industrial chemicals (*see* Figure 1.3).

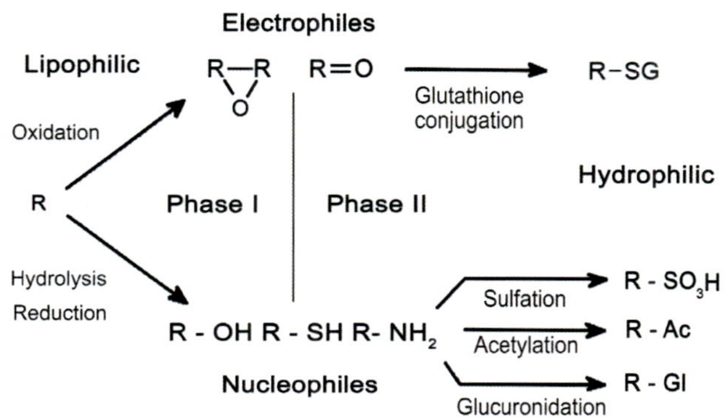

Figure 1.3. *Schematic of xenobiotics.*

Source: By TimVickers – Own work, Public Domain; https://commons.wikimedia.org/w/index.php?curid=4549628.

1.3. Sub-Disciplines

1. **Forensic Toxicology:** It addresses the medical and legal implications of chemical toxicity.
2. **Clinical Toxicology:** The field of clinical toxicology studies medical conditions that result from or are linked to excessive chemical exposure. In other words, toxicology is the study of health issues and disorders caused by or related to hazardous

substances and their causes, diagnoses, treatments, and clinical management(s) (Gossel, 1994).

3. **Nutritional Toxicology:** Nutritional science examines the health effects of various foods, feeds, and dietary practices.
4. **Reproductive Toxicology:** Study of effects of physical or chemical substances on male and female reproductive systems.
5. **Development Toxicology:** Study of the impact of chemicals and medications on the growth and maturation of an organism. Adverse effects can lead to structural abnormalities, growth retardation, loss of function, and even death (Rogers & Kavlock, 1998).
6. **Veterinary Toxicology:** It covers the origin, prognosis, and treatment of confirmed poisonings in wild and domestic animals (Gupta, 2012).
7. **Teratology:** Study of congenital disabilities brought on by hazardous substances during development.
8. **Environmental Toxicology:** In this, pollution prevention and its environmental impacts (food, water, air, or soil) are discussed. Ecotoxicology, marine toxicology, and other disciplines might be among them (Shaw & Chadwick, 1998).
9. **Analytical Toxicology:** Using analytical chemistry techniques to quantitatively and qualitatively estimate the substances involved in the toxicity process.
10. **Aquatic Toxicology:** This focuses on investigating the harmful impacts of chemicals released into fresh and marine water on aquatic life and aquatic ecosystems. The majority of the research focuses on water contamination and its ecological implications.
11. **Ecotoxicology:** A more specific field of study concerning environmental pollution in living organisms' and communities' populations. Ecotoxicology, in its broadest sense, is the study of how pollutants influence organisms besides humans.
12. **Food Toxicology:** It addresses natural pollutants, feed and food additives, and food components' toxic and chemoprotective effects (Shibamoto & Bjeldanes, 2009).
13. **Formal Toxicology:** It addresses formal toxicological investigations required before releasing new medications or substances (e.g., minimum toxic dose and calculation of LD_{50}).
14. **Genetic Toxicology:** It examines how toxicants affect the heritable disease process.
15. **Industrial Toxicology:** It focuses on the clinical evaluation of industry workers and their environment.
16. **Occupational Toxicology:** The potential for negative effects from chemicals in the workplace is assessed, and suggestions for suitable protective and preventative measures are made.
17. **Regulatory Toxicology:** Controlling the availability, use and distribution of chemicals for commercial and therapeutic purposes, as well as administrative activities relating to

the implementation and interpretation of statutory toxicity testing programs are some of the responsibilities that fall under its purview. The Food and Drug Administration (FDA), for instance, is in charge of monitoring the safety of medications, cosmetics, and food additives (Gad, 2001).

18. **Regulation:** Controlling the production, transportation, sale, or disposal of chemicals that have been determined to be harmful through testing procedures or by standards stated in relevant laws is what regulators refer to as regulation.
19. **Toxicodynamics:** It is the study of biochemical and physiological effects of toxins as well as their mode of action.
20. **Toxicokinetics:** A study of how toxins are absorbed, distributed, metabolized, and excreted from the body.
21. **Toxicovigilance:** This is concerned with identifying, investigating, and evaluating diverse hazardous effects in the community to take measures to prevent or control exposures to substances that cause such effects.
22. **Toxicology:** This is concerned with determining the toxicity of compounds derived from plants and animals and those produced by pathogenic organisms/ bacteria.
23. **Toxicoepidemiology:** It is the study of variables influencing toxicity, species at risk, and occurrences of toxicity in organisms and applying this knowledge to develop prevention and control measures.

1.4. Toxicant Types

1.4.1. Poison

It is from the Latin word "POTUS," which means "potentially lethal beverage," that the English word "poison" originates. It is any substance that, when applied to a living body in any way, or when ingested in extremely small doses, either results in a decline in health or results in the complete termination of life. Poison has psychological and legal implications that make manufacturers cautious to use it to describe compounds, especially those that are intended for widespread usage in large quantities, unless it is legally necessary to do so. Even though "toxicant" has the same medical definition, "poison" has some psychological and legal implications. According to Koszucka & Nowak (2019), companies that manufacture products and lawmakers are becoming more receptive to the term "toxicant" (Figure 1.4).

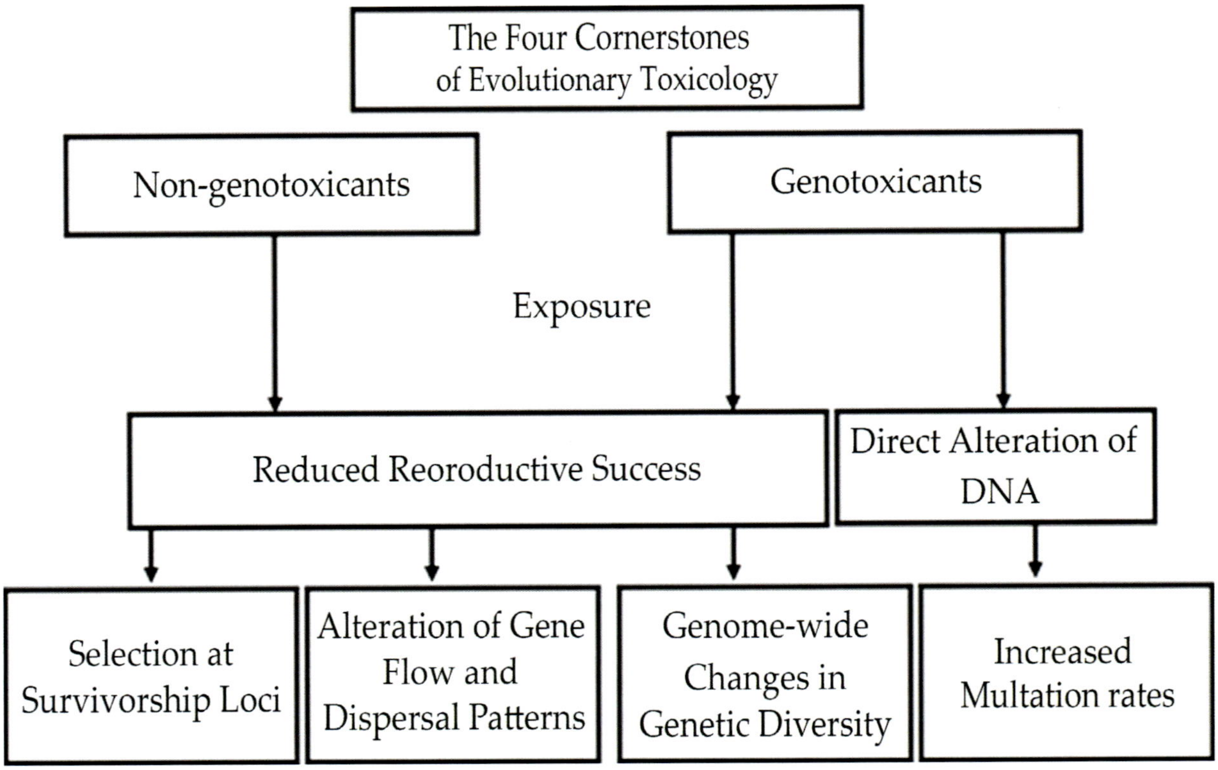

Figure 1.4. *Types of poisons from the clinical point of view.*

Source: *https://www.researchgate.net/.*

1.4.2. Toxicant

Toxicant is another word for poison; it is typically classified as a biotoxin and is produced by living organisms in quantities that are considered to be relatively low. According to Nuwaysir, Bittner, Trent, Barrett, & Afshari (1999), these chemical substances could be bacteriotoxins, which are produced by bacteria, zootoxins, which are produced by lower animals, phytotoxins, which are produced by plants, or mycotoxins, which are produced by fungi.

1.4.3. Endotoxins

Bacterial cells are a potential source for their discovery.

1.4.4. Exotoxins

Biological cells are the source of their production.

1.4.5. Venom

In the process of biting or stinging, a toxic substance is produced in a particular gland and then expelled. Venom is a type of zootoxin. It is, however, transmitted through the act of biting or stinging (Chen & Lu, 2002).

1.4.6. Systemic Toxicant

A toxin that affects the entire body or several organs simultaneously. An example of a systemic toxin is potassium cyanide, which interferes with the ability of a cell to use oxygen. As a result, potassium cyanide has an effect on every cell and organ in the body.

1.4.7. Organ Toxicant

A toxin that can selectively affect particular organs or tissues (also referred to as a tissue toxicant) without causing complete damage to the body as a whole. Benzene, for instance, is an example of a specific organ toxicant because it is extremely toxic to the tissues that are necessary for the formation of blood (Kalina et al., 2020) (Figure 1.5).

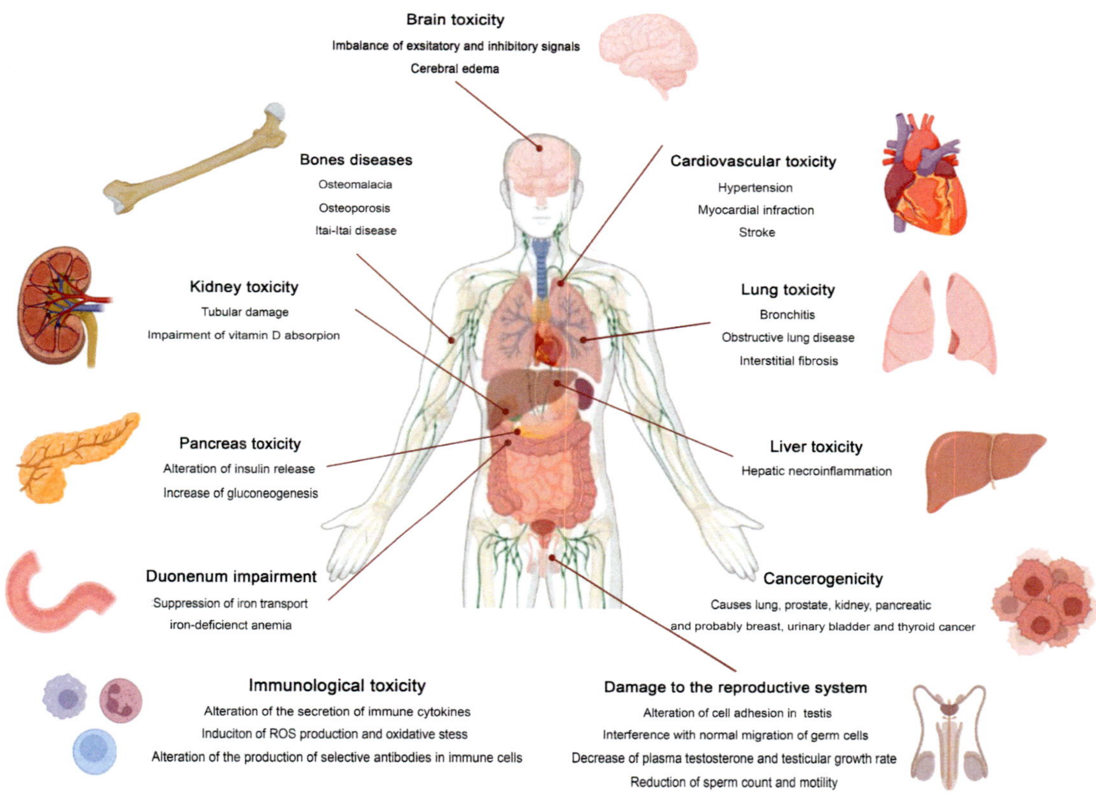

Figure 1.5. *Illustration of organ toxicants-an example of cadmium.*

Source: Peana, M., Pelucelli, A., Chasapis, C. T., Perlepes, S. P., Bekiari, V., Medici, S., & Zoroddu, M. A., (2023). Biological effects of human exposure to environmental cadmium. Biomolecules, 13(1), 36. https://doi.org/10.3390/biom13010036.

1.4.8. Pollutant

According to Min, Liu, He, & Peng (2013), a pollutant is any undesirable solid, liquid, or gaseous substance that is produced in large quantities through the release of harmful substances or their combination. Pollutants are responsible for contaminating the environment and causing pollution.

1.5. Toxic Effects

To compare one substance to another, the phrases "toxic" and "toxicity" are frequently used as relative expressions:

1. **Toxicity:** The biological organism's ability to be poisonous or to cause harm.
2. **Toxicosis:** The disease or condition caused by toxicant exposure. The terms "toxicosis"

and "poisoning" or "intoxication" are frequently used "interchangeably."

3. **Toxic Effects:** Unwanted effects of a toxicant/drug that damage the individual's survival or regular functioning.
4. **Side Effects:** Unwanted side effects caused by medications' typical pharmacological activity. These outcomes could be harmful to the person or not.
5. **Selective Toxicity:** Toxic effects of a substance on one living being without harming another, despite the close relationship between the two (Vineet Kumar, Kumari, Guleria, & Yadav, 2011).
6. **Safety:** Means/implies practical assurance that no harm occurs from using a chemical under defined quantities and conditions of use.
7. **Risk-to-Benefit Ratio:** Even harmful chemicals may be justified if the benefits to many people outweigh the risks.
8. **Risk:** The frequency with which an adverse consequence, like injury or loss, is expected to occur due to exposure to physical or chemical substances under defined conditions.
9. **Risk Assessment:** A quantitative evaluation of the likelihood of harmful outcomes under specified exposure settings (Robertson, Harmon, Tran, Tanaka, & Takahashi, 2003).
10. **Hazard:** A qualitative description of an unpleasant impact caused by a specific chemical or physical substance, regardless of exposure or dose. The phrase "hazard" linked to "risk," but it communicates chance or danger probability, irrespective of exposure and dose. Trait or group of chemical compound properties that, if sufficiently exposed, may have a negative health or ecological effect (Franco, Sánchez-Olea, Reyes-Reyes, & Panayiotidis, 2009).
11. **Tolerance:** A condition or event in which the dose necessary to cause harm increases with repeated exposure. A lowered sensitivity to the negative effects of a chemical produced by previous exposure to that compound or a structurally comparable compound.
12. **Acceptable Risk:** Probability of contracting an illness or suffering damage as a result of drug exposure; it is regarded to be low and acceptable to individuals (Raghunathan, Shaw, & Bagshaw, 2013).
13. **Acceptable Exposure:** Accidental contact with a physical or chemical agent which causes injury.
14. **The Margin of Exposure (MOE):** A critical effect as "No Observed Adverse Effect Level" (NOAEL) expressed as a percentage of the predicted, expected, or calculated concentration or exposure dose.
15. **Threshold Limit Values (TLV):** The level of a substance in the air that suggests nearly all workers can be repeatedly exposed without adverse consequences. These numbers represent a time-weighted concentration based on a 40-week work schedule of seven to eight hours each day (Gunja & Brown, 2012).

1.6. Toxicity with Duration and Frequency of Exposure

1. **Acute Toxicity:** Toxic consequences caused by a single dose, or numerous doses administered over 24 hours.
2. **Subacute Toxicity:** An investigation of toxicant's effects after repeated exposure for thirty days.
3. **Subchronic Toxicity:** It is the study of recurrent toxicant exposure and its consequences throughout one to three months.
4. **Chronic Toxicity:** A study of repeated toxicant exposure and its consequences over three months (Handy, 1994).

1.7. Toxicity of Duration of Induced Effects and Time of Development

1. **Temporary/Transient/Reversible Toxicity:** A toxicity or detrimental effect which lasts for a brief period (e.g., narcotic-produced chemical solvents).
2. **Permanent or Irreversible or Persistent Toxicity:** Toxicity or detrimental effect that lasts throughout an individual's life and is permanent (e.g., skin scarring caused by corrosives).
3. **Delayed Toxicity:** The toxicity or negative influence that has delayed the beginning of action (e.g., several organophosphorus pesticides cause peripheral neuropathy) (Balazs, 1974).
4. **Immediate Toxicity:** Toxicity that occurs shortly after a single exposure to a toxicant (e.g., cyanide poisoning).
5. **Cumulative Toxicity:** Progressive toxicity or a negative effect induced by cumulative incremental harm from subsequent exposures (e.g., ethanol-induced liver fibrosis) (Sledge et al., 2011).

1.8. Dosage Related Terms

A complete or absolute amount or quantity of a chemical that is used or delivered to an individual simultaneously to produce the desired pharmacological or toxicological reaction is referred to as a dose.

1.8.1. Lethal Dose (LD)

A minimum dose such that it causes the death of any animal during the period of observation. It is possible to assign the LD value as a percentage to represent the dose that is necessary to kill 1% (LD_1), 50% (LD_{50}), or 99% (LD_{99}) of the test animals that are part of the population (Pereira, Lawlor, Vigano, Dorgan, & Bruera, 2001).

1.8.2. Lethal Dose 50 (LD_{50})

Also referred to as the median fatal dose (MLD) in some circles. Certain conditions, such as the species, the length of exposure, and the route of exposure, can cause a toxicant dose to kill 50% of the animals. Utilization of this toxicity metric is commonplace.

1.8.3. Lethal Concentration (LC)

One of the components that causes mortality during the observation period is the one that has the lowest concentration in the feed (or water, in the case of fish). Milligrams per kilogram of feed (or water) is the unit of measurement for each ounce.

1.8.4. Lethal Concentration-50 (LC_{50})

There is a chemical concentration in the feed (or water, in the case of fish) that is fatal to 50% of the population where it is present. The primary manifestation of this is acute toxicity that is fatal.

1.8.5. No Observed Effect Level (NOEL)

According to Chahoud et al. (1999), a maximum dose level or concentration of a chemical that does not bring about any changes (alterations) in the functional capacity, development, growth, morphology, or life span of the test animals under the conditions of the exposure.

1.8.6. No Observed Adverse Effect Level (NOAEL)

A greatest dose level/concentration of a chemical which has no observable/detectable effect (alteration) on the growth, development, functional capacity, morphology, or life span of test animals under established conditions of exposure. NOAEL is a NOEL variation specifying that just the effect is negative.

1.8.7. Lowest Observed Adverse Effect Level (LOAEL)

The highest exposure level/dose level/ concentration of substance observed to have an observable/ detectable effect (alteration) on the growth, development, morphology, functional capacity, or life span of test animals under defined conditions of exposure (Pizzo & Benfenati, 2016).

1.8.8. Reference Dose/Reference Concentration (RfD/RfC)

The NOAEL or LOAEL is used as a starting point to compute the oral intake (RfD) or inhalation reference concentration (RfC) of airborne contaminants for noncancerous effects. These values are derived from empirically determined NOAEL or LOAEL values.

1.8.9. Maximum Allowable or Admissible/Acceptable Concentration (MAC)

A regulatory figure defining the maximum concentration of particular atmospheric contaminants permitted in the workplace's ambient air.

1.8.10. Maximum Residue Limit/ Maximum Residue Level (MRL)

A maximum amount of pesticide or grog residue (mainly veterinary medicine) that is legally authorized in or on food commodities and animal feeds. Although both terms possess the same meaning, "maximum residue limit" refers to pesticide residue, and "maximum residue level" refers to drug residue (García-Domenech, de Julián-Ortiz, & Besalú, 2006).

1.8.11. Maximum Tolerated Dose (MTD)

A high amount of drug which generates toxic effects but does not result in death while testing organisms. In chronic toxicity research, MLD has limited toxic effects in test organisms. Still, it shouldn't cause more than a 10% loss in body weight relative to the control group or create overt toxicity (death of cells or organ dysfunction).

1.8.12. Maximum Tolerated Concentration (MTC)

The greatest concentration of a chemical in a medium which generates toxic symptoms but no mortality in the test organism (Horwitz,

Tedesco, Gundberg, Garcia-Ocana, & Stewart, 2003).

1.8.13. Absolute Lethal Dose (LD_{100})

The smallest dose of a medicine that, under certain conditions, kills 100% of the animals exposed. The number of organisms used in its evaluation determines the value.

1.8.14. Absolute Lethal Concentration (LC_{100})

The lowest concentration of a material in an environment medium that is deadly to 100% of exposed species or organisms under specified conditions.

1.8.15. Acceptable Daily Intake (ADI)

An estimated amount of material in drinking water or food that humans can consume every day for a lifetime without experiencing significant health risks. Food additives frequently use the acronym ADI (The term "tolerable daily intake" is used to describe contamination) (Dalal et al., 2016).

1.9. Other Common Terms

1.9.1. Alternative Test

Alternative procedures that provide the same level of information as testing on animals currently in use but involve fewer animals, resulting in less suffering for the animals, or completely eliminating the use of animals. When such methods become available, they ought to be utilized for the purpose of hazard characterization, categorization, and labeling for intrinsic hazards, in addition to the evaluation of chemical safety (Piersma, 2006).

1.9.2. Cheminformatics

There are a few different names for cheminformatics, including chemoinformatics and chemical informatics. In the field of chemistry, the application of computer and information technology to a variety of chemistry-related problems is known as information chemistry. According to Bunin, Siesel, Morales, & Bajorath (2007), pharmaceutical companies, for example, make use of these in silico techniques to generate new drug candidates.

1.9.3. Endpoint Study Record

Strong research summaries of the data derived for particular endpoints are reported using the International Uniform Chemical Information Database (IUCLID) format of technical dossier following the REACH Regulation (Fietkau et al., 2020).

1.9.4. Endpoint

An inherent chemical property or data point that can be observed or measured. It refers to physical-chemical characteristics like a vapor, to the biological effect a substance has on people's health or environment (such as carcinogenicity, irritability, or aquatic toxicity), to degradability, or it can refer to any of these (Long et al., 1990).

1.9.5. In Vitro Test

Means "in glass" or "in a tube," this term describes a test conducted on an organism's external organs, cells, tissues or biochemical systems.

1.9.6. In Vivo Test

The study carried out inside a live thing.

1.9.7. In Silico

A term created as an allegory to well-known expressions in vivo and in vitro. This means "done on a computer or through computer simulation," which refers to scientific study or experiments carried out or created using computer simulation or computer modeling (Wolfe, Long, & Buchman, 1989).

1.9.8. IUCLID Flag

An option in IUCLID software is used to specify the nature of provided data (e.g., experimental data) or their use for legal requirements (e.g., secrecy).

1.9.9. Prediction Model

Theoretical formula, software or algorithm that predicts the chemical substance's hazardous properties or effects based on experimental results obtained by applying test procedure (Small Jr et al., 2018).

1.9.10. QSARs and SARs [Q(SAR)]

Theoretical models that are used to predict, either qualitatively or quantitatively, its physical-chemical, biological (such as (eco) toxicological), and environmental fate features. A SAR is a qualitative relationship that connects the existence or absence of a (sub-) structure to a relevant feature or action. A mathematical model known as a quantitative structure-activity relationship (QSAR) connects one or more quantitative elements to a quantitative measure of an activity or feature (Agrawal & Khadikar, 2001).

1.9.11. Test (or Assay)

An experimental setup designed to learn more about a chemical substance's inherent qualities or negative consequences.

1.9.12. Validated Test

A test in which benefits, performance traits, and restrictions are sufficiently established for a particular purpose.

1.9.13. Validation

The procedure through which a test method's relevance and dependability are assessed to support a particular usage.

1.9.14. Vertebrate Animal

Creatures of the Vertebrata subphylum are chordates with spinal columns and backbones (Kwak, Sim, Kwon, & Choi, 2008).

1.10. Poisoning Sources

Toxins can be introduced into people and other creatures by various actions, including purposeful intake, environmental exposure, occupational exposure, accidental and intentional (suicidal or homicidal) poisoning. If a drug enters the body through the gastrointestinal (GI) tract, skin or lungs, its toxicity may vary (Dabonne et al., 2010).

1.10.1. Accidental Poisoning

Accidental poisoning can happen when animals or people accidentally consume a hazardous substance or are carelessly added to fodder, feed, food or drinking water. Such toxins can be found in both natural and artificial sources. Natural causes include ingesting poisonous plants, getting bitten by or stung by venomous reptiles, eating tainted food, drinking water contaminated with minerals, and more. The sources that humans make include agrochemicals, household goods, and medications (Vishwajeet Kumar, 1991).

1.10.2. Malicious Poisoning

An intentional or criminal killing of a person or an animal using particular toxic or poisonous chemicals is known as malicious poisoning. The likelihood of such poisoning is higher in humans than in animals (Tolpegin, Truex, Gursoy, & Liu, 2020).

1.10.3. Occupational Exposure

Occupational exposure is something that workers frequently experience as a result of the chemical environment in which they inhabit. There are approximately 68,000 to 1,01,000 compounds that are utilized frequently, according to estimates. Both the growth of large cities and the process of industrialization have contributed to the contamination of the air, water, and soil. The synthesis, production, or packaging of such substances, as well as their use in the workplace, exposes workers in the industrial sector to the chemicals in question (Kauppinen et al., 2000). The primary objectives of occupational toxicology are to identify the substance that is causing the problem, to determine the conditions under which it can be safely applied, and to prevent the absorption of substances that are harmful to the body. To define the acceptable levels of ambient air concentrations, guidelines have been developed for several chemicals that are used in the workplace. (Kumar, 2004).

1.11. Duration and Frequency of Exposure

There are four categories of chemical exposure that experimental animals might experience: acute, sub-acute, chronic, and lifelong.

Chemical exposure lasting longer than 24 hours is referred to as acute exposure. Intraperitoneal (IP), intravenous (IV), and subcutaneous injections, oral intubation, and topical application are a few examples of exposure pathways. The term "exposure" often refers to a single dose, but for some marginally hazardous or almost benign drugs, multiple exposures may be given throughout 24 hours. Acute exposure by inhalation is defined as a continuous exposure lasting less than 24 hours, typically 4 hours (Marras et al., 2006).

Sub-acute, sub-chronic, and chronic exposure are the three categories into which repeated exposure falls:

1. Sub-acute exposure is defined as repeated chemical exposure lasting one month or less;
2. Sub-chronic exposure is the recurrent ingestion of a chemical throughout one to three months; and
3. Repeated chemical exposure lasting more than three months is referred to as chronic exposure (usually, this refers to studies with at least one year of repeated dosing) (Ulaganathan, Read, Collins, & Vincent, 2017).

These three forms of repetitive exposure can occur by any route, but the oral route—where a chemical is introduced directly to diet—is the most typical. The frequency and length of exposure are typically not as well-defined in human exposure circumstances as in controlled animal experiments. However, the words used to describe common exposure conditions are essentially the same. As a result, exposures at work or in the environment can be classified as acute (resulting from a single occurrence or episode), sub-chronic (repeatedly occurring over weeks or months), or chronic (repeatedly occurring over a long time, such as years) (Bornstein & D'Agostino, 1992).

1.12. Classifications of Toxicants

The classification of toxic substances can be approached from multiple perspectives, each tailored to different objectives and interests. Given the diversity of hazardous chemicals, an ideal classification system would likely integrate various methods based on several criteria. This complexity arises from the fact that no single classification system can encompass the entire spectrum of toxic agents. Toxic substances can be categorized based on their chemical and biological properties, but exposure characteristics are equally crucial in toxicology (Nendza, Muller, & Wenzel, 2017). For instance, toxins can be classified according to their sources—such as plant toxins, mineral toxicants, animal toxicants, and synthetic toxic substances. They can also be categorized by their physical states, including gaseous toxicants, dusts, liquids, and solids. Another classification focuses on target organs and systems, distinguishing between nephrotoxicants, pulmonary toxicants, neurotoxicants, hepatotoxicants, hematotoxicants, and dermatotoxicants.

Additionally, substances can be sorted by their chemical structure and nature, including nonmetals, metals, acids, alkalies, and organic toxicants like carbon compounds and metallic carbides. Analytical behavior further divides them into volatile toxicants, metalloids, extractive toxicants, and metals. The type of toxicity—whether acute, subacute, chronic, etc.—and specific toxic effects, such as carcinogens, teratogens, and mutagens, also provide valuable classification criteria. Developing a "toxicity rating" system aims to aid medical professionals by offering insights into the potential hazards of various poisons when administered to humans. This rating system typically ranges from one to sixteen, with higher numbers indicating greater toxicity. Such a system helps professionals assess the potency and risks associated with different chemicals, facilitating more informed and effective responses in medical settings.

1.13. Actions of Poisons

Poisons usually act in three ways: locally, remotely, and both locally and remotely.

1. **Locally Acting:** The chemicals are only effective at the location where they are applied, such as the skin or the mucosa (e.g., corrosive poisons).
2. **Remotely Acting:** Some substances don't exert their effect until after they have been absorbed into the circulatory system (e.g., cardiac poisons, narcotic poisons, and so on).
3. **Both Locally and Remotely Acting:** They operate through both remote and local means (e.g., carbolic acid, etc.) (Bajgar, 2004).

1.14. Factors Affecting Toxicology

Xenobiotics are known to have harmful effects on a variety of species, but not all species are equally sensitive to these effects. As an illustration, in contrast to the majority of mammals, rabbits are capable of ingesting substantial quantities of the extremely lethal drug belladonna (Atropa belladonna). A population's exposure to a particular quantity of a toxin may not have the same effects on every individual because there are several factors that can modulate the overall toxic reaction. This is something that is widely known. According to Havenaar & Van den Brink (1997), the age of the substance represents a significant factor in determining the chemical toxicity of the substance. Several factors contribute to the fact that younger people are typically more susceptible to toxicity. One of these factors is a diminished capacity to biotransform and eliminate xenobiotics. There are many factors that can influence how the body reacts to foreign substances (Cao et al., 2020). These factors include environmental factors, personal factors, and even the xenobiotic itself.

The following categories can be used to group some of the factors that can influence chemical toxicity:

- Host factors (factors related to the subject);

- Factors related to toxicants or associated with xenobiotics;
- Environmental conditions.

Hence, individual and non-individual factors may impact how any drug or chemical reacts with the body (Ho Yu, 2000).

1.14.1. Host Factors

1. **The Weight and Size of a Person:** It is crucial in determining the amount of chemical agent needed to trigger a specific response. The chemical concentration in tissues will differ if the chemical in the same amount is administered to people of different sizes, which will change the effect that is caused. Larger people can tolerate a higher dose than smaller people. Therefore, the chemical amount or dosage to be administered or the chemical amount allowed as acceptable daily intake (ADI) is represented as per unit of body weight. This function has been used to establish tolerance thresholds and compute ADI for several chemical agents because metabolism and activity are proportional to body surface area (Virreira Winter, Zychlinsky, & Bardoel, 2016).
2. **Age:** Young animals and infants are particularly vulnerable to relatively harmless toxins later in life. Early life responses differ due to various circumstances, including the blood-brain barrier (BBSs) maturity status, relative inefficiency of some excretory and metabolic pathways, increased vulnerability of some tissues, and others. It is common knowledge that several enzyme systems are not fully formed at birth. The systems for chemical agent excretion or biotransformation are present, although at a much lower level than that of an adult. As a result, this impairment is primarily quantitative (Nemery, 1990).

   In comparison to adults, newborns have much lower activity levels in the oxidative pathways involved in the metabolism of a range of chemical substances. For instance, a lack of glucuronyl transferase activity increases the toxicity of substances that rely on this method of detoxification and buildup of unbound bilirubin, which can cause jaundice. Kidney, brain, and other organ immaturity may also make children more vulnerable to medications or pollutants. Because the BBS is immature, chemical agents of the central nervous system (CNS) may have easier access than in adults (Mehlman & Borek, 1987).
3. **Strains and Species:** The toxicity of a particular substance can be significantly influenced by species differences. When tested on several species, the relative toxicity of some compounds, including endosulfan, varied noticeably. Different forms of biotransformation, which can occur in diverse tissues, frequently cause variations in toxicities. When given to one species, a substance may be quickly converted into a harmless or, occasionally, a more poisonous one; nevertheless, when given to another, the same substance may be digested extremely slowly or even by a different process, leading to another

metabolite (Kalan et al., 2019).

4. **Acute Toxicity:** measurements of different inbred strains of mice have shown that variations in animal strains also cause variations in chemical agent responses. Humans are an incredibly diverse species. Thus, each person's rate of metabolism for any given substance might vary substantially (Lorke, 1983).
5. **Sex:** An animal's gender frequently affects the toxicity of a chemical agent. The direct endocrine influence on significant variations is demonstrated. Castration and estrogen therapy can lessen the nephrotoxic effects of chloroform in male mice; androgen therapy makes female mice more susceptible to these effects. The enzymatic biotransformation of a chemical in certain situations may be affected by sex hormones, which could account for the sex variances. Due to their smaller size than men, women typically need a lower dosage. Medications or chemical agents must be used carefully during pregnancy since they could have teratogenic effects on females due to variations in toxicity due to sex, which is widely documented. It is crucial to remember that some substances expelled during lactation could affect the offspring. Therefore, determining acute toxicity in female and male animals of any species is preferred (Singh et al., 2005).
6. **Feed and Feeding:** Findings of toxicity testing can be impacted by the feed or food's composition. High-carbohydrate and high-protein diets protect against the hepatotoxic effects of chloroform, whereas diets high in fat can make animals more susceptible to those effects. It is worth noting that vitamin C deficiency has been shown to influence drug metabolism in guinea pigs and that mice on a low-protein diet had lower activity of hepatic drug-metabolizing enzyme systems. Animals fed synthetic meals have shown altered reactions in acute poisoning (Speiser, 2001). Even some food items could cause a harmful reaction during pharmacological treatment. For instance, monoamine oxidase inhibitors and cheese with high tyramine content have been shown to produce sympathomimetic effects. These results suggest that a typical and nutritionally sufficient meal must be offered in toxicity research. Yet, there is a lot of interest in toxicity research in animals with some nutritional deficiencies (e.g., protein). For instance, oral toxicity testing usually sees a decrease in the absorption of chemicals in the animal feed before intubation. Thus, it is common to withhold the feed for 16–18 hours before intubation to assume equal absorption. Yet, the catabolic effects of hunger may also affect the outcomes of poisoning. Overnight hunger is a popular practice for pragmatic reasons. Before and after the dose, water is available at no charge (Van Huis, 2013).
7. **Changes in the Internal Environment:** It is known that

several physiological factors, including physical exercise, stress, an animal's hormonal status, and deterioration of internal organs, can affect a compound's toxicity, and toxicity tests are carried out on healthy animals. Changes in body composition or metabolism may affect toxicological reactions during major surgery, as well as during pregnancy and lactation (Coley & Kershaw, 2010).

8. **Chemical Toxicity Alteration:** It is triggered by a substance administered before the one being studied, which is crucial. For instance, some substances may cause an increase in the production of liver microsomal enzymes and affect the metabolism of another substance. Chemical agents can also prevent the metabolism of drugs or other chemicals, displace a chemical's protein binding, or prevent a chemical's renal clearance (Horzmann & Freeman, 2016).

9. **Pathologic Conditions:** Because animals or people react to the same chemical in various ways when they are healthy compared to when they are unwell, chemical agents are frequently modified to a very substantial level. Any one of these conditions will significantly increase medication or chemical toxicity (Kim et al., 2007).

10. **Habitually Used Drugs:** Humans who regularly take some psychoactive substances have been shown to either increase or lessen their susceptibility to harmful medication reactions. Caffeine is widely utilized in beverages like coffee, tea, and sodas containing nicotine and alcohol. Caffeine is also frequently abused for social purposes. The sensitivity of humans to toxic amounts of pharmaceuticals and other chemicals may be impacted by habitual, and especially excessive, usage of these compounds (Adler & Lotecka, 1973).

11. **Idiosyncratic Reaction/Toxicity:** On occasion, toxicity that is unique to a person or manifests in a small number of people but not in the general population has been noted. Idiosyncratic toxicity is rare, occurring in as few as 1 in 1,00,000 people to as many as 1 in 10. Idiosyncratic drug reactions frequently happen after drug sensitization and subsequent preexposure. Certain medications, including amoxicillin clavulanic acid, can cause clinical indications to appear 3–4 weeks after a 1-–2-week course of treatment. However, the onset is sped up with a subsequent challenge. Halothane, diclofenac, phenytoin, and sulfonamides are just a few of the medications that are thought to produce immune-mediated idiosyncratic reactions in people. Skin reactions to chemicals or medications taken systemically have frequently been recorded, including urticaria, bronchial asthma, angioneurotic edema, and anaphylactic shock (Knowles, Uetrecht, & Shear, 2000).

    Hemolysis can occur in people who lack the enzyme glucose-6-phosphate dehydrogenase when they consume specific medications or meals. Although having a long latency period (up to 12 months), some idiosyncratic drug reactions occasionally occur, and their responses to a subsequent challenge are unpredictable. They are categorized as idiosyncratic nonimmune-mediated reactions. Troglitazone, ketoconazole, valproate, disulfiram, amiodarone, and isoniazid are a few examples of medications that have been linked to this particular unique reaction. Nonetheless, some allergic mechanisms may be involved (Uetrecht, 2007).

1.14.2. Factors Related to Toxicant

The toxicant's physical condition and chemical characteristics, such as:

- Water solubility;
- Vegetable oil solubility;
- The suspending medium;
- The size of the particle;
- Rates of breakdown of chemical compositions;
- The chemical agent's chemical stability;
- The crystal form;
- The gritty nature of inert chemicals used in large doses (Mak & Tay, 2014).

For example, fine particles are more easily absorbed than coarse particles (in the case of poisons with irritant qualities, such as zinc phosphide and -naphthylthiourea). However, coarse particles are more difficult to absorb. As a result of their ability to reach a larger portion of the gastric mucosa, smaller particles have the potential to cause protective vomiting. In alkaline solutions, certain compounds can be easily converted into dichlorvos, which has an oral LD_{50} in rats that is eight times lower than the original substance. According to van Straalen & Timmermans (2002), dichlorvos is available in the form of a powder that can be wettable for the management of external parasites. Furthermore, solvents and other components that are incorporated into commercial preparations have the potential to influence the overall toxicity of the active principle. When nonpolar solvents are taken into consideration, particularly when cutaneous exposure is taken into account, it is possible that the rate at which lipophilic toxins are absorbed is significantly increased (Overstreet, 2021).

Itineraries and the speed of administration: It is the route that is the most rapid in delivering a substance to the bloodstream that is associated with the highest level of toxicity. Parenteral administration of the majority of xenobiotics results in a faster and more comprehensive bioavailability than oral administration, which frequently leads to a lower cumulative lethal dose (LD_{50}). A significant influence on the potentially harmful intravenous dosage is the rate of injection. According to the findings of Perng et al. (2019), the digestive tract can have a variety of effects on the absorption of an ingredient. It is possible to gain insight into the amount of a substance that is absorbed by comparing the parenteral and oral LD_{50} variations. In addition, by ingesting poisons, one may undergo first-pass metabolism, which, depending on the circumstances, may lead to almost complete detoxification. According to Faustman, Silbernagel, Fenske, Burbacher, & Ponce (2000), pyrethrum-based pesticides are practically harmless in mammalian species because of the significant amount of gut hydrolysis that occurs. However, fish are not safe to consume because there is a possibility of significant molecular ingestion through the gills during fish consumption. Drug-drug interactions can occur when a person has had previous or coincidental contact with other compounds. By either increasing (enzyme inducers) or decreasing (enzyme inhibitors) the expression or activity of hepatic as well as extrahepatic phase I and phase II enzyme systems involved in biotransformation reactions, a wide variety of chemicals, such as pesticides, plant toxins, drugs, and environmental pollutants, can modulate the toxicity of several xenobiotics. Such chemicals include pesticides, plant toxins, drugs, and environmental pollutants.

To achieve this goal, the expression or activity of these enzyme systems can be either increased or decreased, respectively. Therefore, the simultaneous administration of two or more compounds that have different structures may result in an effect that is additive, potentiation, antagonism, negative summation, or summation. According to Rossignol, Genuis, & Frye (2014), an additive effect takes place when two agents act on the same tissue or organ, and the impact developed is an algebraic sum of the activities of both of the agents.

In the event that the substance induces enzymes, the process is typically sluggish and necessitates continuous exposure to the molecule or molecules that induce the enzymes. The modification of the biotransformation capacity that is specified for a particular toxicant may have a variety of clinically meaningful outcomes, depending on the nature of the toxicant that is being discussed and the metabolite(s) that are produced as a result of the toxicant. If the parent molecule is the cause of any harmful effects, then it is anticipated that the level of overall toxicity will decrease. On the other hand, the opposite is true if one or more (re)active metabolites produced during biotransformation reactions are the cause of toxic injury (Mak & Tay, 2014).

On the other hand, it is believed that enzyme inhibition has beneficial effects in toxicant poisonings that require metabolic activity; when certain conditions are met, inhibitors may be utilized therapeutically. Cimetidine is recommended for the treatment of acetaminophen toxicosis in dogs and cats because of its inhibitory effects on the CYP-mediated synthesis of reactive metabolite NAPQI. This metabolite is responsible for severe liver damage in animals that have been poisoned (Liess & Beketov, 2011).

Enzyme inhibition can increase the harmful efficacy of compounds that act directly (that is, without the need for metabolic activation), and it can also provide a rationale for explaining multiple drug-drug interactions.

It is also possible for drugs to interact with one another in the bloodstream. Several anticoagulant rodenticides, including bromadiolone, warfarin, and brodifacoum, have plasma half-lives that are relatively longer than average. This is because these drugs have a high affinity for plasma proteins.

A final point to consider is that the co-administration of certain medications can potentially alter the toxicity of certain toxins by acting at the receptor level. Medications that can block neuromuscular activity by acting on nicotinic receptors, such as d-tubocurarine or succinylcholine, have the potential to increase the toxicity of carbamates or organophosphates, for instance. In contrast, the opposite is true when the subject is exposed to parasympatholytic agents like atropine, which is commonly used in clinical practice as an antagonist (Sabater, Guasch, Romaní, & Muñoz, 2002).

Allowance for: It has been generally established that the harmful reaction of an animal to a dose of medicine that has been administered can either decrease, remain unchanged, or increase during subsequent administrations of the same amount. On the other hand, hyper-susceptibility refers to an increase in harmful responses, whereas tolerance refers to a decrease in harmful responses. This is a common method for developing tolerance to a drug after repeated administration, according to Babich & Stotzky (1983). High enzyme activity or enzyme induction, which are both involved in the process of drug detoxification and elimination, is a common method. Also known to be the cause of tolerance is a reduction in the end-organ sensitivity to the harmful effects of the drug. In normal albino rats, for instance, chlorpromazine has the effect of lowering the central nervous system and decreasing locomotor activity. An increase in excitatory feedback to regions that were previously depressed by the drug is the result of repeated administration of chlorpromazine. Additionally, the sensitivity of those regions to the depressive effects of the drug gradually decreases as the drug is administered more frequently. The abrupt discontinuation of medication results in a significant increase in brain activity, locomotor activity, and insomnia (Roex, Van Gestel, Van Wezel, & Van Straalen, 2000). This is because the depressive effect of the drug no longer balances the excitatory feedback that it normally provides.

1.14.3. Environmental Conditions

An environment can have an impact on how animals and humans react to substances. In an environment of laboratory animals employed in toxicity testing, there are three essential elements:

1. An existence of other animal species, with humans being the most prevalent of these. Depending on the researcher's methods, the animals used in experiments can acquire feelings that range from hostility to apathy to affection. The disposition of the animal can influence adverse reactions it has to drugs (Gordon, 2003).
2. An existence of other creatures of the same species. A harmful reaction to certain substances can be influenced by the presence of another female or male of the same species, most likely owing to hostility or fear.
3. Physical environment: A physical setting where a toxicity test is conducted has a significant impact on the toxic reaction (e.g., light, relative humidity, temperature, etc.). Similarly, the temperature has been shown to affect the LD_{50} of numerous compounds in rats (change in LD_{50} values at 37°C & 26°C). In inhalation toxicity experiments, a warm, humid environment has been shown to improve skin absorption and affect toxicity (Pietrock & Marcogliese, 2003). The toxicity is influenced by the day's dark and light cycles, the number of animals in cages, the cage's architecture, and seasonal fluctuations. Because it is rarely possible to examine the effects of all variations in environmental factors, it is important to note the circumstances of an experiment so that the cause of variance may be explained when the experiment is repeated and produces different results (Bednarska & Laskowski, 2009).

By uncoupling mitochondrial oxidative phosphorylation, for instance, high ambient temperatures have been shown to increase the toxicity of chlorophenols and nitrophenols, which in turn generate a greater amount of heat production. On the other hand, the rodenticide and aviicide chloralose can cause fatal hypothermia in cats by acting on hypothalamic thermoreceptors (Hallam, Clark, & Jordan, 1983).

Because of this, exposure to toxins can result in a variety of outcomes depending on several different conditions. Most of the time, the variation in the toxic reaction is caused by different expressions of proteins or enzymes that are involved in the kinetics of the poison. These expressions can change depending on the food, species, breed, and physiopathological characteristics of previous or concurrent exposure to many foreign chemicals. The recent significant advancements in molecular techniques have made it possible for researchers to gain insight into many of the mechanisms that are behind many of the discrepancies in reaction to foreign substances, which previously had no explanation (Bonde & Storgaard, 2002).

A Closer Look

Organic Toxicants

Organic toxicants, also known as organic pollutants, are chemical substances that can cause adverse effects on living organisms and the environment. These compounds, often synthetic, include pesticides, herbicides, industrial chemicals, and byproducts of various manufacturing processes. One of the most notorious groups of organic toxicants is persistent organic pollutants (POPs), which include substances like polychlorinated biphenyls (PCBs), dioxins, and certain pesticides such as DDT. These compounds are characterized by their long-term persistence in the environment, bioaccumulation in the food chain, and potential for significant health impacts. POPs can travel long distances from their source through air and water, leading to widespread environmental contamination. The impact of organic toxicants on human health can be profound. They are often linked to a range of chronic conditions, including cancers, reproductive disorders, immune system suppression, and endocrine disruption. For example, PCBs have been associated with neurodevelopmental deficits in children, while dioxins are potent carcinogens. The mechanism by which these toxicants exert their effects often involves disruption of cellular processes, DNA damage, and interference with hormone signaling pathways. Environmental exposure to these toxicants can occur through various routes, including ingestion of contaminated food and water, inhalation of polluted air, and direct skin contact. Wildlife is also at risk, with many species experiencing population declines and disruptions in reproductive success due to exposure to organic toxicants. Birds of prey, marine mammals, and fish are particularly vulnerable due to their position at the top of the food chain, where bioaccumulation of these substances is most pronounced. Addressing the issue of organic toxicants involves a multi-faceted approach. Regulatory measures are critical in controlling the production, use, and disposal of these harmful substances. International agreements, such as the Stockholm Convention on Persistent Organic Pollutants, aim to eliminate or restrict the production and use of the most dangerous POPs. Additionally, efforts to remediate contaminated sites, promote alternative, less harmful chemicals, and enhance public awareness are essential components of mitigating the impact of organic toxicants. Advances in environmental science and toxicology are crucial in understanding the behavior, distribution, and long-term effects of these pollutants. Innovative techniques in monitoring and analysis allow for better detection and quantification of organic toxicants in various environmental matrices. Furthermore, research into the development of bioremediation strategies, using microorganisms or plants to degrade or detoxify harmful compounds, offers promising avenues for reducing environmental contamination. Public health initiatives also play a vital role in managing the risks associated with organic toxicants. Educating communities about the sources and dangers of these substances, promoting safer agricultural practices, and advocating for stronger regulatory frameworks are key strategies in protecting human health and the environment. By fostering collaboration between scientists, policymakers, and the public, it is possible to address the threat posed by organic toxicants and work towards a healthier, more sustainable future.

Summary

The purpose of this chapter is to provide an overview of the various disciplines and types of toxicology, as well as the historical background and significance of modern toxicology throughout the scientific community. This chapter provides an overview of the history of toxicology, beginning with the utilization of poisons in ancient times and progressing all the way up to the establishment of toxicology as a respected scientific field in the 20th century. When it comes to understanding the effects of environmental and occupational exposures to chemicals and other toxic agents on human health, this chapter places a strong emphasis on the important role that toxicology plays.

This chapter provides an overview of the various subfields that fall under the umbrella of toxicology, such as environmental toxicology, forensic toxicology, clinical toxicology, and regulatory toxicology. This chapter provides an overview of the various categories of toxicology, including acute toxicity, chronic toxicity, genotoxicity, and reproductive toxicity, among others. This chapter explains the various effects of toxicity, such as neurotoxicity, systemic toxicity, and toxicity of the target organ. Within the scope of toxicology, this chapter introduces several essential terms, including dose-response relationship, threshold dose, LD_{50}, and NOAEL. Taking everything into consideration, the chapter offers a thorough introduction to toxicology and lays the groundwork for further research in the field.

References

1. Bagheri, M., Roshanaei, G., Asgari, G., Chavoshi, S., & Ghasemi, M. (2020). Application of carbon-doped nano-magnesium oxide for catalytic ozonation of real textile wastewater: Fractional factorial design and optimization. *Desalination and Water Treatment, 175*, 79–89.
2. Cai, L., Chen, J., Liu, Z., Wang, H., Yang, H., & Ding, W. (2018). Magnesium oxide nanoparticles: Effective agricultural antibacterial agent against *Ralstonia solanacearum*. *Frontiers in Microbiology, 9*, 790.
3. Cai, L., Liu, M., Liu, Z., Yang, H., Sun, X., Chen, J., Xiang, S., & Ding, W. (2018). MgONPs can boost plant growth: Evidence from increased seedling growth, morpho-physiological activities, and Mg uptake in tobacco (*Nicotiana tabacum* L.). *Molecules, 23*, 3375.
4. Cai, L., Wei, X., Feng, H., Fan, G., Gao, C., Chen, H., & Sun, X. (2021). Antimicrobial mechanisms of g-C3N4 nanosheets against the oomycetes *Phytophthora capsici*: Disrupting metabolism and membrane structures and inhibiting vegetative and reproductive growth. *Journal of Hazardous Materials, 417*, 126121.
5. Caten, C. E., & Jinks, J. L. (1968). Spontaneous variability of single isolates of *Phytophthora infestans*. I. Cultural variation. *Canadian Journal of Botany, 46*, 329–348.
6. Chen, F., Aqeel, M., Maqsood, M. F., Khalid, N., Irshad, M. K., Ibrahim, M., Akhter, N., Afzaal, M., Ma, J., Hashem, M., et al. (2022). Mitigation of lead toxicity in *Vigna radiata* genotypes by silver nanoparticles. *Environmental Pollution, 308*, 119606.
7. Chen, J., Sun, L., Cheng, Y., Lu, Z., Shao, K., Li, T., Hu, C., & Han, H. (2016). Graphene oxide-silver nanocomposite: Novel agricultural antifungal agent against *Fusarium graminearum* for crop disease prevention. *ACS Applied Materials and Interfaces, 8*, 24057–24070.
8. Chen, J., Wu, L., Lu, M., Lu, S., Li, Z. Y., & Ding, W. (2020). Comparative study on the fungicidal activity of metallic MgO nanoparticles and macroscale MgO against soilborne fungal phytopathogens. *Frontiers in Microbiology, 11*, 365.
9. Chhipa, H. (2019). Applications of nanotechnology in agriculture. In V. Gurtler, A. S. Ball, & S. Soni (Eds.), *Methods in Microbiology* (Vol. 46, pp. 115–142). Academic Press.
10. Dimkpa, C. O., Mclean, J. E., Britt, D. W., & Anderson, A. J. (2013). Antifungal activity of ZnO nanoparticles and their interactive effect with a biocontrol bacterium on growth antagonism of the plant pathogen *Fusarium graminearum*. *BioMetals, 26*, 913–924.
11. Ding, Y., Zhang, G. J., Wu, H., Hai, B., Wang, L., & Qian, Y. (2001). Nanoscale magnesium hydroxide and magnesium oxide powders: Control over size, shape, and structure via hydrothermal synthesis. *Chemistry of Materials, 13*, 435–440.
12. Donici, A., Bunea, C. I., Călugăr, A., Hărşan, E., & Bora, F. D. (2019). Investigation of the copper content in vineyard soil, grape, must and wine in the main vineyards of Romania: A preliminary study. *Bulletin of University of Agricultural Sciences and Veterinary Medicine Cluj-Napoca. Horticulture, 76*(2), 241–250.
13. El-Batal, A. I., Balabel, N. M. A., Attia, M. S., & El-Sayyad, G. S. (2019). Antibacterial and antibiofilm potential of mono-dispersed stable copper oxide nanoparticles-streptomycin nano-drug: Implications for some potato plant bacterial pathogen treatment. *Journal of Cluster Science, 31*, 1021–1040.

14. Hassan, S. E. D., Fouda, A., Saied, E., Farag, M. M. S., Eid, A. M., Barghoth, M. G., Awad, M. A. A., Hamza, M. F., & Awad, M. F. (2021). *Rhizopus oryzae*-mediated green synthesis of magnesium oxide nanoparticles (MgO-NPs): A promising tool for antimicrobial, mosquitocidal action, and tanning effluent treatment. *Journal of Fungi, 7*, 372.

15. Hassanisaadi, M., Barani, M., Rahdar, A., Heidary, M., Thysiadou, A., & Kyzas, G. Z. (2022). Role of agrochemical-based nanomaterials in plants: Biotic and abiotic stress with germination improvement of seeds. *Plant Growth Regulation, 97*, 375–418.

16. He, Y., Ingudam, S., Reed, S., Gehring, A., Strobaugh Jr., T. P., & Irwin, P. (2016). Study on the mechanism of antibacterial action of magnesium oxide nanoparticles against foodborne pathogens. *Journal of Nanobiotechnology, 14*, 54.

17. Huang, L., Li, D. Q., Lin, Y., Wei, M., Evans, D. G., & Duan, X. (2005). Controllable preparation of nano-MgO and investigation of its bactericidal properties. *Journal of Inorganic Biochemistry, 99*, 986–993.

18. Imada, K., Sakai, S., Kajihara, H., Tanaka, S., & Ito, S. (2015). Magnesium oxide nanoparticles induce systemic resistance in tomato against bacterial wilt disease. *Plant Pathology, 65*, 551–560.

19. Ivanov, A. A., Ukladov, E. O., & Golubeva, T. S. (2021). *Phytophthora infestans*: An overview of methods and attempts to combat late blight. *Journal of Fungi, 7*, 1071.

20. Jayarambabu, N., Sivakumari, B., Venkateswararao, K. T., & Prabhu, Y. T. (2016). Enhancement of growth in maize by biogenic-synthesized MgO nanoparticles. *International Journal of Pure and Applied Zoology, 4*, 262–270.

21. Joe, A., Park, S. H., Shim, K. D., Kim, D. J., Jhee, K. H., Lee, H. W., Heo, C. H., Kim, H. M., & Jang, E. S. (2017). Antibacterial mechanism of ZnO nanoparticles under dark conditions. *Journal of Industrial and Engineering Chemistry, 45*, 430–439.

22. Judelson, H. S., & Blanco, F. (2005). The spores of *Phytophthora*: Weapons of the plant destroyer. *Nature Reviews Genetics, 3*, 47–58.

23. Kasemets, K., Ivask, A., Dubourguier, H. C., & Kahru, A. (2009). Toxicity of nanoparticles of ZnO, CuO and TiO_2 to yeast *Saccharomyces cerevisiae. Toxicology in Vitro, 23*, 1116–1122.

24. Khan, A. M., Shabbier, D., Ahmad, P., Khandaker, M. U., Faruque, M. R. I., & Din, I. U. (2020). Biosynthesis and antibacterial activity of MgO-NPs produced from *Camellia sinensis* leaves extract. *Materials Research Express, 8*, 015402.

25. Kim, D., Langmead, B., & Salzberg, S. L. (2015). HISAT: A fast spliced aligner with low memory requirements. *Nature Methods, 12*, 357–360.

26. Klopfenstein, D. V., Zhang, L., Pedersen, B. S., Ramírez, F., Warwick Vesztrocy, A., Naldi, A., Mungall, C. J., Yunes, J. M., Botvinnik, O. B., Weigel, M., et al. (2018). GOATOOLS: A Python library for Gene Ontology analyses. *Scientific Reports, 8*, 10872.

27. Kumar, A., & Kumar, J. (2008). On the synthesis and optical absorption studies of nano-size magnesium oxide powder. *Journal of Physics and Chemistry of Solids, 69*, 2764–2772.

28. Kumar, D., Reddy, V. B., Mishra, B. G., Rana, R., Nadagouda, M. N., & Varma, R. S. (2007). Nanosized magnesium oxide as catalyst for the rapid and green synthesis of substituted 2-amino-2-chromenes. *Tetrahedron, 63*, 3093–3097.

29. Kumar, S., Li, G., Yang, J., Huang, X., Ji, Q., Liu, Z., Ke, W., & Hou, H. (2021). Effect of salt stress on growth, physiological parameters, and ionic concentration of water dropwort (*Oenanthe javanica*) cultivars. *Frontiers in Plant Science, 12*, 660409.

30. Kumari, M., Shukla, S., Pandey, S., Giri, V. P., Bhatia, A., Tripathi, T., Kakkar, P., Nautiyal, C. S., & Mishra, A. (2017). Enhanced cellular internalization: A bactericidal mechanism more relative to biogenic nanoparticles than chemical counterparts. *ACS Applied Materials & Interfaces, 9*, 4519–4533.

31. Li, B., & Dewey, C. N. (2011). RSEM: Accurate transcript quantification from RNA-Seq data with or without a reference genome. *BMC Bioinformatics, 12*, 323.

32. Li, J., Chang, X., Chen, X., Gu, Z., Zhao, F., Chai, Z., & Zhao, Y. (2014). Toxicity of inorganic nanomaterials in biomedical imaging. *Biotechnology Advances, 32*, 727–743.

33. Li, W., Wang, C., Yao, Y., Wu, C., Luo, W., & Zou, Z. (2020). Photocatalytic materials: An Apollo's arrow to tumor cells. *Trends in Chemistry, 2*, 1126–1140.

34. Lipovsky, A., Tzitrinovich, Z., Friedmann, H., Applerot, G., Gedanken, A., & Lubart, R. (2009). EPR study of visible light-induced ROS generation by nanoparticles of ZnO. *The Journal of Physical Chemistry C, 113*, 15997–16001.

35. Liu, B., Xue, Y., Zhang, J., Han, B., Zhang, J., Suo, X., & Mu, L. (2017). Visible-light-driven TiO2/Ag3PO4 heterostructures with enhanced antifungal activity against agricultural pathogenic fungi *Fusarium graminearum* and mechanism insight. *Environmental Science: Nano, 4*, 255–264.

36. Makhluf, S. B. D., Dror, R., Nitzan, Y., Abramovich, Y., Jelinek, R., & Gedanken, A. (2005). Microwave-assisted synthesis of nanocrystalline MgO and its use as a bacteriocide. *Advanced Functional Materials, 15*, 1708–1715.

37. Medina, E., Kim, S. H., Yun, M., & Choi, W. G. (2021). Recapitulation of the function and role of ROS generated in response to heat stress in plants. *Plants, 10*, 371.

38. Mohammadpour, R., Dobrovolskaia, M. A., Cheney, D. L., Greish, K. F., & Ghandehari, H. (2019). Subchronic and chronic toxicity evaluation of inorganic nanoparticles for delivery applications. *Advanced Drug Delivery Reviews, 144*, 112–132.

39. Ogunyemi, S. O., Zhang, M., Abdallah, Y., Ahmed, T., Qiu, W., Ali, M. A., Yan, C., Yang, Y., Chen, J., & Li, B. (2020). The bio-synthesis of three metal oxide nanoparticles (ZnO, MnO2, and MgO) and their antibacterial activity against the bacterial leaf blight pathogen. *Frontiers in Microbiology, 11*, 588326.

40. Pacilly, F. C. A., Groot, J. C. J., Hofstede, G. J., Schaap, B. F., & van Bueren, E. T. L. (2016). Analysing potato late blight control as a social-ecological system using fuzzy cognitive mapping. *Agronomy for Sustainable Development, 36*, 1–18.

41. Parizi, M. A., Moradpour, Y., Roostaei, A., Khani, M., Negahdari, M., & Rahimi, G. (2014). Evaluation of the antifungal effect of magnesium oxide nanoparticles on *Fusarium oxysporum* F. Sp. lycopersici, pathogenic agent of tomato. *European Journal of Experimental Biology, 4*, 3.

42. Pertea, M., Pertea, G., Antonescu, C., Chang, T. C., Mendell, J. T., & Salzberg, S. L. (2015). String Tie enables improved reconstruction of a transcriptome from RNA-seq reads. *Nature Biotechnology, 33*, 290–295.

43. Petrov, V., Hille, J., Mueller-Roeber, B., & Gechev, T. S. (2015). ROS-mediated abiotic stress-induced programmed cell death in plants. *Frontiers in Plant Science, 6*, 69.

44. Pritchard, J. K., Stephens, M., Rosenberg, N. A., & Donnelly, P. (2000). Association mapping in structured populations. *American Journal of Human Genetics, 67*, 170–181.

45. Raghupathi, K. R., Koodali, R. T., & Manna, A. C. (2011). Size-dependent bacterial growth inhibition and mechanism of antibacterial activity of zinc oxide nanoparticles. *Langmuir, 27*, 4020–4028.

46. Schepers, H., Kessel, G. J. T., Lucca, F., Förch, M. G., van den Bosch, G. B. M., Topper, C. G., & Evenhuis, A. (2018). Reduced efficacy of fluazinam against *Phytophthora infestans* in the Netherlands. *European Journal of Plant Pathology, 151*, 947–960.

47. Stoimenov, P. K., Klinger, R. L., Marchin, G., & Klabunde, K. J. (2002). Metal oxide nanoparticles as bactericidal agents. *Langmuir, 18*, 6679–6686.

48. Sukhanova, A., Bozrova, S., Sokolov, P., Berestovoy, M., Karaulov, A., & Nabiev, I. (2018). Dependence of nanoparticle toxicity on their physical and chemical properties. *Nanoscale Research Letters, 13*, 44.

49. Sun, Y., Oberley, L. W., & Li, Y. (1988). A simple method for clinical assay of superoxide dismutase. *Clinical Chemistry, 34*, 497–500.

50. Tremblay, V., Mclaren, D. L., Kim, Y. M., Strelkov, S. E., Conner, R. L., Wally, O. S. D., & Bélanger, R. R. (2021). Molecular assessment of pathotype diversity of *Phytophthora sojae* in Canada highlights declining sources of resistance in soybean. *Plant Disease, 105*, 4006–4013.

51. Vleeshouwers, V. G. A. A., Raffaele, S., Vossen, J. H., Champouret, N., Oliva, R., Segretin, M. E., Rietman, H., Cano, L. M., Lokossou, A., Kessel, G., et al. (2011). Understanding and exploiting late blight resistance in the age of effectors. *Annual Review of Phytopathology, 49*, 507–531.

52. Wang, Y., Cao, A., Jiang, Y., Zhang, X., Liu, J. H., Liu, Y., & Wang, H. (2014). Superior antibacterial activity of zinc oxide/graphene oxide composites originating from high zinc concentration localized around bacteria. *ACS Applied Materials & Interfaces, 6*, 2791–2798.

53. Xie, C., Mao, X., Huang, J., Ding, Y., Wu, J., Dong, S., Kong, L., Gao, G., Li, C. Y., & Wei, L. (2011). KOBAS 2.0: A web server for annotation and identification of enriched pathways and diseases. *Nucleic Acids Research, 39*, 316–322.

Chapter

2

DIFFERENT CLASSES OF TOXICANTS AND THEIR CHARACTERISTICS: AN OVERVIEW

Contents

Introduction

The classification of toxic substances is a complex and nuanced process that varies based on the specific needs and preferences of the entities undertaking the classification. This variability arises because there is no universally accepted system that encompasses all types of hazardous chemicals. As such, the most effective approach often involves integrating multiple classification systems that take into account a variety of characteristics. These characteristics can be biological, chemical, and even include factors related to the visibility and detectability of the toxins.

Toxic substances can be categorized based on a multitude of criteria. One common method involves classifying toxins by their origin. This includes categories such as mineral toxins derived from inorganic sources, toxins produced by animals, those originating from plants, and synthetically created man-made toxins. Another approach classifies toxins based on their physical state, distinguishing among solids, liquids, gases, and particulates, which affects how these toxins interact with the environment and living organisms.

Focusing on the effects of toxins, classification can also be by the target organ or system they primarily affect. Examples include hepatotoxic substances that damage the liver, hematotoxic substances that affect the blood, pulmotoxic agents impacting the lungs, and nephrotoxic substances that impair kidney function. Multiple instances of such classification are evident, with some toxins affecting several systems or organs simultaneously.

The chemical nature or structure of toxins also plays a crucial role in their classification. This can range from broad categories such as metals and non-metals to more specific groupings like acids, alkalis, carbonates, other carbon compounds (excluding carbon oxides), cyanides, and metal carbides. Additionally, the analytical behavior of toxicants provides another layer of classification, differentiating among extractive toxicants, volatile substances, and various forms of metalloids and metals.

The types of toxic effects—whether acute, chronic, or subacute—also form a basis for categorizing toxins. This extends to more specific toxicological effects such as teratogenicity, carcinogenicity, mutagenicity, and clastogenicity, which describe the potential of substances to cause birth defects, cancer, mutations, and chromosome breakages, respectively.

Moreover, toxins are classified by their uses, such as in pesticides (insecticides, rodenticides, herbicides, fungicides) and as food additives. Each category involves distinct regulatory considerations and health implications. The mode of action of the toxin, which explains how the toxin exerts its effect at the molecular or cellular level, is another critical aspect of classification.

Finally, environmental and health impacts play a significant role in the classification of toxic substances. These factors are crucial for understanding the broader implications of toxin exposure on public health and ecosystems, guiding the development of safety regulations and preventive measures.

Orientation and Directional Terms

Term	Definition	Illustration
Air Pollutants	Substances in the air that are harmful to human health or the environment, including gases, particulates, and biological molecules.	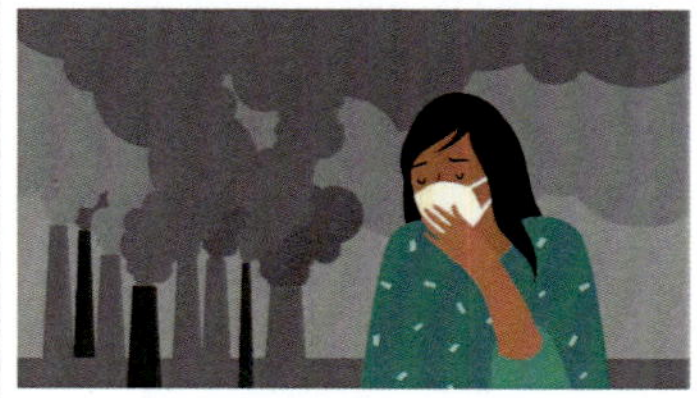
Lead	A toxic heavy metal that can cause severe health problems, especially in children, including developmental and neurological damage.	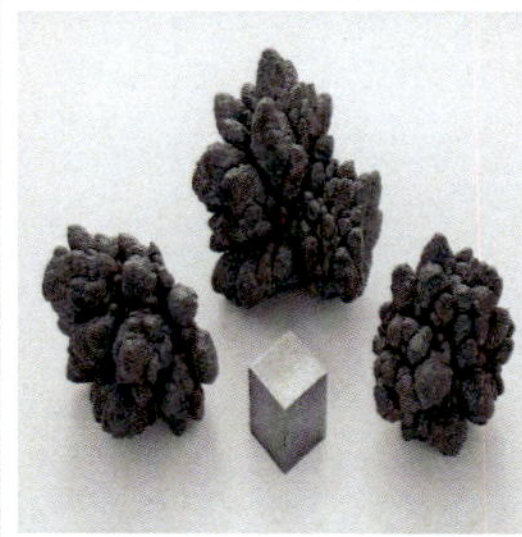
Arsenic	A toxic metalloid element that can cause cancer and skin lesions, and can affect various organs in the body.	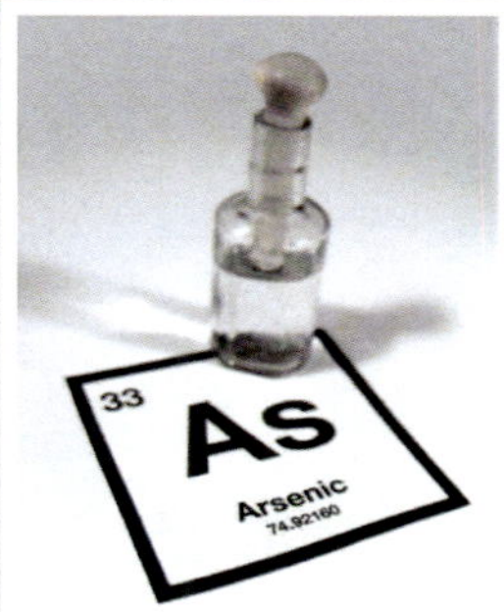
Cadmium	A heavy metal that can lead to kidney damage, bone weakening, and respiratory issues; it is commonly found in industrial settings.	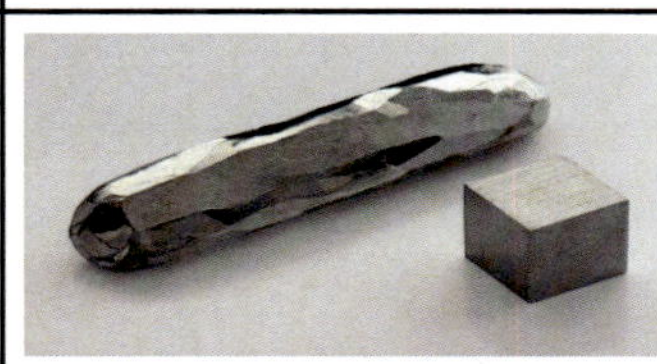
Mercury	A heavy metal that is highly toxic, affecting the nervous system and causing various health problems, often found in contaminated water and soil.	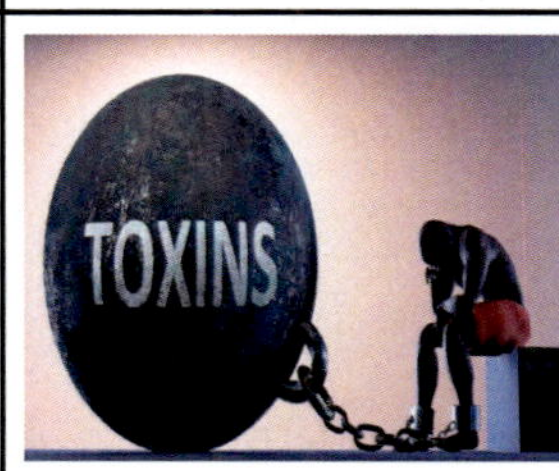

2.1. Toxicants Originating from Air Pollution: Sources, Characteristics, and Health Impacts

Air pollution most likely began when people started using wood for heating and cooking. For thousands of years, fireplaces were used in such a way that living spaces were full of smoke. Combustion products and culinary odors were diverted from living spaces and vented outdoors with the construction of chimneys (Giudice, 2016; Ostrosky-Wegman & Gonsebatt, 1996). Coal smoke became a nuisance in cities after soft coals were found and used as fuel. By the 13th century, fuel smoke became a problem in London, and in 1273 Edward I enacted the first Clean Air Act, banning coal burning during sessions of the National Assembly: "It is clear to all in the tone of my voice, and any man therefore convicted of coal burning shall lose his head." Despite this and subsequent royal decrees, smoke pollution continues to be a problem in London (Goldizen et al., 2016) (Figure 2.1).

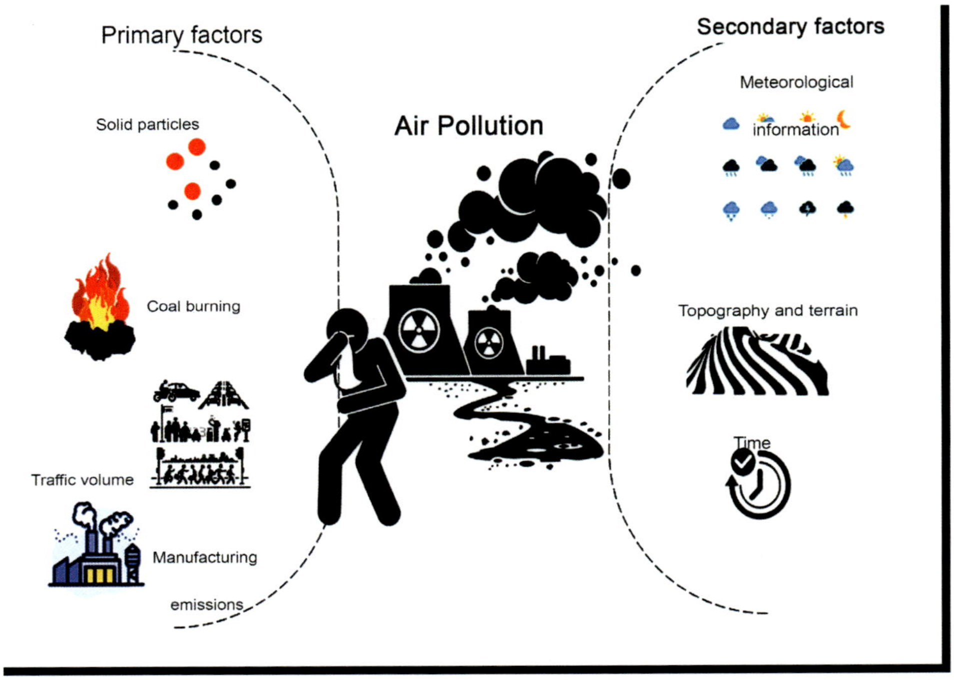

Figure 2.1. *Illustration of pollution sources in the air.*

Source: Mengara, A. G., Kim, Y., Yoo, Y., & Ahn, J., (2020). Distributed deep features extraction model for air quality forecasting. Sustainability, 12(19), 8014. https://doi.org/10.3390/su12198014.

Air pollution has steadily worsened with the increase in domestic and industrial coal consumption, especially in large cities. The most notable development in the 20th century was the huge increase in the number of vehicles, which rose from almost nothing at the turn of the century to 1 million in just a few years (Pinkerton & Joad, 2006). Until well after the Second World War, only minimal measures were taken to regulate air quality in some industrialized countries. Two serious cases of air pollution, in which human deaths were caused by excessive levels of pollutants, motivated action. In 1948, an event occurred in Donora, a tiny steel mill area in western Pennsylvania. In late October, heavy smog formed in the region and a meteorological inversion prevented the pollutants from leaving the area. The effects of the pollution were directly responsible for twenty-one deaths. The story of "Donora" drew attention to the problem of air pollution in the United States (Gordon, 2003; Colombo, 2020).

2.1.1. Types of Air Pollutants

What is the definition of clean air? Pollution-free air would be an idea of what the air would look like if there were no humans and their activities on the planet so that natural sources such as forest fires and volcanoes would not pollute the air. Since humans have been polluting the atmosphere for centuries, the actual structure of "unpolluted" air is unclear. Terpenes from trees, smoke from forest fires and gasses and smoke from volcanoes are all organic pollutants. Table 2.1 shows the elements that are considered clean air in the absence of pollution (Curtis et al., 2006) (Figure 2.2).

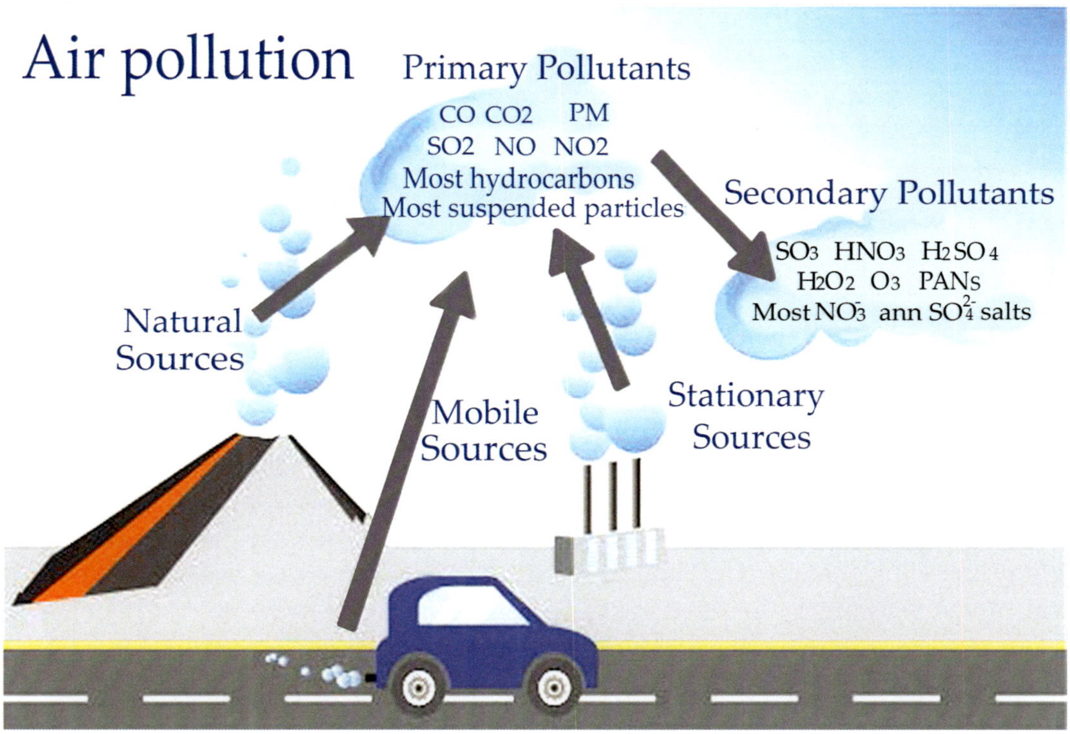

Figure 2.2. *Schematic of pollutant types in the air.*

Source: https://assets-global.website-files.com/.

1. **Gaseous Pollutants:** These substances include gasses at room temperature and atmospheric pressure as well as vapors that evaporate from solids or liquids. Hydrocarbons, carbon monoxide (CO), hydrogen sulfide (H_2S), nitrogen oxides (NxOy), ozone (O_3) and other oxidizing agents, sulfur oxides (SxOy) and CO_2 are some of the most dangerous pollutants (Stuck, 1977).

Table 2.1. *Gaseous Components of Normal Dry Air*

Component	Percentage by Volume (%)
Nitrogen (N_2)	78.08
Oxygen (O_2)	20.95
Argon (Ar)	0.93
Carbon dioxide (CO_2)	0.04
Neon (Ne)	0.0018
Helium (He)	0.0005
Methane (CH_4)	0.00017
Krypton (Kr)	0.0001
Hydrogen (H_2)	0.00005
Xenon (Xe)	0.000009
Ozone (O_3)	Trace amounts
Nitrous oxide (N_2O)	Trace amounts
Other trace gases	Trace amounts

Source: (Ravindra et al., 2008)

Table 2.1 lists the major and trace gases found in normal dry air, excluding water vapor which varies in concentration depending on the humidity and environmental conditions. Pollutant concentrations are often measured in micrograms per cubic meter (g/m^3) and parts per million (ppm) per volume for toxic gasses, where 1 ppm corresponds to one part pollutant per million parts (106) of air (Tian et al., 2019).

Particulate pollutants: Air can contain fine particles or liquid. Below are some examples of different types of particles (Guo et al., 2019):

1. **Dust:** Particles with a diameter of about 100 m that come directly from the chemicals used (e.g., sawdust, coal dust, cement dust, ash, grain dust).
2. **Vapors:** Suspended particles with a diameter of 1 m are usually released during mechanical or chemical processes (e.g., lead and zinc oxides).
3. **Mists:** Liquid droplets suspended in the air with a radius of less than 2.0 m (e.g., sulphuric acid mist).
4. **Smoke:** Improper combustion of fossil fuels produces solid particles (size range 0.05–1.0 m).
5. **Aerosol:** Solids (diameter range 0.05–1.0 m) are produced when fossil fuels are burned improperly.

2.1.2. Examples of Air Pollutants

Acute pollution events such as those in London and Donora provide the most data on the effects of air pollution on humans. Chemical irritation of the pulmonary system can lead to illness, with particularly sensitive groups of people being much more affected:

1. Extremely young infants with underdeveloped circulatory and respiratory systems.
2. Elderly people whose cardiovascular and pulmonary systems are in poor condition; (Kim et al., 2014).
3. People who suffer from cardiovascular diseases such as asthma, emphysema, or cardiovascular disease and who smoke are also more susceptible to air pollution.

The combined effect of particulate matter and sulfur dioxides (SO_2) appears to be responsible in most cases; no single pollutant appears to be to blame (Schradee et al., 2014).

Table 2.2 provides an overview of some of the most common air pollutants and their origin and consequences (Mauderly & Samet, 2009).

1. **Carbon Monoxide:** This rapidly interacts with hemoglobin (Hb) to form carboxyhemoglobin (COHb), which impedes tissue oxygenation. The sensitivity of hemoglobin

to CO is about 210 times greater than its oxygen demand. A COHb level of 5% in the blood, which corresponds to equilibrium at about 45 ppm CO, is associated with cardiovascular consequences (Harkov, 1982; Hofmann, 1995). Headaches, dizziness, nausea, and breathing problems can occur at levels of 100 ppm. An acute concentration of 1,000 ppm is always fatal. Carbon monoxide concentrations have been observed to reach 400 parts per million (ppm) during heavy traffic congestion; in addition, smoking increases the total weight of CO in the body more than in non-smokers. The long-term consequences of low concentrations of CO are not known, but it is likely to exacerbate heart and respiratory diseases (Goldstein & Carruth, 2003).

2. **Sulfur Oxides:** These are a type of sulfur compound. Sulfur dioxide appears to be a widespread pollutant, mainly from the industrial combustion of coal, with soft coal having the highest sulfur content. Sulfur oxides adhere to air particles and enter the lungs where they are poorly excreted. SO_2 reacts quickly with fluids in the airways and produces sulfurous acid, which causes inflammation of the mucous membranes and constriction of the bronchial tubes. This inflammation makes the airways more susceptible to certain other toxic elements in the air (Krupa & Legge, 2000).

Table 2.2. *Some of the Most Important Air Pollutants, Their Common Sources, and Their Effects on Health and the Environment*

Pollutant	Common Sources	Effects
Carbon monoxide (CO)	Vehicles, industrial processes, residential wood burning.	Reduces oxygen delivery to organs, potentially fatal.
Sulfur dioxide (SO_2)	Power plants, industrial processes.	Causes respiratory problems and acid rain.
Nitrogen oxides (NOx)	Vehicles, power plants, industrial processes.	Respiratory problems, forms ground-level ozone, contributes to smog.
Particulate matter (PM)	Construction sites, unpaved roads, fields, smokestacks.	Respiratory and cardiovascular diseases, reduces visibility.
Ozone (O_3)	Reaction of NOx and volatile organic compounds in sunlight.	Respiratory issues, damages vegetation.
Lead (Pb)	Old paint, industrial processes.	Affects nervous system, harmful to child development.
Volatile organic compounds (VOCs)	Solvents, paints, vehicle emissions.	Forms ozone and smog, various health effects.

Source: (Colman, 2021)

3. **Nitrogen Oxides (NO_2):** A lung irritant found in photochemical smog, has been associated with pulmonary edema and hemorrhage. Although nitrogen oxides can contribute to acid deposition, it is their role in the formation of photochemical smog and ozone that is of particular concern.

4. **Ozone:** The photochemical reaction of ultraviolet (UV) light on nitrogen dioxide during

smog produces a very unpleasant and oxidizing gas. The resulting ozone can lead to lung congestion, edema, and bleeding (Castell et al., 2005; Shen, 2015).

$$NO_2 + \text{UV light} \quad NO + O^{\check{z}}$$

$$O\check{z} + O_2 \quad O_3$$

At this stage, it is important to distinguish between "good" and "bad" ozone. Tropospheric ozone is toxic and is found between zero and ten miles directly above the earth's crust. Stratospheric ozone, which is located about 30 miles above the earth's crust and is benign, is essential for shielding incoming UV light (Nicas & Lomax, 1999). The most recent concern is the depletion of the stratospheric ozone layer. It is estimated that a 1% decrease in the stratospheric ozone layer will increase the number of UV rays reaching the earth's crust by 2%, causing a 10% increase in skin cancer. Chlorofluorocarbons (CFCs) are considered to be one of the main causes of ozone depletion in the stratosphere. By reacting with UV radiation, chlorine is extracted from the CFC components in the earth's atmosphere, which can damage stratospheric ozone through self-perpetuating reactive species (Winner et al., 1991).

$$Cl + O_3 \quad ClO + O_2$$

$$ClO + O \quad Cl + O_2$$

Every chlorine atom may damage up to 10,000 layers of ozone before even being inactivated by methane and nitrogen dioxide. International agreements are progressively phasing out the use of CFC chemicals (Nazaroff & Weschler, 2004).

2.2. Water and Soil Pollutants

With three quarters of the earth's surface covered by water and much of the rest covered by soil, it is not surprising that both soil and water are the final discharges of most man-made pollutants. Until recently, the main concern with water pollution was disease-related health effects, and this is still the case in most poor countries. However, in the United States and other industrialized nations, treatment methods have virtually eradicated bacterial pathogens from the water system, and the focus has shifted to chemical pollutants (Milner et al., 2011).

2.2.1. Examples of Water and Soil Pollutants

There are three types of metals that are hazardous to the environment (Menzer & Nelson, 1991):

- Metals that have been linked to cancer;
- Metals that spread freely in the soil; and
- Metals that are passed through the food chain (Henschler & Lehnert, 1994).

2.2.2. Lead

Lead (Pb) and Arsenic are the two heavy metals that pose the biggest health risk when consumed via groundwater. The major sources of lead in drinking water include lead pipes and lead soldering. Leakage of lead through soil polluted by the fallout from leaded petrol, as well as leakages of lead from dangerous sites, are further causes for worry. Lead poisoning is a regular occurrence in children, particularly in elderly residential units and inner-city residences, where youngsters may ingest lead-contaminated paint colors (Fowler et al., 1999).

2.2.3. Arsenic

The dissolution of inorganic toxic elements formerly used in pesticide sprays, the burning of oil and coal containing arsenic, and the dissolution of mining waste and smelting effluents pose a risk to arsenic-contaminated drinking water. Irregular skin pigmentation, blocked noses, hyperkeratosis, and stomach complaints can be symptoms of high long-term exposure. Lower levels of prolonged exposure pose the greatest risk of cancer. Chronic exposure to arsenic has been associated with malignant diseases of the skin, lymph glands and lungs in epidemiological studies (Monn, 2001).

2.2.4. Cadmium

Contamination with metals has several serious consequences, including the accumulation of metals in the tissues of aquatic organisms, leading to higher metal concentrations in the food chain. Concerns about prolonged exposure to cadmium grew when the disease itai-itai (achy-painful) was discovered in certain parts of Japan. In places where rice is contaminated with high levels of cadmium, the disease manifests as a mixture of severe kidney damage and severe bone and joint disease. This pollution comes from irrigating the land with water containing cadmium from industrial sources. Cadmium poisoning has also been linked to the consumption of cadmium-containing fish caught in rivers near smelters in Japan (Manning & Keane, 1988).

2.2.5. Mercury

In the 1950s and 1960s, mercury-containing waste from the chemical and plastics industries was dumped into Minamata Bay in Japan. Bacteria in the underwater sediments converted the mercury into easily absorbable methylmercury (MeHg).

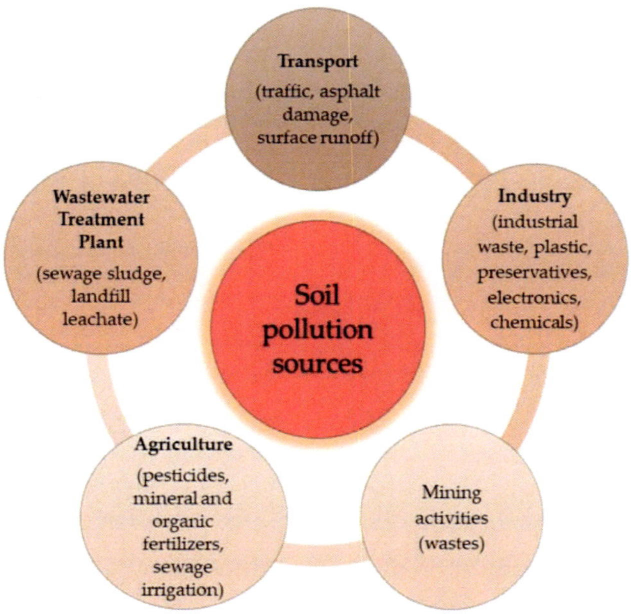

Figure 2.3. *Soil contamination and subterranean water pollution.*

Source: Wołejko, E., Wydro, U., Odziejewicz, J. I., Koronkiewicz, A., & Jabłońska-Trypuć, A., (2022). Biomonitoring of soil contaminated with herbicides. Water, 14(10), 1534. https://doi.org/10.3390/w14101534.

The consumption of fish and shellfish by the local population led to several cases of mercury poisoning, often referred to as Minamata disease. By 1970, mercury poisoning was blamed for at least 107 deaths, and 800 cases of Minamata disease were documented. Although the women appeared to be in good health, many of the children of these mothers, who had already eaten infected fish, showed cerebral palsy and mental deficits (Scow & Johnson, 1996) (Figure 2.3).

Since the mid-1960s, phosphates and nitrates, two important nutrients, have steadily increased in natural rivers. Fertilizers, wastewater treatment plant discharges, sewerage and manure leachate are all causes of nitrate pollution. Fertilizer nitrates run off quickly from the soil and it is estimated that up to 40% of applied nitrates enter water bodies via drainage and leachate. Fertilizer phosphates, on the other hand, are preferentially absorbed or bound to sand grains, so that only 20 to 25% of the nitrates applied reach the water. Another source of phosphates are phosphate-containing detergents, which have recently been the subject of much media coverage (Mostert et al., 2010).

Excess nutrients can lead to "algal blooms" or eutrophication in lakes, estuaries, ponds, and very slow-flowing rivers, so the increase in such nutrients, especially phosphates, is of environmental concern. The algal bloom reduces light penetration and prevents the water from being re-oxygenated by the atmosphere. When a thick algal bloom dies, microbial decomposition occurs, leading to an anaerobic environment and the death of a variety of aquatic life. As watercourses are constantly being washed away and algae do not concentrate, high levels of phosphate and algal blooms are rarely a problem (Havlikova & Kroeze, 2006).

Oils or petroleum are ubiquitous contaminants in today's environment, be it from the waste oil of individual vehicles or from spills from oil transporters. Oil spills at sea are also the cause of many bird deaths. Only a small percentage of heavily polluted birds recover after manual oil removal or feeding. The oil also builds up on sand and rocks, making the sites unusable until an expensive clean-up is completed. Crabs, mussels, shrimps, and barnacles, for example, are damaged by the toxic hydrocarbons they ingest. The long-term consequences for aquatic species are not yet fully known, and they could be more harmful than previously thought (Hirano & Tamae, 2011).

Other widespread groundwater pollutants are volatile organic compounds (VOCs). These include petroleum products and halogenated solvents, commonly known as VOCs. Both categories of chemicals are used in significant quantities in a variety of sectors, including rust removers, laundries, paints, and the armed forces. Hydrocarbons used to be stored in underground tanks that eroded or leaked to the surface. Trichloroethylene, vinyl chloride, toluene, xylene, benzene, chloroform, ethylbenzene, tetrachloroethylene, 1,1,1-trichloroethane, trans-1,2-dichloroethane, and dichloromethane are among the 11 VOCs on the EPA's National Priorities List (Loureiro et al., 2018).

In some regions of the world, some levels of radiation of natural origin, such as radon, cause radioactive fallout, but the pollution of ground and surface water by radiation compounds resulting from the manufacture of nuclear weapons and the production of nuclear fuel is of particular concern. Due to government monitoring, most of these sites have gone unnoticed (Copaciu et al., 2016).

Most freshwater lakes and rivers are heavily contaminated with acids found in rainfall or mine runoff. Acids are particularly dangerous as they can lower the pH of water to lethal levels and release harmful metals into solutions

(Havugimana et al., 2017). Every year, the number of PCB-containing organic chemicals detected as water and soil pollutants increases. These include PCBs, phenols, solvents, cyanides, plasticizers, and a variety of other industrial compounds. PCBs are known by-products of plastic, lubricant, rubber, and paper manufacturing and have traditionally been used as coolants in power transformers. They are lipid-soluble, stable, and degrade slowly in tissues. Because of these properties, they accumulate in large quantities in fish and waterfowl; in 1969, PCBs were blamed for the deaths of thousands of seabirds in the Irish Sea (Crouau et al., 1999).

Due to industrial accidents and the extensive use of 2,4,5-T herbicides, dioxin in the form of the extremely dangerous TCDD (2,3,7,8-tetrachlorodibenzo-p-dioxin) has contaminated large areas of soil and water. Small amounts of TCDD have been found as a pollutant in the production of herbicides. The herbicide Agent Orange was used extensively by the US Army in Vietnam as a dispersant (Zhang & Zhang, 2022). TCDD is one of the most toxic synthetic chemicals to laboratory animals, with LD_{50} values of 0.022 mg/kg for male mice, 0.045 mg/kg for female rats and 0.0006 mg/kg for female guinea pigs (the most sensitive species studied). In addition, it is fetotoxic in pregnant rats at doses as low as 1/400 of the LD_{50} and has been shown to cause birth defects at concentrations as low as 1 to 3 ng/kg. TCDD has been shown to be carcinogenic in mice and rats, with the liver being the organ most severely affected. While TCDD does not appear to be particularly acutely harmful to humans, chronic low-level exposure is thought to contribute to sexual abnormalities and carcinogenic effects (Cakmak et al., 2018).

2.3. Occupational Toxicology

Examples of industrial toxins: Exposure to carcinogens is mostly due to lifestyle factors such as tobacco smoking, although occupation is also an important source of carcinogen exposure (Costa et al., 2017) (Figure 2.4).

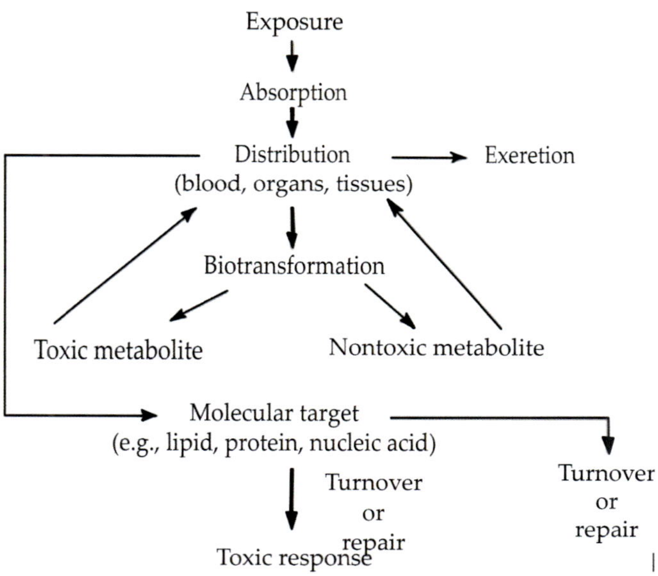

Figure 2.4. *Illustration of occupational toxicology.*

Source: https://ars.els-cdn.com/.

Cadmium appears to be a cumulative toxicant to humans with a biological midlife of up to 30 years. Over 70% of cadmium in the blood is bound to red blood cells; cadmium accumulates primarily in the kidney and liver, where it binds to metallothionein. The kidney would be the critical target organ in humans after long-term cadmium poisoning, with elevated protein urine being the first recognizable sign of kidney damage (Zawadzki et al., 2016).

Chromium toxicity is caused by hexavalent chromium, which is rapidly absorbed by the lungs and digestive tract (GI), but less so by the skin. Dermatitis, nasal septum, ulcers on arms and hands, perforation of mucous membranes (possibly caused by chromic acid), throat, and liver infections and bronchitis are all symptoms of occupational chromium (Cr^{6+}) exposure. Chromate is a carcinogen that causes bronchial carcinomas; workers in chromating plants have a 20-fold higher risk of lung cancer than the general population. Trivalent chromium compounds are only weakly assimilated. Chromium is a non-accumulative chemical that is rapidly excreted in the urine after ingestion (Zhang et al., 2021).

Since lead is a common toxic substance in the environment, the healthy level of lead in the body depends on the circumstances of exposure. Only about half of the lead produced in the lungs is absorbed, while only about 10% of ingested lead enters the bloodstream. Although lead is no longer a major hazard in the workplace, environmental contamination is still ubiquitous (Ng & Amini, 2021). Lead inhibits the formation of porphyrins and heme, and numerous methods for screening for lead toxicity take advantage of this relationship by looking for suppression of the enzyme aminolevulinic acid dehydratase (AAD) or the presence of aminolevulinic acid (ALA) and coproporphyrin in urine (UCP). The metabolism of inorganic lead is closely linked to that of calcium, and excess lead can be stored in the bones and remain there for years. Fatigue, sleep disturbances, anemia, colic, and neuritis are all symptoms of inorganic lead poisoning. Severe lead poisoning can lead to encephalopathy, mental retardation and, in rare cases, visual impairment in children (Lichtfouse, 2009).

Mercury is widely used in science and electrical equipment, with the chlor-alkali sector using the most mercury for electrolytic chlorine and sodium hydroxide synthesis. This sector is one of the main causes of mercury pollution around the world. However, MeHg toxicity is the most common cause of mercury poisoning, especially as a result of eating infected seafood (Franssen et al., 1997). The entry and absorption pathways for organic and inorganic mercury are different. Metallic mercury in industry is mainly absorbed by inhalation, with about 80% of inhaled mercury being absorbed as vapor; metallic mercury is less readily absorbed via the gastrointestinal tract. When exposed to inorganic mercury salts, they accumulate mainly in the kidneys and brain. Organic mercury particles can be absorbed by any route. Inflammation of the mouth, muscle tremors (hatter), mental irritability and kidney disease characterized by proteinuria are all symptoms of occupational mercury consumption. Occupational mercurialism, on the other hand, is no longer a serious problem (Zhukova et al., 2011).

In the second half of the 19th century, benzene was used extensively as a rubber latex agent in the rubber industry. The volatile nature of benzene, which made it so attractive to the industry, also led to high solvent concentrations in the atmosphere. Benzene-based rubber types of cement were used in the processing and packaging industry as well as in shoe manufacturing. Although the toxicity of benzene was pointed out as early as 1897 and further findings and warnings were published in the 1920s, the excellent solvent properties of benzene led to its wider use. When benzene was used as a toner solvent in the printing industry in the 1930s, incidents of benzene toxicity occurred. Today, benzene consumption exceeds 11 billion liters of water per year (Preuss et al., 2003).

Benzene appears to be an inhaled steroid and affects the hematopoietic cells in the bone marrow. The number of red blood cells, white blood cells and platelets decreases over time, and a mixture of these signs can also be observed. Aplastic anemia and severe damage to the bone marrow are the result of prolonged exposure to benzene. Leukemia has been associated with benzene exposure (Frigerio et al., 2019).

2.4. Metallic Toxins

Since most metals usually occur naturally in rocks, soil, ores, air, and water, their concentrations are often low and widespread. Human impact is the most significant of human exposure and toxicological significance, as it increases metal concentrations at the site of human activities (Levander, 1977).

For most of human history, metals were used to make tools, machines, and other objects, and mining provided metals for these applications. Metal concentrations in the environment have been increased by these activities. More recently, metals have found a variety of applications in industry, medicine, and agriculture. These activities have led to increased exposure, not only for professionals dealing with metals, but also for the end users of the various products (Khan et al., 2011).

Despite the enormous variety of toxic metals and toxic properties, many metals exhibit a wide range of toxicological characteristics. The following section briefly describes some of the most important issues. To develop its toxicity, a metal must penetrate the cell surface and then enter the cell. If the metal is always present in a lipid-soluble form, such as MeHg, it can easily cross the membrane; if it is bound to proteins, such as cadmium-metallothionein, the metal is taken up into the cell by endocytosis; other metals (e.g., lead) are absorbed by passive diffusion. Metal toxicity is generally the result of interactions between the free metal and cellular targets. Specific metabolic activities and/or different cell membranes are often used as targets (Sharma et al., 2019).

2.4.1. Lead

Lead is one of the most commonly used hazardous metals due to its long history and wide use. Exposure can occur through air, water, and food. Major industrial uses such as fuel additives and paint pigments have been phased out in the United States, while other uses, such as batteries, are not really an issue. Lead from pipes and ceramic tiles in food containers are two other sources of lead (Klaine et al., 2008).

Inorganic lead (Pb) can enter the body through the gastrointestinal tract, respiratory system and skin. Inorganic lead is more effectively absorbed from the gastrointestinal tract of children than adults, readily crosses the placenta and penetrates the BBS of children. Lead is generally distributed in the blood, kidneys, and liver; however, with prolonged exposure, up to 95 of the body's lead load is detected in bone cells (Flora et al., 2006).

The hematological system and also the neurological system are the main targets of lead poisoning. Many enzymes involved in heme synthesis are susceptible to lead degradation, with ALAD and heme synthetase being the two most susceptible (HS). Although clinical anemia is not detected until lead exposure is significant, biochemical consequences can be seen at lower levels. Therefore, restriction of ALAD or the presence of ALA in the urine can be used as a sign of lead poisoning (Ju-Nam & Lead, 2008). Lead poisoning can also affect the neurological system, which is particularly important in infants and young children whose nervous systems are still growing. Children may exhibit hyperactivity, poor attention span, mental impairment and impaired vision even with moderate exposure. Encephalopathy may affect adults and children to a greater extent. Lead causes cerebral edema and neuronal degeneration by damaging the arterioles and capillaries. Ataxia, coma, convulsions, and stupor are clinical signs of this damage (Flora et al., 2006).

The reproductive organs are another mechanism that is damaged by lead. Lead poisoning can lead to reproductive toxicity in both men and women, as well as miscarriages and malformed children (Handy et al., 2008; Fabrega et al., 2011).

2.4.2. Mercury

Mercury (Hg_0), organic methylmercury (CH_3Hg), inorganic mercury (Hg^+) and mercury salts (Hg^{2+}) as well as dimethylmercury (CH_3HgCH_3) and organic methylmercury molecules (CH_3Hg) are all found in nature. Respiration almost completely absorbs pollutants in the form of mercury vapor, while ingested elemental mercury is also not rapidly absorbed and is therefore generally harmless. Elemental mercury can pass through the BBS and enter the neurological system once ingested. Most people who are exposed to elemental mercury do so at work (Schroeder & Munthe, 1998).

Exposure to organic mercury compounds is of greater concern due to environmental pollution. Through the action of sulfate-reducing microbes, inorganic mercury can be converted to organic mercury, producing MeHg, an extremely toxic form that can easily permeate membranes. Thus, many large outbreaks of mercury poisoning have resulted from the consumption of seafood contaminated with MeHg or seeds treated with mercury fungicides (Harris et al., 2003). In the 1950s and 1960s, mercury-containing waste from a Japanese chemical and plastics plant was dumped into Minamata Bay. Bacteria in the aquaculture sediments converted the mercury into absorbable MeHg. The consumption of fish and seafood by local residents led to numerous cases of mercury poisoning or Minamata disease. Mercury poisoning was blamed for at least 107 deaths by 1970, with 800 symptoms of Minamata disease detected. Many babies born to mothers who were fed contaminated fish showed neurological paralysis and mental deficits, even though their mothers appeared healthy. Organic mercury primarily affects the neurological system, with the brains of pre-born children being more susceptible to mercury toxicity than those of adults (Clarkson, 1997).

The renal tubule cells are the primary uptake site for inorganic mercury salts, which are primarily nephrotoxic. Mercury interacts with the amino groups of membrane proteins and causes oliguria, uremia, and anuria by impairing the stability of the membrane (Langford & Ferner, 1999).

2.4.3. Cadmium

Cadmium occurs naturally mainly in zinc and lead ores and is emitted in the vicinity of mines and smelters that process these ores. Cadmium is used in industry as a pigment in paints and plastics as well as in electroplating, alloys, and alkaline batteries (e.g., nickel-cadmium batteries) (Bidari et al., 2013). Groundwater pollution from smelting and industry and the use of wastewater as fertilizer for food crops are the main sources of cadmium exposure in the environment. The main sources of cadmium in food are cereal products, grains, and green leafy vegetables. Itai-Itai disease, caused by the consumption of cadmium-contaminated rice in Japan, has already been mentioned (Chapter 4,

Section 4.2.2) (Telisman et al., 1986) (Figure 2.5). Most of the acute effects of cadmium exposure are caused by local inflammation. Nausea, abdominal pain and vomiting are the most common symptoms after ingestion. Pneumonia and respiratory edema may occur as a result of inhalation. As cadmium is gradually excreted from the body with a half-life of around 30 years, the chronic effects are of particular concern. As a result, even small amounts of exposure can lead to a considerable accumulation of cadmium (Cambar et al., 1983). The kidneys would be the main organ affected by prolonged exposure, with the distal tubules being the predominant primary site. Cadmium is largely associated with the metal-binding protein metallothionein, which is produced in the liver and circulatory system. CMT is effectively taken up into the body by the tubule cells after glomerular filtration in the kidney, where it accumulates in the lysosomes. The CMT complex is then degraded, releasing Cd+2, which restricts lysosomal action and causes cell damage (Piotrowski et al., 1974).

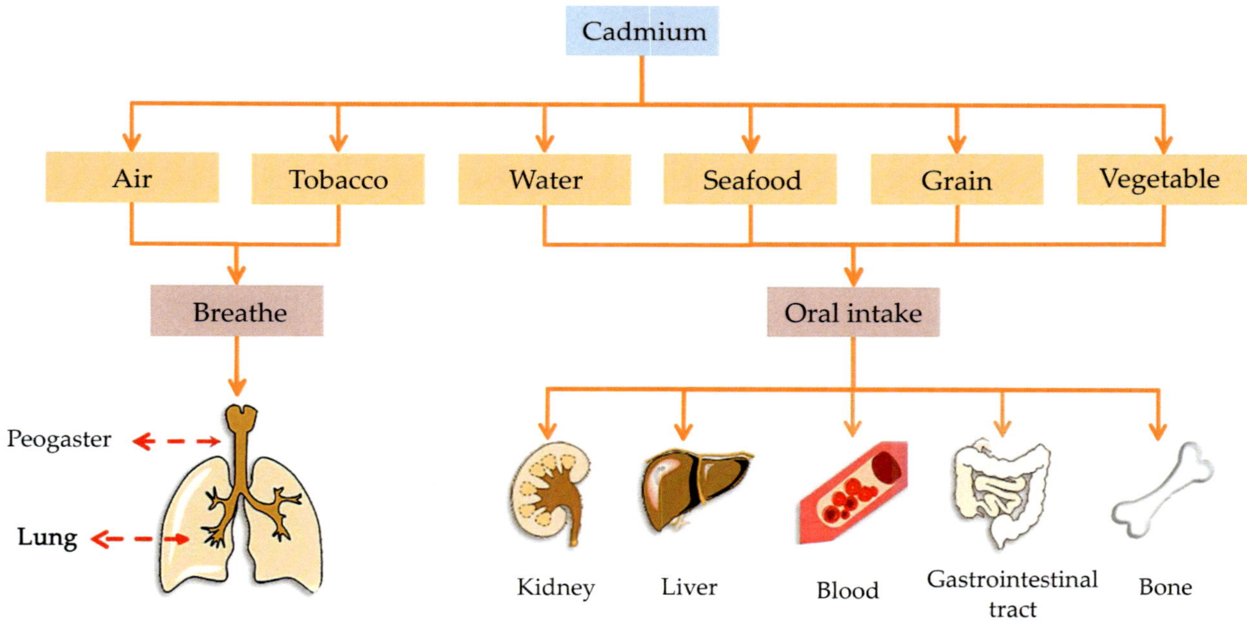

Figure 2.5. *Effects of cadmium exposure on the immune system and immunoregulation.*

Source: Wang, Z., Sun, Y., Yao, W., Ba, Q., & Wang, H., (2021). Effects of cadmium exposure on the immune system and immunoregulation. Front Immunol., 12, 695484. doi: 10.3389/fimmu.2021.695484. PMID: 34354707; PMCID: PMC8330548.

2.4.4. Chromium

Mining, industrial use and smelting pose a risk to the environment, as chromium occurs naturally in ores. Stainless steel, various alloys and paints all contain chromium. The levels of this metal in air, food and water are generally very low, and worker exposure is the most common cause of human exposure. Chromium occurs in a variety of oxidation states, ranging from Cr+2 to Cr+6, but only the trivalent (Cr+3) and hexavalent (Cr+6) forms are biologically relevant (Rai et al., 1989). Although the trivalent molecule is more common, the hexavalent version is more important in industry. Hexavalent chromium is also absorbed faster through cell membranes than trivalent chromium, although the latter is not soluble in water. The hexavalent form is actually converted to the trivalent form, which can form complexes with internal macromolecules and cause toxicity. Chromium is a proven human carcinogen that causes lung cancer in workers exposed to it. The carcinogenicity of chromium (Cr+6) in the lung is thought to be caused by the degradation of chromium (Cr+6) to Cr+3 and the formation of intermediates that lead to bronchogenic carcinoma (Kimbrough et al., 1999).

2.4.5. Arsenic

Arsenic concentrations in water and air are generally low, and the main source of human exposure is food. However, in some places in South America and Taiwan, the water contains significant amounts of this metalloid, causing hyperkeratosis of the skin including hyperpigmentation in the inhabitants. Higher levels of exposure have led to a more severe condition known as "blackfoot disease" or gangrene of the lower extremities. Skin cancer can also occur in these locations (Oremland & Stolz, 2003).

Pesticides account for about 80% of arsenic compounds. Other applications include glassware, pigments, and paints. Arsenic gas is used in the electronics industry. There are three types of arsenic compounds:

i. Pentavalent, As^{+5}, organic or arsenate compounds (e.g., alkyl arsenates);

ii. Trivalent, As^{+3}, inorganic or arsenate compounds (e.g., sodium arsenate, arsenic trioxide); and

iii. Arsine gas, a colorless gas resulting from the action of acids on arsenic.

Arsenic-containing gas is the most toxic form of arsenic and has a TLV-TWA of 0.05 ppm (Braman & Foreback, 1973). Arsenic is converted by microbes into dimethyl arsenate, which can accumulate in fish and seafood, endangering, and contaminating humans. Arsenic compounds can also be found as contaminants in well water. Arsenite molecules (As+3) are lipophilic and can be absorbed through food, inhalation or skin contact. Arsenic is distributed throughout the entire systemic organism within 24 hours of ingestion, where it attaches itself to SH groups of the protein metabolism. Only a tiny percentage makes it beyond the BBS. Arsenic can also be used to restore phosphorus in bone tissue and has a long shelf life. Acute gastrointestinal symptoms occur thirty minutes to two hours after acute poisoning. Symptoms such as vomiting, bloody and watery diarrhea, stomach pain and burning pain in the esophagus are among the symptoms. Vasodilation, cardiovascular depression, cerebral edema, edema and proximal neuropathic pain are possible side effects. Jaundice and renal failure are symptoms of advanced intoxication. Blood Failure of blood flow failure usually leads to death within 24 to 4 days (Nordstrom, 2002).

Diarrhea, hyperkeratosis, abdominal pain, and hyperpigmentation are common symptoms of chronic exposure. Spherical sensory neuropathic pain is often the result. Delayed changes include gangrene of the limbs, anemia, skin, nasal tissue, and lung cancer (Meharg & Hartley-Whitaker, 2002).

2.5. Agricultural Chemicals

Pesticides have been used for thousands of years to destroy or control pests. The Chinese used arsenic to control insects, while the ancient Romans used common salt to control weeds and the Chinese used sulfur to control pests. In the 1800s, the insecticidal properties of pyrethrin (compounds found in the flowers of the chrysanthemum *Pyrethrum cineraefolium*) were discovered (Hallberg, 1987). The Chinese and the natives of South America used the roots of some Derris plant species (*D. eliptica* and *Lonchocarpus* spp.) against fish poisoning. Rotenone, the active component of the plant, was discovered around 1895 and was initially used to control insects. Paris green, a combination of arsenic and copper salts, was another substance produced in the 1800s for pest control. Bordeaux mixture, a mixture of lime and copper sulfate, was used to control fungi (Mann et al., 2009).

2.5.1. Pesticides

However, it was not until the 19th century that the pesticidal substances we know today were developed. Petroleum oils, which are obtained from unrefined crude oil, were first used in the 1920s to treat scale insects and red crawlers. In the 1940s, chlorinated hydrocarbon insecticides such as DDT and phenoxy acid herbicides such as 2,4-D were introduced. Red squill, a natural active ingredient extracted from the bulb of the red orchid, Urginea (Scilla) Maritima, proved useful in controlling rodents (Hallberg, 1987).

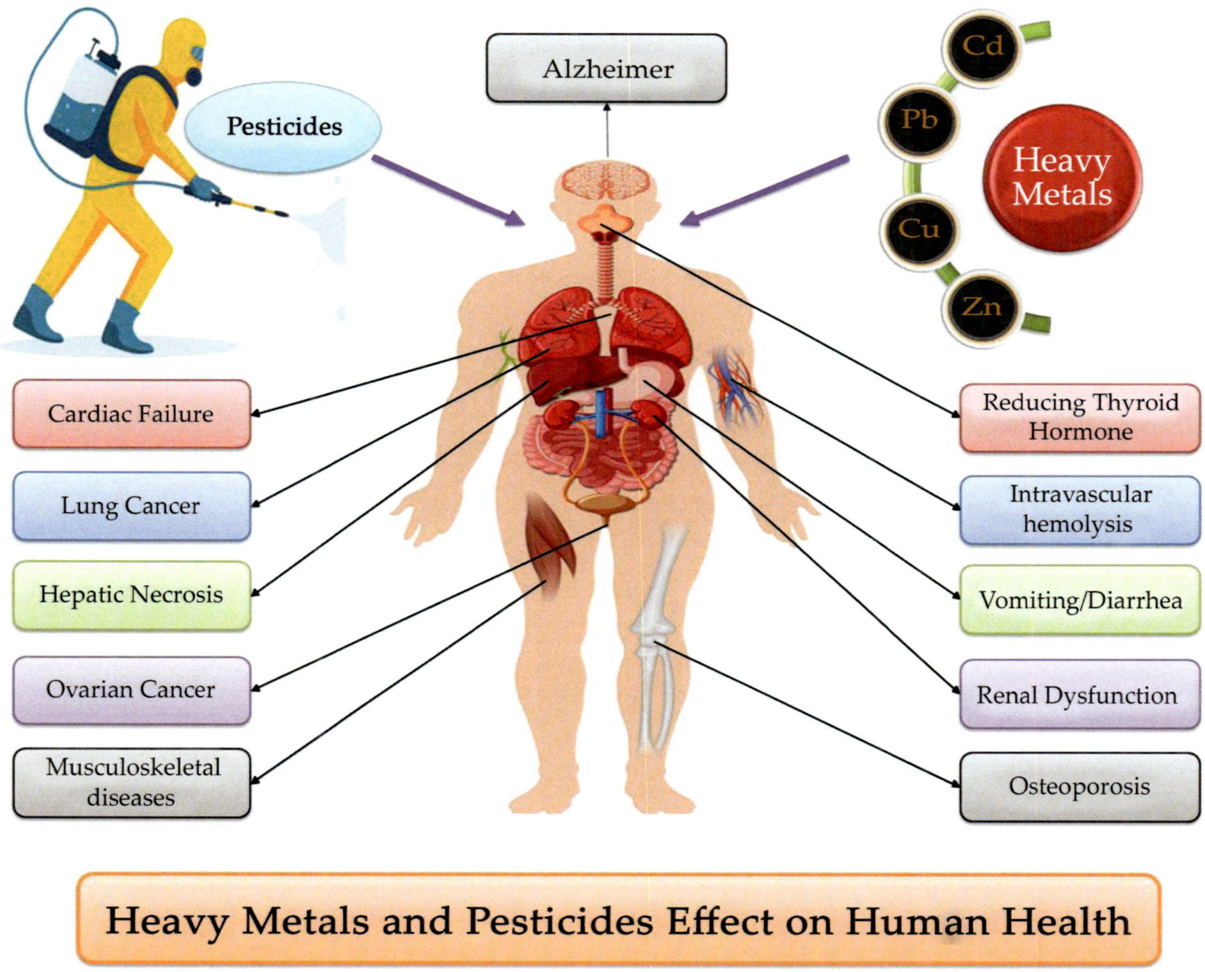

Figure 2.6. *Illustration of pesticides in terms of their effects.*

Source: Alengebawy, A., Abdelkhalek, S. T., Qureshi, S. R., & Wang, M. Q., (2021). Heavy metals and pesticides toxicity in agricultural soil and plants: Ecological risks and human health implications. Toxics, 9(3), 42. https://doi.org/10.3390/toxics9030042.

For many years, triazine herbicides such as atrazine, which came onto the market in the late 1950s, dominated the global herbicide industry. Due to their low toxicity, increased persistence compared to pyrethrins and low application rates, synthetically produced pyrethrins or pyrethroid insecticides (e.g., resmethrin) were and are widely used as insecticides. As older chemicals lose popularity due to pest resistance or negative health effects, families of fungicides, herbicides, and insecticides continue to be introduced to the global market (Gupta & Crissman, 2013) (Figure 2.6).

Pesticides are unique among environmental pollutants in that they are used with the intention of destroying living things. Ideally, pesticides must be highly selective, i.e., they must eliminate the target species while causing little harm to non-target species. Most insecticides, on the other hand, are not so selective (Nielsen, 1987). When deciding for or against the use of pesticides, the benefits must be weighed against the risks to health and the environment. Preventing vector-borne diseases, increasing agricultural production and reducing urban pests are all benefits of pesticides. Environmental contamination, particularly the translocation of pesticides in the environment, poses a significant risk of pesticides entering the food supply and environmental water systems. Persistence in the ecosystem and the possibility of biomagnification are two factors that must be considered (Grant, 1982).

2.5.2. Herbicides

Herbicides are the most commonly used insecticides for weed control. According to recent statistics from the U.S. Environmental Protection Agency (EPA), herbicides accounted for 578 million pounds of pesticides used in the U.S. in 1997, or about 47% of all pesticides used. To eliminate or reduce weed populations, these types of herbicides can be applied to crops in a variety of ways. Examples include pre-sowing integration and pre- and post-sowing treatments. Herbicides that are applied in small quantities are largely non-phytotoxic to crops and therefore ecologically safe and are still under development. Some of the new families, such as the imidazolinones, block the enzyme acetohydroxy acid synthesis, which is responsible for the production of branched-chain amino acids in plants. These herbicides are harmless to animals, fish, birds and insects, as this enzyme is found exclusively in plants (Moreland, 1980).

Herbicides that have been used for years can damage the environment. Chlorophenoxy herbicides such as 2,4,5-T (2,4,5-trichlorophenoxyacetic acid) and 2,4D (2,4-dichlorophenoxyacetic acid) are systemic herbicides that have been used to suppress foliage plants since about the 1940s. These chemicals are not very toxic when ingested (Kudsk & Streibig, 2003).

During the Vietnam War, the US military used a combination of 2,4,5-T and 2,4-D known as Agent Orange as a pure defoliant, and allegations by military personnel of long-lasting health effects have sparked a fierce debate. TCDD (2,3,7,8-tetrachlorodibenzo-dioxin), a pollutant formed during the production process, has been recognized as the chemical of greatest toxicological concern (Morrison et al., 1992). In laboratory animals, TCDD is one of the most toxic synthetic chemicals known. In male rats the lethal dose (LD) was 0.022 mg/kg, in female guinea pigs (the most sensitive species studied) 0.0006 mg/kg. In pregnant mice, TCDD is harmful to developing embryos at doses as low as 1/400 of the LD_{50} and has been reported to cause birth defects at concentrations as low as 1 to 3 ng/kg body weight. TCDD has been shown to be carcinogenic in rats and mice, with the liver being the most severely affected organ.

In exposed animals, this substance has also been shown to alter the immune system and increase susceptibility (Ashton & Crafts, 1973).

The potential for environmental contamination continues to come from herbicide families that have been in use for years. The chlorophenoxy herbicides such as 2,4D (2,4-dichlorophenoxyacetic acid) and 2,4,5-T (2,4,5-trichlorophenoxyacetic acid) are systemic compounds used to control broadleaf plants and have been in use since the 1940s. The oral toxicity of these compounds is low.

Triazines, a class of herbicides, continue to be of concern to environmentalists and toxicologists because they contaminate surface and groundwater supplies that become public drinking water. Atrazine [6-chloro-N-ethyl-N'-(1-methylethyl)-1,3,5-triazine-2,4-diamine] is a corn herbicide with an MCL of 3.0 g/L and is used primarily on corn. This pesticide has been detected in surface and groundwater resources around the world at levels ranging from 1 to >130 g/L (Gianessi, 2013). Together with cyanazine [2–4-chloro-6-(methylamino)-1,3,5-triazine-2ylamino-2-methylpropanenitrile] and simazine (6-chloro-N,Ndiethyl-1,3,5-triazine-2,4-diamine), it has an MCL of 4.0 g/L. The use of cyanazine was phased out in 2001, with no further use permitted after 2002. Although generally harmless (atrazine, for example, has an oral LD_{50} of 3,100 mg/kg (rat)), the main concern with these chemicals is their carcinogenic potential, and the US Environmental Protection Agency has classified all three triazines as probable known human carcinogens (Category C) (Fedtke & Duke, 2005).

2.5.3. Fungicides

Every year, molds cause millions of dollars in agricultural losses in the USA. In addition, recent research has found that toxins and other airborne organics produced by molds inside homes are likely the cause of a variety of negative health effects. Fungicides are substances that have been developed to counteract such losses and negative health effects, and some of these groups have been around for a long time (Qu et al., 2021).

Chlorothalonil (tetrachloroisophthalonitrile) is a widely used fungicide that is often used in urban areas. It is quite inexpensive and controls about 140 different types of organisms. Due to its widespread use, this chemical is often detected in surface waters that enter public water supply systems. In the formulation available to the public, it is largely harmless (Audus, 1964; Walker, 2002).

The dithiocarbamates, sulfur compounds of dithiocarbamic acid, which include the metallic diethyldithiocarbamate, are a class of fungicides that should be avoided. Mancozeb (a coordination product of zinc ions and manganese ethylene bisdithiocarbamate), Maneb (manganese ethylene bisdithiocarbamate) and Zineb (manganese ethylene bisdithiocarbamate) belong to the latter category (zinc ethylene bisdithiocarbamate). All are excellent fungicides that are used on grapes, sugar beet and ornamental plants, among others. They are hydrolyzed and produce recognized carcinogens such as ethylthiourea but are largely harmless (ETU) (Gianessi & Reigner, 2007).

2.5.4. Rodenticides

This family of chemicals is used to keep rodents out of grain stores and other food storage facilities, where they cause annual losses of 20 to 30%. Fleas contain both germs and other organisms, and all of these pests transmit disease in the form of fleas (Knight et al., 1997). Warfarin [3-(-acetonylbenzyl)-4-hydroxycoumarin], an anticoagulant, is one of the rodenticides that has been used for years. With an oral LD_{50} of only 3.0 mg/kg, it is a potent poison (rat). The rats injure it when they move through narrow passages, which leads to slight bleeding. Anticoagulants prevent the formation of blood clots, so the animals die in agony within a week. People who are sensitized to this family of chemicals are treated with vitamin K and, in cases of severe poisoning, with blood donations (Bartett et al., 2001).

Some rodenticides are harmful to animals and are often only used in conjunction with an attractant such as peanut butter that overcomes bait aversion. Fluoroacetamide is a fast-acting poison with an ingestible LD_{50} of 15 mg/kg in rats. This substance is available in the form of bait pellets or granules. Some fast-acting poisons are ANTU ('-naphthylthiourea), strychnine, and thallium saltswere on the market for many years. Most rodenticides have a limited use and are only administered by qualified pest controllers. Poisoning by rodenticides in humans is mainly caused by accidental or suicidal ingestion of the chemicals (Bartlett et al., 2002).

2.5.5. Fumigants

Fumigants are highly toxic gasses that are used to secure stored goods, especially grain, and to eliminate soil worms. Storage facilities, freight vehicles and homes infested with parasites such as the grain weevil are treated with these agents. Due to the risk of inhalation and rapid diffusion into the respiratory tract, special care must be taken when handling and using this family of pesticides. All fumigants are designated as restricted-use substances that may only be used by authorized users (Murphy, 2002).

Methyl bromide is one of the strongest fumigants. It is used to disinfect warehouses and sterilize the soil when applied under a ground cover as it destroys insects, worms, and weed seeds. When inhaled in large quantities, this molecule causes respiratory problems, heart attacks and central nervous system effects. The LC_{50} value for inhalation of air (rat) is 0.06 mg/L (15 min) and 7,900 ppm (1.5 h) (human). Under the Environmental Quality Act, methyl bromide has already been classified as an ozone-depleting substance and is to be phased out by 2005 (Watt et al., 2005).

Another soil/room fumigant that has been used for a long time is chloropicrin (trichloronitromethane). It has an LC_{50} of 150 ppm when inhaled (15 minutes). Consequently, it is very toxic when inhaled, can damage the heart and can also cause significant damage to the eyes (Murphy, 2018).

2.6. Food Additives and Contaminants

Chemicals can be added to foods for various purposes, e.g., as antibacterial, antioxidant or antifungal preservatives, to change physical properties, especially during production, to change taste, color, and odor. In general, flavor enhancers have been shown to be safe and do not cause long-term harm. However, most of them were introduced to the market when toxicological studies were less advanced and some of them have since been shown to be harmful.

Table 2.3 illustrates the many forms of natural food additives (Ibekwe et al., 2001; Joint et al., 2007). Later we will discuss inorganic substances, of which nitrate and nitrite are the most important. Hundreds, if not thousands, of food ingredients are used worldwide, several of which are not adequately tested. The possibility of synergistic effects between these drugs has still not been thoroughly investigated. Not all food toxins are man-made; numerous organically occurring toxins in the human diet, such as carcinogens and genetic mutations, are well recognized (Price, 1985).

Table 2.3. *Examples of Organic Chemicals Commonly Used as Food Additives, Along with Their Typical Uses*

Chemical Name	Type of Additive	Common Use
Acetic acid	Preservative, acidulant	Vinegar, pickles, condiments
Citric acid	Acidulant, preservative	Beverages, canned fruits, ice creams
Ascorbic acid (Vitamin C)	Antioxidant	Fruit juices, cereals
Sodium benzoate	Preservative	Soft drinks, salads, jams
Sucrose (table sugar)	Sweetener	Baked goods, beverages, desserts
Lecithin	Emulsifier	Chocolate, bakery products, dressings
Sodium bicarbonate (baking soda)	Leavening agent	Baked goods, cakes, cookies
Monosodium glutamate (MSG)	Flavor enhancer	Soups, snacks, seasonings

Source: (Saltmarsh, 2019)

2.7. Toxins

2.7.1. Microbial Toxins

Microbiologists commonly refer to toxic chemicals produced by microorganisms that have a certain molecular weight and antigenic properties as "microbial toxins,"" while pollutants produced by microorganisms that do not meet these requirements are vaguely referred to as poisons. Most of the former are proteins or mucoproteins with various enzymatic capabilities. Tetanus toxin, botulinum toxin or diphtheria toxin are among the most dangerous chemicals known. Bacterial toxins can be extremely dangerous to mammals and affect a number of body systems such as the nervous and cardiovascular systems. The scope of this book does not allow for a complete description of their chemical makeup or mode of action (Gupta et al., 2021).

In addition, bacteria produce a wide range of toxic compounds. Again, similar substances can be used for good reasons; for example, the insecticidal properties of *Bacillus thuringiensis*, which are related to the toxin, have long been used in the agricultural industry (Rajkovic, 2014) (Figure 2.7).

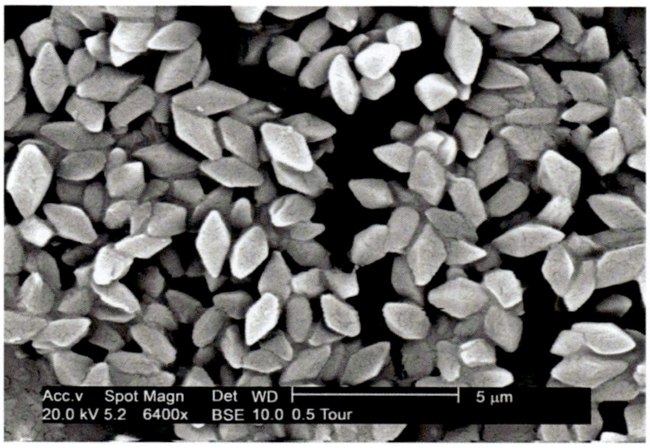

Figure 2.7. *Illustration of bacterial toxins.*

Source: By Jim Buckman is credited and the original uploader is P.R. Johnston. – w:en:Image:Bacillus thuringiensis.JPG, Public Domain; https://commons.wikimedia.org/w/index.php?curid=2471877.

2.7.2. Mycotoxins

The large category of fungi has a wide range of chemical compositions and biological activities that cannot be dealt with in a short time. Mycotoxins are not a distinct chemical group as they do not share common molecular characteristics (Richard, 2007).

Mycotoxins detected in the human diet or even in the feeding of domestic animals are of particular interest. *Claviceps* sp. produces ergot alkaloids, *Aspergillus* sp. produces aflatoxins and similar substances, and various fungal species, especially *Fusarium* sp. produce trichothecenes (Coulombe Jr., 1993).

Ergot alkaloids are known to have a central nervous system and vasoconstrictive effect. They have been associated in the past with severe infections and convulsive illnesses caused by ergot (St. Anthony's fire), but such outbreaks no longer occur in humans due to a better understanding of the causes and a more varied diet. Therefore, ergot infections in animals are still common. Abortifacients have also been made from these chemicals. The ergot alkaloids contain compounds of ergotin, with the amides of lysergic acid being the most potent (Pitt, 2000; Schatzmayr et al., 2006).

Aflatoxins are produced by Aspergillus species, in particular *A. flavus*, a widespread fungus found in cereals, maize, nuts, and other foods. They were first linked to poultry diseases such as turkey X and were later shown to increase the risk of cancer in humans in animal and epidemiologic studies. To develop its carcinogenic effect, aflatoxin B1, the most dangerous of the aflatoxins, must be enzymatically activated (Speijers & Speijers, 2004).

Trichothecenes are a group of sesquiterpenoid fungal metabolites that are mainly produced by Trichoderma and Fusarium fungi. They are generally acutely toxic, have bactericidal, insecticidal, and fungicidal effects to cause diarrhea, anorexia, and ataxia in animals. They have been linked to natural poisoning in humans and animals, including abakabi disease in Japan and stachybotryotoxicosis in the former Soviet Union, and are at the center of a heated debate about whether they could be used as chemical weapons. Mycotoxins can also have a positive effect. The mycotoxin avermectin is currently causing quite a stir, both as an insecticide and for the control of nematode parasites in pets (van Egmond et al., 2007).

2.7.3. Algal Toxins

Algal toxin is a broad term that refers to a variety of compounds produced by diatoms, cyanobacteria (blue-green bacteria) and dinoflagellates. The toxins produced by these marine and freshwater microorganisms often accumulate in nearby shellfish and fish, leading to animal and human illnesses as well as blatant fish kills. Unlike many microbiological toxins, algal toxins are often heat-resistant and therefore unaffected by cooking, increasing the risk of human exposure and harm. Many of the most common algal toxins that cause human poisoning worldwide are listed here (Van Dolah, 2000).

Amnesic Shellfish Poisoning (ASP): When four people died after eating infected shellfish, the disease was first identified on Prince Edward Island, Canada, in 1987. It is caused by domoic acid, which is produced by numerous species of Pseudo-nitzschia diatoms. Mussels, crabs, and clams from the Pacific coast of the United States of America are the main causative agents (Collins, 1978).

Paralytic Shellfish Poisoning (PSP): was originally recognized as a threat in 1942 when three people and several seabirds died after eating shellfish on the Columbia River on the west coast of the USA. The largely determined family (saxitoxin + 18 related chemicals) produced by many Alexandrium dinoflagellate species is the cause. Mussels, fish, clams, crabs, and mussels from the Pacific Northwest and North Atlantic are the most contaminated (Carmichael, 1986).

Neurotoxic shellfish poisoning (NSP): is caused by an ebb tide generator originally discovered in Florida in 1880, but there are older historical allusions. It causes people to become ill for several days. Humans are not affected by NSP, but it has been reported to harm fish, marine animals, invertebrates, and seabirds. The brevetoxin group (brevetoxin + 10 related chemicals) produced by the dinoflagellate Karenia brevis aka Gymnodinium breve causes the disease. Shellfish and other filter feeders from the Gulf Coast and southeastern Atlantic, particularly North Carolina, are the main causative agents (Falconer, 1998).

Diarrheic shellfish poisoning (DSP): The first forms of human toxicity were discovered in the 1960s. It leads to an illness lasting several days but is not fatal. The causative agents are chemicals from the okadaic acid group (okadaic acid + 4 similar drugs), which are produced by numerous dinophysis dinoflagellate species. Mussels, clams, and other shellfish from the warm and cold temperate zones of the Pacific and Atlantic Oceans, especially in Japan and Europe, are the main culprits. Only two cases of DSP have been reported in North America (Shilo, 1967).

Ciguatera fish poisoning (CFP): CFP is a highly toxic tropical-subtropical seafood that affects up to 50,000 people annually and is the most commonly reported foodborne illness of chemical origin in the United States. It was first recognized in 1511, but is the most commonly reported foodborne illness of chemical origin in the U.S., grouper, snapper), and it lasts for many days or even weeks, but is rare. It is caused by the ciguatoxin group (ciguatoxin + 3 or more similar chemicals) produced by various dinoflagellate taxa, including Gambierdiscus, Prorocentrum, and Ostreopsis. Herbivorous tropical reef fishes are among the most vulnerable species to pollution (Rositano et al., 2001).

Cyanobacteria (blue-green bacteria) toxins: Poisoning by cyanobacteria was first recorded in the late 1800s. Poisoning in humans is rare, but cattle, other animals, aquatic invertebrates, birds and fish are frequently killed. It is affected by a variety of biotoxins, including cytotoxins produced by cyanobacteria such as Anabaena, Aphanizomenon, Nodularia, Oscillatoria, and Microcystis, including anatoxin, microcystin, and nodularin. All eutrophic freshwater rivers, ponds, and streams are at risk from pollution (McNabb et al., 2005).

Ambush Predator (*Pfiesteria piscicida* and Toxic Pfiesteria Complex) toxins: The very first specimens of this genus were discovered in North Carolina estuaries in 1991. They were thought to produce a toxin that has been linked to several massive fish kills and is believed to be harmful to humans. However, the toxin or toxins have not yet been discovered, and toxicity studies are sometimes inconclusive. *Pfiesteria piscicida* and *Pfiesteria shumway* are and possibly numerous other undiscovered, unnamed dinoflagellate taxa related to the potentially toxic Pfiesteria complex that produces this toxin. Massive fish kills in North Carolina and Maryland and potential human health problems are the main concerns. The range could expand from the Gulf of Mexico to Atlantic estuarine waters, including Florida, Maryland, Delaware, and North Carolina, and possibly to Europe (Lawton & Codd, 1991).

2.8. Solvents

Solvents are often found in the workplace but can also be present in the household. In addition to dermatological effects such as degreasing or local irritation, many also have systemic harmful effects such as effects on the CNS or, as in the case of benzene, on plasma components. Petroleum and other hydrocarbon chemicals are examples of industrial solvents, which are usually complex mixtures of nitrogen- and sulfur-containing organic compounds (Zuccato et al., 2000).

Some of the most common solvents are listed below:

1. **Aliphatic Hydrocarbons, such as Hexane:** These chemicals can have a linear or branched chain and are often found in mixtures.
2. **Halogenated Aliphatic Hydrocarbons:** Methylene dichloride, carbon tetrachloride and chloroform are very good examples, but chlorinated ethylenes are also commonly used (Di Carlo et al., 1999).
3. **Aliphatic Alcohols:** Ethanol and methanol are typical examples.
4. **Glycols and Glycol Ethers:** Antifreezes containing propylene glycols and ethylene, for example, expose the population to significant amounts of propylene glycols and ethylene. Glycol ethers, such as methyl cellosolve, are also frequently used.
5. **Aromatic Hydrocarbons:** Benzene is the most dangerous substance, although other chemicals such as toluene are also sometimes used (Gabathuler, 2010).

2.9. Therapeutic Drugs

Even though pharmacology studies the therapeutic properties of substances, almost all therapeutic drugs can be toxic and have negative consequences at a certain dosage. The type of toxic reaction, the dose required to elicit the reaction and the ratio between the prescribed dose and the toxic dose all influence the risk to the individual. All the variables that affect the toxicity of many other xenobiotics, such as individual (genetic) variations, diet, age, and the availability of many other exogenous chemicals, affect the toxicity of drugs (Khan et al., 2021).

Even when the risk of a drug for dangerous health risks has been assessed, it must be weighed against the likely benefit. If this is the only therapy for an otherwise fatal disease, the use of an extremely risky drug with only limited tolerance between therapeutic and toxic doses may be acceptable. However, when safer substances are available or when the disease to be treated is minor, a reasonably safe drug may be inappropriate (Robinson & Kolb, 2004).

Melphalan, nitrogen mustard, methotrexate, adriamycin, an antitumor antibiotic, and an antimetabolite are all examples of cytotoxic drugs used in cancer therapy that contain carcinogens. Diethylstilbestrol (DES), a formerly widely used drug, has been associated with cervical and vaginal cancer in the children of women exposed to it (Finney, 1971).

Other pharmacologic side effects can be associated with virtually any organ system. Subacute myelo-optic neuropathy (SMON), which was common in Japan in the 1960s, was thought to be a harmful symptom of chloroquine (Enterovioform), an antidiarrheal agent. Drugs can also cause teratogenesis, with thalidomide being the most worrying case. Skin reactions (dermatitis) are a typical adverse effect of drugs, with topically administered corticosteroids being one example (Piomelli et al., 2000).

Chlorpromazine-induced agranulocytosis, methyldopa-induced hemolytic anemia and methotrexate-induced megaloblastic anemia are just a few examples of blood toxicity. Ocular toxicity has been reported, ranging from thioridazine-induced retinotoxicity to systemic corticosteroid-induced glaucoma (Schooltink & Rose-John, 2002).

2.10. Drugs of Abuse

At some point, every drug is toxic. Illegal drugs, on the other hand, either have no therapeutic purpose or are used in higher doses than necessary for treatment. Although some illicit substances primarily affect upper neurological functions such as mood, reaction time, and coordination, many others cause physical dependence and have catastrophic physical consequences, including fatal overdoses (Leshner & Koob, 1999). Central nervous depressants such as ethanol, secobarbital, and methaqualone (Quaalude); central nervous stimulants such as narcotics, caffeine, methamphetamine (speed), and nicotine; opioids such as meperidine (Demerol) and heroin; and hallucinogens such as lysergic acid diethylamide (LSD), tetrahydrocannabinol (THC), and phencyclidine (PCP). Most drugs of abuse are produced in illegal and inadequately equipped facilities without quality assurance, which further complicates their toxicological relevance. As a result, many of the end products are contaminated with chemicals whose toxicity is unknown but potentially lethal. Figure 2.8 shows the structures of some of these compounds (Stein & Tallman, 2016).

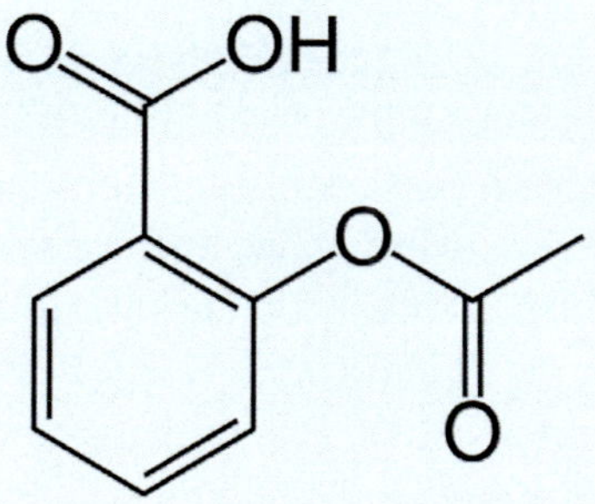

Figure 2.8. *Chemical structures of asprin.*

Source: By Originally User:Benjah-bmm27 – SVG conversion of File:Aspirin-skeletal.png, Public Domain; https://commons.wikimedia.org/w/index.php?curid=791572.

2.11. Combustion Products

While many air pollutants are also the result of natural or anthropogenic combustion, polycyclic aromatic hydrocarbons are among the most harmful to health. They are found in exhaust fumes from wood, coal, petroleum, and cigarettes, as well as in fried foods, and are derived from natural product lines such as petroleum and coal (Baumgartner et al., 1989). These are typically associated with incomplete combustion of fossil fuel components and are detected, for example, in smoke from wood, oil, coal, and cigarettes. Since some of these compounds are carcinogenic, they have been thoroughly investigated with regard to their metabolization, DNA linkages and other elements of chemical carcinogenesis. Some of them are heterocyclic, i.e., they contain another ring with nitrogen.

2.12. Cosmetics

Occasionally, allergic reactions and skin irritations are the most common side effects of today's cosmetics. The very toxic and carcinogenic or aromatic ammonia dyes and the organometallic compounds used in earlier eras are no longer used (Nelson et al., 2014).

Bromates, which are used in certain cold wave neutralizers, and ethanol, which is often used as a solvent in hair dyes and perfumes, can be very toxic if ingested (Ajwa et al., 2002). The ingestion of thioglycerin and thioglycolates, which are contained in cold wave lotions and depilatories, as well as sodium hydroxide, which is contained in hair straighteners, is harmful. The risk of systemic toxicity from cosmetics appears to be low when used as intended, as the ingredients that have now been shown to be harmful have been removed and the quantities ingested are small (Moeller et al., 1998).

A Closer Look

Lead Toxicity

Lead toxicology is a critical area of study within environmental health and toxicology due to the pervasive nature and severe impact of lead exposure on human health. Lead, a naturally occurring heavy metal, has been utilized extensively in various industries, including paint, plumbing, gasoline, and batteries, leading to widespread environmental contamination. Exposure to lead occurs primarily through ingestion or inhalation of lead-containing dust, water, soil, or paint. Once in the body, lead is absorbed into the bloodstream and distributed to organs such as the brain, liver, kidneys, and bones, where it can be stored for extended periods. The toxic effects of lead are most profound in children, as their developing nervous systems are particularly vulnerable. Lead exposure in children can result in cognitive deficits, behavioral issues, and reduced IQ, as well as developmental delays and learning disabilities. In adults, chronic lead exposure is associated with hypertension, renal dysfunction, reproductive issues, and neurological impairments. One of the primary mechanisms by which lead exerts its toxic effects is through its ability to mimic and disrupt the action of calcium, a vital element in numerous physiological processes. Lead interferes with neurotransmitter release, mitochondrial function, and cellular signaling pathways, leading to cellular damage and apoptosis. Additionally, lead induces oxidative stress by generating reactive oxygen species (ROS) and depleting antioxidant defenses, further contributing to cellular injury. The body's ability to excrete lead is limited, with most of the absorbed lead being stored in bones and teeth, where it can remain for decades and be mobilized back into the bloodstream during periods of physiological stress, such as pregnancy or osteoporosis. Diagnosing lead poisoning involves measuring blood lead levels (BLLs), with levels above 5 micrograms per deciliter considered a cause for concern by the Centers for Disease Control and Prevention (CDC). Treatment of lead poisoning includes chelation therapy, which involves the administration of chelating agents that bind to lead and facilitate its excretion from the body. However, chelation therapy is not without risks and is typically reserved for cases with significantly elevated BLLs. Preventing lead exposure is paramount and involves measures such as eliminating lead-based paint in homes, using lead-free plumbing materials, and reducing industrial emissions. Public health policies and regulations have significantly reduced lead exposure in many countries, but it remains a persistent issue in low- and middle-income regions where regulatory enforcement is lax, and environmental lead contamination is widespread. Addressing lead toxicity requires a comprehensive approach, involving rigorous environmental monitoring, public education, and robust regulatory frameworks to minimize lead exposure and protect vulnerable populations. Ongoing research is essential to better understand the mechanisms of lead toxicity, develop more effective treatments, and establish safer exposure limits. Overall, lead toxicology underscores the need for continued vigilance and proactive measures to mitigate the impact of this insidious toxin on global public health.

Summary

- This chapter offers a detailed examination of various toxic substances and their implications for human health. It is structured to address several educational objectives, guiding readers through the complex landscape of toxicology. The chapter begins by categorizing toxic substances into distinct classes, including metals, agricultural chemicals, food additives, and substances related to drug abuse. Each class is explored in terms of its source, exposure routes, and health effects.
- The narrative then moves into the environmental context of these toxins, discussing how soil, air, and water pollution contribute to human exposure and detailing the resultant health consequences. This discussion is critical for understanding the pervasive nature of these substances in our environment and their pathways to affecting human health.
- Particularly, the chapter sheds light on the dual nature of metal toxins, outlining both their beneficial uses in various industries and their potential harmful effects when mismanaged or overly abundant in the environment. Similarly, the role of agrochemicals in enhancing food production is balanced with a caution about their misuse and overuse, which can lead to significant environmental and health issues.
- Furthermore, the chapter explains the role of food additives in the food industry, discussing both their necessity for preserving the quality and safety of food and the risks associated with their overuse or the presence of unintended contaminants. The broader concept of toxins, including their classification, mechanisms of action, and impacts on health, is elaborated to provide a thorough understanding of their potential dangers.
- In addressing drug abuse, the chapter highlights the severe health impacts associated with addictive substances, discussing both the immediate and prolonged consequences of their use. The addictive nature of these substances, coupled with their widespread health ramifications, underscores the critical need for effective regulation and public health interventions.
- The chapter offers a comprehensive overview of various classes of toxicants, emphasizing the necessity for informed regulatory policies and management practices. These measures are essential to mitigate the adverse effects of toxic substances on public health, ensuring a safer environment for current and future generations.

References

1. Abbott Chalew, T. E., Galloway, J. F., & Graczyk, T. K. (2012). Pilot study on effects of nanoparticle exposure on *Crassostrea virginica* hemocyte phagocytosis. *Marine Pollution Bulletin, 64*, 2251–2253.
2. Abdel-Latif, H. M. R., Dawood, M. A. O., Menanteau-Ledouble, S., & El-Matbouli, M. (2020). Environmental transformation of N-TiO_2 in the aquatic systems and their ecotoxicity in bivalve mollusks: A systematic review. *Ecotoxicology and Environmental Safety, 200*, 110776.

3. Adams, E., & Bruhl, C. A. (2020). Fungicide exposure induces sensitivity differences in aquatic life stages of European common frogs (*Rana temporaria*). *South American Journal of Herpetology, 54*, 331–336.
4. Adams, M. S., & Stauber, J. L. (2004). Development of a whole-sediment toxicity test using a benthic marine microalga. *Environmental Toxicology and Chemistry, 23*, 1957–1968.
5. Adan, A., Kiraz, Y., & Baran, Y. (2016). Cell proliferation and cytotoxicity assays. *Current Pharmaceutical Biotechnology, 17*, 1213–1221.
6. Al-Khazrajy, O. S. A., & Abdallh, M. (2020). Sorption and degradation of ranitidine in soil: Leaching potential assessment. *Chemosphere, 259*, 127495.
7. Al-Thomali, A. W., Tag, H. M., Mohammadein, A., El-Shenawy, N. S., & El-Naggar, M. S. (2022). Mercaptophos impacts on redox status biomarkers of common carp (*Cyprinus carpio*) as an endocrine disruptor. *Aquaculture Reports, 22*, 100959.
8. Álvarez-Alarcón, N., Osorio-Méndez, J. J., Ayala-Fajardo, A., Garzón-Méndez, W. F., & Garavito-Aguilar, Z. V. (2021). Zebrafish and *Artemia salina* in vivo evaluation of the recreational 25C-NBOMe drug demonstrates its high toxicity. *Toxicology Reports, 8*, 315–323.
9. Amadi, C. N., Frazzoli, C., & Orisakwe, O. E. (2020). Sentinel species for biomonitoring and biosurveillance of environmental heavy metals in Nigeria. *Journal of Environmental Science and Health Part C Toxicology and Carcinogenesis, 38*, 21–60.
10. Anastas, P. T., & Warner, J. C. (1998). *Green Chemistry: Theory and Practice*. Oxford University Press.
11. Ansell, G. R., Frewin, A. J., Gradish, A. E., & Scott-Dupree, C. D. (2021). Contact toxicity of three insecticides for use in tier I pesticide risk assessments with *Megachile rotundata* (Hymenoptera: Megachilidae). *PeerJ, 9*, e10744.
12. Antón, V., Muñoz-Embid, J., Gascón, I., Artal, M., & Lafuente, C. (2017). Thermophysical characterization of furfuryl esters: Experimental and modeling. *Energy & Fuels, 31*, 4143–4154.
13. Araújo, C. V. M., Tornero, V., Lubián, L. M., Blasco, J., van Bergeijk, S. A., Cañavate, P., Cid, Á., Franco, D., Prado, R., Bartual, A., et al. (2010). Ring test for whole-sediment toxicity assay with a benthic marine diatom. *Science of the Total Environment, 408*, 822–828.
14. Ariba, H., Wang, Y., Devouge-Boyer, C., Stateva, R. P., & Leveneur, S. (2020). Physicochemical properties for the reaction systems: Levulinic acid, its esters, and γ-valerolactone. *Journal of Chemical & Engineering Data, 65*, 3008–3020.
15. Arreguin Rebolledo, U., Nandini, S., Sarma, S. S. S., & Escobar-Sánchez, O. (2020). Effect of salinity and temperature on the acute and chronic toxicity of arsenic to the marine rotifers *Proales similis* and *Brachionus ibericus*. *Marine Pollution Bulletin, 157*, 111341.
16. Azelmad, K., Hamadi, F., Mimouni, R., El Boulani, A., Amzil, K., & Latrache, H. (2018). Physicochemical characterization of *Pseudomonas aeruginosa* isolated from catering substratum surface and investigation of their theoretical adhesion. *Surfaces and Interfaces, 12*, 26–30.
17. Bae, J. H., Kim, S., Amr, I. T., Seo, J., Jang, D., Bamagain, R., Fadhel, B. A., Abu-Aisheh, E., & Lee, H. K. (2022). Evaluation of physicochemical properties and environmental impact of environmentally amicable Portland cement/metakaolin bricks exposed to humid or CO_2 curing condition. *Journal of Building Engineering, 47*, 103831.
18. Bagherifam, S., Brown, T. C., Fellows, C. M., & Naidu, R. (2019). Derivation methods of soils,

water and sediments toxicity guidelines: A brief review with a focus on antimony. *Journal of Geochemical Exploration, 205*, 106348.

19. Baker, K. N. (1985). Laboratory and field experiments on the responses by two species of woodland salamanders to malathion-treated substrates. *Archives of Environmental Contamination and Toxicology, 14*, 685–691.

20. Baysal, A., Saygin, H., & Ustabasi, G. S. (2018). Influence of environmental media on carbon nanotubes and graphene nanoplatelets towards bacterial toxicity. *Archives of Environmental Protection, 44*, 85–98.

21. Bermudez, E., Mangum, J. B., Wong, B. A., Asgharian, B., Hext, P. M., Warheit, D. B., & Everitt, J. I. (2004). Pulmonary responses of mice, rats, and hamsters to subchronic inhalation of ultrafine titanium dioxide particles. *Toxicological Sciences, 77*, 347–357.

22. Bernal, M. H., Solomon, K. R., & Carrasquilla, G. (2009). Toxicity of formulated glyphosate (Glyphos) and Cosmo-Flux to larval and juvenile Colombian frogs. *Journal of Toxicology and Environmental Health, Part A, 72*, 966–973.

23. Białk-Bielińska, A., Maszkowska, J., Mrozik, W., Bielawska, A., Kołodziejska, M., Palavinskas, R., Stepnowski, P., & Kumirska, J. (2012). Sulfadimethoxine and sulfaguanidine: Their sorption potential on natural soils. *Chemosphere, 86*, 1059–1065.

24. Boğa, A., Binokay, S., & Sertdemir, Y. (2009). The toxicity and teratogenicity of gibberellic acid (GA3) based on the frog embryo teratogenesis assay-Xenopus (FETAX). *Turkish Journal of Biology, 33*, 181–188.

25. Boonpeng, C., Sriviboon, C., Polyiam, W., Sangiamdee, D., Watthana, S., & Boonpragob, K. (2018). Assessing atmospheric pollution in a petrochemical industrial district using a lichen-air quality index (LiAQI). *Ecological Indicators, 95*, 589–594.

26. Bopp, S. K., Kienzler, A., Richarz, A. N., van der Linden, S. C., Paini, A., Parissis, N., & Worth, A. P. (2019). Regulatory assessment and risk management of chemical mixtures: Challenges and ways forward. *Critical Reviews in Toxicology, 49*, 174–189.

27. Boyd, W. A., McBride, S. J., Rice, J. R., Snyder, D. W., & Freedman, J. H. (2010). A high-throughput method for assessing chemical toxicity using a Caenorhabditis elegans reproduction assay. *Toxicology and Applied Pharmacology, 245*, 153–159.

28. Boyd, W. A., Smith, M. V., Co, C. A., Pirone, J. R., Rice, J. R., Shockley, K. R., & Freedman, J. H. (2016). Developmental effects of the ToxCastTM phase I and phase II chemicals in Caenorhabditis elegans and corresponding responses in zebrafish, rats, and rabbits. *Environmental Health Perspectives, 124*, 586–593.

29. Bracher, G. A., & Bider, J. R. (1982). Changes in terrestrial animal activity of a forest community after an application of Aminocarb (Matacil). *CalEcotox, 60*, 1981–1997.

30. Brito, R. O., Marques, E. F., Silva, S. G., do Vale, M. L., Gomes, P., Araújo, M. J., Rodriguez-Borges, J. E., Infante, M. R., Garcia, M. T., Ribosa, I., et al. (2009). Physicochemical and toxicological properties of novel amino acid-based amphiphiles and their spontaneously formed catanionic vesicles. *Colloids and Surfaces B: Biointerfaces, 72*, 80–87.

31. Brühl, C. A., Pieper, S., & Weber, B. (2011). Amphibians at risk? Susceptibility of terrestrial amphibian life stages to pesticides. *Environmental Toxicology and Chemistry, 30*, 2465–2472.

32. Bundschuh, M., Zubrod, J. P., Wernicke, T., Konschak, M., Werner, L., Brühl, C. A., Baudy, P.,

& Schulz, R. (2021). Bottom-up effects of fungicides on tadpoles of the European common frog (*Rana temporaria*). *Ecology and Evolution, 11*, 4353–4365.

33. Burton, G. A. (1991). Assessing the toxicity of freshwater sediments. *Environmental Toxicology and Chemistry, 10*, 1585–1627.

34. Campbell, K. S., Keller, P. G., Heinzel, L. M., Golovko, S. A., Seeger, D. R., Golovko, M. Y., & Kerby, J. L. (2022). Detection of imidacloprid and metabolites in northern leopard frog (*Rana pipiens*) brains. *Science of the Total Environment, 813*, 152424.

35. Cantanhêde, S. M., de Carvalho, I. S. C., Hamoy, M., Corrêa, J. A. M., de Carvalho, L. M., Barbas, L. A. L., de Assis Montag, L. F., & Amado, L. L. (2022). Evaluation of cardiotoxicity in Amazonian fish *Bryconops caudomaculatus* by acute exposure to aluminum in an acidic environment. *Aquatic Toxicology, 242*, 106044.

36. Chang-Ming, Y., Xing-Jun, W., & He-Hui, Z. (2002). Biodegradation of acetanilide herbicides acetochlor and butachlor in soil. *Journal of Environmental Sciences, 14*, 524–529.

37. Chen, Q., Jin, L., Zhong, Y., & Ji, G. (2022). Effects of enrofloxacin on the epiphytic algal communities growing on the leaf surface of *Vallisneria natans*. *Antibiotics, 11*, 1020.

38. Chen, S. C., & Chung, K. T. (2000). Mutagenicity and antimutagenicity studies of tannic acid and its related compounds. *Food and Chemical Toxicology, 38*, 1–5.

39. Chung, S., Kim, S. H., Seo, Y., Kim, S. K., & Lee, J. Y. (2017). Quantitative analysis of cell proliferation by a dye dilution assay: Application to cell lines and cocultures. *Cytometry Part A, 91*, 704–712.

40. Clippinger, A. J., Raabe, H. A., Allen, D. G., Choksi, N. Y., van der Zalm, A. J., Kleinstreuer, N. C., Barroso, J., & Lowit, A. B. (2021). Human-relevant approaches to assess eye corrosion/irritation potential of agrochemical formulations. *Cutaneous and Ocular Toxicology, 40*, 145–167.

41. Conti, M. E., & Cecchetti, G. (2001). Biological monitoring: Lichens as bioindicators of air pollution assessment—A review. *Environmental Pollution, 114*, 471–492.

42. Cormier, B., Cachot, J., Blanc, M., Cabar, M., Clérandeau, C., Dubocq, F., Le Bihanic, F., Morin, B., Zapata, S., Bégout, M. L., et al. (2022). Environmental microplastics disrupt swimming activity in acute exposure in *Danio rerio* larvae and reduce growth and reproduction success in chronic exposure in *D. rerio* and *Oryzias melastigma*. *Environmental Pollution, 308*, 119721.

43. Daimari, R., Bhuyan, P., Hussain, S., Nayaka, S., Mazumder, M. A. J., & Hoque, R. R. (2021). Anatomical, physiological, and chemical alterations in lichen (*Parmotrema tinctorum* (Nyl.) Hale) transplants due to air pollution in two cities of Brahmaputra Valley, India. *Environmental Monitoring and Assessment, 193*, 1–12.

44. De Oliveira Gonçalves, A. L., Gebara, R. C., da Silva Mansano, A., Rocha, G. S., & da Graça Gama, M. (2022). Individual and combined effects of manganese and chromium on a freshwater Chlorophyceae. *Environmental Toxicology and Chemistry, 41*, 1004–1015.

45. De Viana, C. O., Vaz, R. P., Cano, A., Santos, A. P., Cançado, L. G., Ladeira, L. O., & Junior, A. C. (2015). Physiological changes of the lichen *Parmotrema tinctorum* as result of carbon nanotubes exposition. *Ecotoxicology and Environmental Safety, 120*, 110–116.

46. Deblonde, T., & Hartemann, P. (2013). Environmental impact of medical prescriptions: Assessing the risks and hazards of persistence, bioaccumulation and toxicity of pharmaceuticals. *Public Health, 127*, 312–317.

47. Do Amaral VilasBoas, L., Senra, M. V. X., Fernandes, K., da Anunciação Gomes, A. M., Pedroso Dias, R. J., Pinto, E., & Fonseca, A. L. (2020). In vitro toxicity of isolated strains and cyanobacterial bloom biomasses over *Paramecium caudatum* (*Ciliophora*): Lessons from a non-metazoan model organism. *Ecotoxicology and Environmental Safety, 202*, 110937.

48. Doyle, J. J., Ward, J. E., & Wikfors, G. H. (2018). Acute exposure to TiO_2 nanoparticles produces minimal apparent effects on oyster, *Crassostrea virginica* (Gmelin), hemocytes. *Marine Pollution Bulletin, 127*, 512–523.

49. Dumont, E. R., Elger, A., Azéma, C., Castillo Michel, H., Surble, S., & Larue, C. (2021). Cutting-edge spectroscopy techniques highlight toxicity mechanisms of copper oxide nanoparticles in the aquatic plant *Myriophyllum spicatum*. *Science of the Total Environment, 803*, 150001.

50. Duo, L., Yin, L., Zhang, C., & Zhao, S. (2019). Ecotoxicological responses of the earthworm *Eisenia fetida* to EDTA addition under turfgrass growing conditions. *Chemosphere, 220*, 56–60.

51. Elofsson, R., & Klemm, N. (1972). Monoamine-containing neurons in the optic ganglia of crustaceans and insects. *Zeitschrift für Zellforschung und Mikroskopische Anatomie, 133*, 475–499.

52. Eluk, D., Nagel, O., Gagneten, A., Reno, U., & Althaus, R. (2021). Toxicity of fluoroquinolones on the cladoceran *Daphnia magna*. *Water Environment Research, 93*, 2914–2930.

53. Evans, S. J., Clift, M. J. D., Singh, N., Wills, J. W., Hondow, N., Wilkinson, T. S., Burgum, M. J., Brown, A. P., Jenkins, G. J., & Doak, S. H. (2019). In vitro detection of in vitro secondary mechanisms of genotoxicity induced by engineered nanomaterials. *Particle and Fibre Toxicology, 16*, 8.

54. Fan, X., Wang, C., Wang, P., Hu, B., & Wang, X. (2018). TiO_2 nanoparticles in sediments: Effect on the bioavailability of heavy metals in the freshwater bivalve *Corbicula fluminea*. *Journal of Hazardous Materials, 342*, 41–50.

55. Fan, X., Wang, P., Wang, C., Hu, B., & Wang, X. (2017). Lead accumulation (adsorption and absorption) by the freshwater bivalve *Corbicula fluminea* in sediments contaminated by TiO_2 nanoparticles. *Environmental Pollution, 231*, 712–721.

56. Fekete-Kertész, I., Ullmann, O., Csizmár, P., & Molnár, M. (2018). *Tetrahymena pyriformis* phagocytic activity test for rapid toxicity assessment of aquatic micropollutants. *Periodica Polytechnica Chemical Engineering, 62*, 167–174.

57. Ferreira, T., Hansel, F. A., Maia, C. M. B. F., Guiotoku, M., Cunha, L., & Brown, G. G. (2021). Earthworm-biochar interactions: A laboratory trial using *Pontoscolex corethrurus*. *Science of the Total Environment, 777*, 146147.

58. Flynn, R. W., Hoover, G., Iacchetta, M., Guffey, S., de Perre, C., Huerta, B., Li, W., Hoverman, J. T., Lee, L., & Sepúlveda, M. S. (2022). Comparative toxicity of aquatic per- and polyfluoroalkyl substance exposure in three species of amphibians. *Environmental Toxicology and Chemistry, 41*, 1407–1415.

59. Flynn, R. W., Hoskins, T. D., Iacchetta, M., de Perre, C., Lee, L. S., Hoverman, J. T., & Sepúlveda, M. S. (2021). Dietary exposure and accumulation of per- and polyfluoroalkyl substances alters growth and reduces body condition of post-metamorphic salamanders. *Science of the Total Environment, 765*, 142730.

60. Garczynska, M., Paczka, G., & Kostecka, J. (2019). Influence of neonicotinoids on selected characteristics of the earthworm *Dendrobaena veneta* (Rosa) in laboratory conditions. *Journal of Ecological Engineering, 20*, 217–224.

61. Garralaga, M. P., Lomba, L., Leal-Duaso, A., Gracia-Barberán, S., Pires, E., & Giner, B. (2022). Ecotoxicological study of bio-based deep eutectic solvents formed by glycerol derivatives in two aquatic bio models. *Green Chemistry, 24*, 5228–5241.

62. Gemeda, F. T., Guta, D. D., Wakjira, F. S., & Gebresenbet, G. (2020). Physicochemical characterization of effluents from industries in Sabata Town of Ethiopia. *Heliyon, 6*, e04624.

63. Gendron, A. (2013). Amphibian ecotoxicology. In *Encyclopedia of Aquatic Ecotoxicology* (pp. 21–38). Springer, Berlin/Heidelberg, Germany.

64. Ghaedi, A. (2015). Predicting the cytotoxicity of ionic liquids using QSAR model based on SMILES optimal descriptors. *Journal of Molecular Liquids, 208*, 269–279.

65. Giner, B., Aldea, M. E., Martín, S., Gascón, I., & Lafuente, C. (2003). Viscosities of binary mixtures of isomeric butanols or isomeric chlorobutanes with 2-methyltetrahydrofuran. *Journal of Chemical & Engineering Data, 48*, 1296–1300.

66. Giner, B., Artigas, H., Carrión, A., Lafuente, C., & Royo, F. M. (2003). Excess thermodynamic properties of isomeric butanols with 2-methyl-tetrahydrofuran. *Journal of Molecular Liquids, 108*, 303–311.

67. Giner, B., Gascón, I., Artigas, H., Royo, F. M., & Lafuente, C. (2005). Surface behavior of the 1-bromobutane with isomeric butanol mixtures. *Journal of Physical Chemistry B, 109*, 23096–23102.

68. Giner, B., Gascón, I., Villares, A., Cea, P., & Lafuente, C. (2006). Densities and viscosities of the binary mixtures of tetrahydrofuran with isomeric chlorobactenes at 298.15 K and 313.15 K. *Journal of Chemical & Engineering Data, 51*, 1321–1325.

69. Giner, B., Lafuente, C., Lapeña, D., Errazquin, D., & Lomba, L. (2020). QSAR study for predicting the ecotoxicity of NADES towards *Aliivibrio fischeri*. Exploring the use of mixing rules. *Ecotoxicology and Environmental Safety, 191*, 110004.

70. Giner, B., Royo, F. M., Lafuente, C., & Galindo, A. (2007). Intermolecular potential model parameters for cyclic ethers and chloroalkanes in the SAFT-VR approach. *Fluid Phase Equilibria, 255*, 200–206.

71. Giner, I., Montaño, D., Haro, M., Artigas, H., & Lafuente, C. (2009). Study of isobaric vapor–liquid equilibrium of some cyclic ethers with 1-chloropropane: Experimental results and SAFT-VR modelling. *Fluid Phase Equilibria, 278*, 62–67.

72. Gooderham, N. J., Cohen, S. M., Eisenbrand, G., Fukushima, S., Guengerich, F. P., Hecht, S. S., Rietjens, I. M. C. M., Rosol, T. J., Bastaki, M., Linman, M. J., et al. (2020). The safety evaluation of food flavoring substances: The role of genotoxicity studies. *Critical Reviews in Toxicology, 50*, 1–27.

73. Gowri, S., & Thangaraj, R. (2020). Studies on the toxic effects of agrochemical pesticide (Monocrotophos) on physiological and reproductive behavior of indigenous and exotic earthworm species. *International Journal of Environmental Health Research, 30*, 212–225.

74. Gradish, A. E., van der Steen, J., Scott-Dupree, C. D., Cabrera, A. R., Cutler, G. C., Goulson, D., Klein, O., Lehmann, D. M., Lückmann, J., O'Neill, B., et al. (2019). Comparison of pesticide exposure in honey bees (Hymenoptera: Apidae) and bumble bees (Hymenoptera: Apidae): Implications for risk assessments. *Environmental Entomology, 48*, 12–21.

75. Greenstein, D., Bay, S., Anderson, B., Chandler, G. T., Farrar, J. D., Keppler, C., Phillips, B.,

Ringwood, A., & Young, D. (2008). Comparison of methods for evaluating acute and chronic toxicity in marine sediments. *Environmental Toxicology and Chemistry, 27*, 933–944.

76. Gu, W., Li, X., Du, M., Ren, Z., Li, Q., & Li, Y. (2021). Identification and regulation of ecotoxicity of polychlorinated naphthalenes to aquatic food chain (Green Algae-Daphnia Magna-Fish). *Aquatic Toxicology, 233*, 105774.
77. Guler, U. A., & Solmaz, B. (2022). Biosorption of tetracycline and cephalexin onto surfactant-modified waste biomass using response surface methodology and ecotoxicological assessment: Phytotoxicity and biotoxicity studies. *Water, Air, and Soil Pollution, 233*, 117.
78. Gutiérrez-Lovera, C., Martínez-Val, J., Cabezas-Sainz, P., López, R., Rubiolo, J. A., & Sánchez, L. (2019). In vivo toxicity assays in zebrafish embryos: A pre-requisite for xenograft preclinical studies. *Toxicology Mechanisms and Methods, 29*, 478–487.
79. Guzzella, L. (1998). Comparison of test procedures for sediment toxicity evaluation with *Vibrio fischeri* bacteria. *Chemosphere, 37*, 2895–2909.
80. Haag, E. S., Fitch, D. H. A., & Delattre, M. (2018). From "the worm" to "the worms" and back again: The evolutionary developmental biology of nematodes. *Genetics, 210*, 397–433.
81. Hagiwara, A., & Yoshinaga, T. (2018). Rotifers: Aquaculture, ecology, gerontology, and ecotoxicology. In *Springer* (pp. 149–176). Berlin/Heidelberg, Germany.
82. Hardwick, R. N., Betts, C. J., Whritenour, J., Sura, R., Thamsen, M., Kaufman, E. H., & Fabre, K. (2020). Drug-induced skin toxicity: Gaps in preclinical testing cascade as opportunities for complex in vitro models and assays. *Lab on a Chip, 20*, 199–214.
83. Harlow, P. H., Perry, S. J., Widdison, S., Daniels, S., Bondo, E., Lamberth, C., Currie, R. A., & Flemming, A. J. (2016). The nematode *Caenorhabditis elegans* as a tool to predict chemical activity on mammalian development and identify mechanisms influencing toxicological outcome. *Scientific Reports, 6*, 22965.
84. Hasany, S. M., & Chaudhary, M. H. (1996). Sorption potential of Haro River sand for the removal of antimony from acidic aqueous solution. *Applied Radiation and Isotopes, 47*, 467–471.
85. He, M., Mei, C. F., Sun, G. P., Li, H. B., Liu, L., & Xu, M. Y. (2016). The effects of molecular properties on ready biodegradation of aromatic compounds in the OECD 301B CO_2 evolution test. *Archives of Environmental Contamination and Toxicology, 71*, 133–145.
86. He, M., Xiong, X., Wang, L., Hou, D., Bolan, N. S., Ok, Y. S., Rinklebe, J., & Tsang, D. C. W. (2021). A critical review on performance indicators for evaluating soil biota and soil health of biochar-amended soils. *Journal of Hazardous Materials, 414*, 125378.
87. He, R., Guo, D., Lin, C., Zhang, W. G., & Fan, J. (2022). Enantioselective bioaccumulation, oxidative stress, and thyroid disruption assessment of cis-metconazole enantiomers in zebrafish (*Danio rerio*). *Aquatic Toxicology, 248*, 106205.
88. He, X., Han, M., Zhan, W., Liu, F., Guo, D., Zhang, Y., Liang, X., Wang, Y., & Lou, B. (2022). Mixture effects of imidacloprid and difenoconazole on enzymatic activity and gene expression in small yellow croakers (*Larimichthys polyactis*). *Chemosphere, 306*, 135551.
89. Heddle, J. A., Hite, M., Kirkhart, B., Mavournin, K., MacGregor, J. T., Newell, G. W., & Salamone, M. F. (1983). The induction of micronuclei as a measure of genotoxicity. A report of the U.S. Environmental Protection Agency Gene-Tox Program. *Mutation Research, 123*, 61–118.

90. Heinrich, U., Fuhst, R., Rittinghausen, S., Creutzenberg, O., Bellmann, B., Koch, W., & Levsen, K. (1995). Chronic inhalation exposure of Wistar rats and two different strains of mice to diesel engine exhaust, carbon black, and titanium dioxide. *Inhalation Toxicology, 7*, 533–556.

91. Henson-Ramsey, H., Kennedy-Stoskopf, S., Levine, J. F., Taylor, S. K., Shea, D., & Stoskopf, M. K. (2008). Acute toxicity and tissue distributions of malathion in *Ambystoma tigrinum*. *Archives of Environmental Contamination and Toxicology, 55*, 481–487.

92. Hernández-Altamirano, R., Mena-Cervantes, V. Y., Perez-Miranda, S., Fernández, F. J., Flores-Sandoval, C. A., Barba, V., Beltrán, H. I., & Zamudio-Rivera, L. S. (2010). Molecular design and QSAR study of low acute toxicity biocides with 4,4 -dimorpholyl-methane cores obtained by microwave-assisted synthesis. *Green Chemistry, 12*, 1036–1048.

93. Hirano, T., Ishida, T., Oh, K., & Sudo, R. (2007). Biodegradation of chlordane and hexachlorobenzenes in river sediment. *Chemosphere, 67*, 428–434.

94. Honnen, S. (2017). *Caenorhabditis elegans* as a powerful alternative model organism to promote research in genetic toxicology and biomedicine. *Archives of Toxicology, 91*, 2029–2044.

95. Horibe, A., Odashima, S., Hamasuna, N., Morita, T., & Hayashi, M. (2018). Weight of contribution of in vitro chromosomal aberration assay for evaluation of pesticides: Experience of risk assessment at the food safety commission of Japan. *Regulatory Toxicology and Pharmacology, 95*, 133–141.

96. Horie, Y., & Takahashi, C. (2021). Development of an in vivo acute bioassay using the marine medaka *Oryzias melastigma*. *Environmental Monitoring and Assessment, 193*, 725.

97. Huang, W., Song, B., Liang, J., Niu, Q., Zeng, G., Shen, M., Deng, J., Luo, Y., Wen, X., & Zhang, Y. (2021). Microplastics and associated contaminants in the aquatic environment: A review on their ecotoxicological effects, trophic transfer, and potential impacts to human health. *Journal of Hazardous Materials, 405*, 124187.

98. Hunt, P. R. (2017). The *C. elegans* model in toxicity testing. *Journal of Applied Toxicology, 37*, 50–59.

99. Hunt, P. R., Olejnik, N., Bailey, K. D., Vaught, C. A., & Sprando, R. L. (2018). *C. elegans* development and activity test detects mammalian developmental neurotoxins. *Food and Chemical Toxicology, 121*, 583–592.

100. Hunt, P. R., Olejnik, N., & Sprando, R. L. (2012). Toxicity ranking of heavy metals with screening method using adult *Caenorhabditis elegans* and propidium iodide replicates toxicity ranking in rat. *Food and Chemical Toxicology, 50*, 3280–3290.

101. Ilyas, H., Masih, I., & van Hullebusch, E. D. (2020). Pharmaceuticals' removal by constructed wetlands: A critical evaluation and meta-analysis on performance, risk reduction, and role of physicochemical properties on removal mechanisms. *Journal of Water and Health, 18*, 253–291.

102. Inami, K., Okazawa, M., & Mochizuki, M. (2009). Mutagenicity of aromatic amines and amides with chemical models for cytochrome P450 in Ames assay. *Toxicology in Vitro, 23*, 986–991.

103. Jeong, C. B., Kang, H. M., Lee, M. C., Byeon, E., Park, H. G., & Lee, J. S. (2019). Effects of polluted seawater on oxidative stress, mortality, and reproductive parameters in the marine rotifer *Brachionus koreanus* and the marine copepod *Tigriopus japonicus*. *Aquatic Toxicology, 208*, 39–46.

104. Jiang, J., Zhang, C., Wang, L., Wang, X., He, H., Wu, S., & Zhao, X. (2022). Insights into the combined effects of environmental concentration of difenoconazole and tebuconazole on zebrafish early life stage. *Science of The Total Environment, 830*, 154687.

105. Judson, R. S., Houck, K. A., Kavlock, R. J., Knudsen, T. B., Martin, M. T., Mortensen, H. M., Reif, D. M., Rotroff, D. M., Shah, I., Richard, A. M., et al. (2010). In vitro screening of environmental chemicals for targeted testing prioritization: The ToxCast project. *Environmental Health Perspectives, 118*, 485–492.

106. Jurjanz, S., Fournier, A., Clostre, F., Godard, E., & Feidt, C. (2020). Control of poultry contamination in chlordecone-contaminated areas of the French West Indies. *Environmental Science and Pollution Research International, 27*, 41117–41121.

107. Kalčíková, G., Zagorc-Končan, J., & Gotvajn, A. Ž. (2012). *Artemia salina* acute immobilization test: A possible tool for aquatic ecotoxicity assessment. *Water Science and Technology, 66*, 903–908.

108. Khan, I., & Umar, R. (2019). Environmental risk assessment of coal fly ash on soil and groundwater quality, Aligarh, India. *Groundwater for Sustainable Development, 8*, 346–357.

109. Kolle, S. N., & Landsiedel, R. (2021). Human-derived in vitro models used for skin toxicity testing under REACH. *Handbook of Experimental Pharmacology, 265*, 3–27.

110. Kolle, S. N., Sullivan, K. M., Mehling, A., van Ravenzwaay, B., & Landsiedel, R. (2012). Applicability of in vitro tests for skin irritation and corrosion to regulatory classification schemes: Substantiating test strategies with data from routine studies. *Regulatory Toxicology and Pharmacology, 64*, 402–414.

111. Kolle, S. N., van Ravenzwaay, B., & Landsiedel, R. (2017). Regulatory accepted but out of domain: In vitro skin irritation tests for agrochemical formulations. *Regulatory Toxicology and Pharmacology, 89*, 125–130.

112. Kostopoulou, V., Carmona, M. J., & Divanach, P. (2012). The rotifer *Brachionus plicatilis*: An emerging bio-tool for numerous applications. *Journal of Biological Research, 17*, 97.

113. Kouadria, N., Alioua Berrebbah, A., Belhoucine, F., Bouredja, N., & Aitkaci, M. (2021). Cellular impact of metal trace elements on the lichen *Lobaria pulmonaria* (L.) Hoffm. (1796), a bio indicator of atmospheric pollution and identification of its antioxidant response. *Applied Ecology and Environmental Research, 19*, 4721–4738.

114. Krell, B., Moreira-Santos, M., & Ribeiro, R. (2011). An estuarine mudsnail in situ toxicity assay based on postexposure feeding. *Environmental Toxicology and Chemistry, 30*, 1935–1942.

115. Kudsk, P., Mathiassen, S., Cedergreen, N., Mathiassen, S. K., & Streibig, J. C. (2007). Combination effects of herbicides on plants and algae: Do species and test systems matter? *Pest Management Science, 63*, 282–295.

116. Kumar, P., Nagarajan, A., & Uchil, P. D. (2018). Analysis of cell viability by the MTT assay. *Cold Spring Harbor Protocols, 2018*, 469–471.

117. Kuramochi, H., Takigami, H., Scheringer, M., & Sakai, S. ichi (2014). Estimation of physicochemical properties of 52 non-PBDE brominated flame retardants and evaluation of their overall persistence and long-range transport potential. *Science of the Total Environment, 491–492*, 108–117.

118. Kwak, J. I., & An, Y. J. (2022). Length- and polymer-dependent ecotoxicities of microfibers to

the earthworm *Eisenia andrei*. *Comparative Biochemistry and Physiology Part C: Toxicology & Pharmacology, 257*, 109354.

119. Labine, L. M., Oliveira Pereira, E. A., Kleywegt, S., Jobst, K. J., Simpson, A. J., & Simpson, M. J. (2022). Comparison of sub-lethal metabolic perturbations of select legacy and novel perfluorinated alkyl substances (PFAS) in *Daphnia magna*. *Environmental Research, 212*, 113582.

120. Lapeña, D., Errazquin, D., Lomba, L., & Giner, B. (2020). Ecotoxicity and biodegradability of pure and aqueous mixtures of deep eutectic solvents: Glyceline, ethaline, and reline. *Environmental Science and Pollution Research, 28*, 8812–8821.

121. Laurent, A., Harkema, J. R., Andersen, E. W., Owsianiak, M., Vea, E. B., & Jolliet, O. (2017). Human health no-effect levels of TiO_2 nanoparticles as a function of their primary size. *Journal of Nanoparticle Research, 19*, 130.

122. Lee, K. P., Trochimowicz, H. J., & Reinhardt, C. F. (1985). Pulmonary response of rats exposed to titanium dioxide (TiO_2) by inhalation for two years. *Toxicology and Applied Pharmacology, 79*, 179–192.

123. Lehutso, R. F., & Thwala, M. (2021). Assessment of nano pollution from commercial products in water environments. *Nanomaterials, 11*, 2537.

124. Leiva-Presa, À., & Jenssen, B. M. (2006). Effects of p,p -DDE on retinoid homeostasis and sex hormones of adult male European common frogs (*Rana temporaria*). *Journal of Toxicology and Environmental Health, Part A, 69*, 2051–2062.

125. Lescano, M. R., Masin, C. E., Rodríguez, A. R., Godoy, J. L., & Zalazar, C. S. (2020). Earthworms to improve glyphosate degradation in bio beds. *Environmental Science and Pollution Research International, 27*, 27023–27031.

126. Leung, M. C. K., Williams, P. L., Benedetto, A., Au, C., Helmcke, K. J., Aschner, M., & Meyer, J. N. (2008). *Caenorhabditis elegans*: An emerging model in biomedical and environmental toxicology. *Toxicological Sciences, 106*, 5–28.

127. Lewis, J. L., Agostini, G., Jones, D. K., & Relyea, R. A. (2021). Cascading effects of insecticides and road salt on wetland communities. *Environmental Pollution, 272*, 116006.

128. Li, P., Wu, H., Wang, Y., Peng, W., & Su, W. (2020). Toxicological evaluation of naringin: Acute, sub chronic, and chronic toxicity in Beagle dogs. *Regulatory Toxicology and Pharmacology, 111*, 104580.

129. Li, R., Meng, Z., Sun, W., Wu, R., Jia, M., Yan, S., Tian, S., Zhu, W., & Zhou, Z. (2020). Bioaccumulation and toxic effects of penconazole in earthworms (*Eisenia fetida*) following soil exposure. *Environmental Science and Pollution Research International, 27*, 38056–38063.

130. Liu, T., Wang, P., Lu, Y., Zhou, G., Diao, J., & Zhou, Z. (2012). Enantioselective bioaccumulation of soil-associated fipronil enantiomers in *Tubifex tubifex*. *Journal of Hazardous Materials, 219–220*, 50–56.

131. Liu, Y. H., Lv, Y. Z., Huang, Z., Guan, Y. F., Huang, J. W., Zhao, J. L., & Ying, G. G. (2021). Uptake, elimination, and toxicokinetic of selected pharmaceuticals in multiple tissues of Nile tilapia (*Oreochromis niloticus*) exposed to environmentally relevant concentrations. *Ecotoxicology and Environmental Safety, 226*, 112874.

132. Loll, A., Reinwald, H., Ayobahan, S. U., Göckener, B., Salinas, G., Schäfers, C., Schlich, K., Hamscher, G., & Eilebrecht, S. (2022). Short-term test for toxicogenomic analysis of ecotoxic modes of action in *Lemna minor*. *Environmental Science & Technology, 56*(19), 11504–11515.

133. Lomba, L., Lapeña, D., Ros, N., Aso, E., Cannavò, M., Errazquin, D., & Giner, B. (2020). Ecotoxicological study of six drugs in *Aliivibrio fischeri*, *Daphnia magna*, and *Raphidocelis subcapitata*. *Environmental Science and Pollution Research International, 27*(9), 9891–9900.

134. Lomba, L., Ribate, M. P., Zaragoza, E., Concha, J., Garralaga, M. P., Errazquin, D., García, C. B., & Giner, B. (2021). Deep eutectic solvents: Are they safe? *Applied Sciences, 11*(19), 10061.

135. Lomba, L., Ribate, M. P., Zuriaga, E., García, C. B., & Giner, B. (2019). Acute and subacute effects of drugs in embryos of *Danio rerio*: QSAR grouping and modelling. *Ecotoxicology and Environmental Safety, 172*, 232–239.

136. Lopes Andrade, A. W., Dias Ribeiro Figueiredo, D., TorequlIslam, M., Viana Nunes, A. M., da Conceição Machado, K., Uddin, S. J., Ahmed Shilpi, J., Rouf, R., de Carvalho Melo-Cavalcante, A. A., & David, J. M. (2019). Toxicological evaluation of the biflavonoid, agathisflavone in albino Swiss mice. *Biomedicine & Pharmacotherapy, 110*, 68–73.

137. Lorite, G. S., Rocha, J. M., Miilumäki, N., Saavalainen, P., Selkälä, T., Morales-Cid, G., Gonçalves, M. P., Pongrácz, E., Rocha, C. M. R., & Toth, G. (2017). Evaluation of physicochemical/microbial properties and life cycle assessment (LCA) of PLA-based nanocomposite active packaging. *LWT–Food Science and Technology, 75*, 305–315.

138. Luzak, B., Siarkiewicz, P., & Boncler, M. (2022). An evaluation of a new high-sensitivity PrestoBlue assay for measuring cell viability and drug cytotoxicity using EA. Hy926 endothelial cells. *Toxicology in Vitro, 83*, 105407.

139. Ma-Hock, L., Burkhardt, S., Strauss, V., Gamer, A. O., Wiench, K., Van Ravenzwaay, B., & Landsiedel, R. (2009). Development of a short-term inhalation test in the rat using nano-titanium dioxide as a model substance. *Inhalation Toxicology, 21*(2), 102–118.

140. Makaras, T., & Stankevičiūtė, M. (2022). Swimming behaviour in two ecologically similar three-spined (*Gasterosteus aculeatus* L.) and nine-spined sticklebacks (*Pungitius pungitius* L.): A comparative approach for modelling the toxicity of metal mixtures. *Environmental Science and Pollution Research International, 29*(11), 14479–14496.

141. Marisa, I., Marin, M. G., Caicci, F., Franceschinis, E., Martucci, A., & Matozzo, V. (2015). In vitro exposure of haemocytes of the clam *Ruditapes philippinarum* to titanium dioxide (TiO_2) nanoparticles: Nanoparticle characterization, effects on phagocytic activity and internalization of nanoparticles into hemocytes. *Marine Environmental Research, 103*, 11–17.

142. Marisa, I., Matozzo, V., Martucci, A., Franceschinis, E., Brianese, N., & Marin, M. G. (2018). Bioaccumulation and effects of titanium dioxide nanoparticles and bulk in the clam *Ruditapes philippinarum*. *Marine Environmental Research, 136*, 179–189.

143. Marquart, H. (2016). Practical guide for SME managers and REACH coordinators: How to fulfil your information requirements at tonnages 1–10 and 10–100 tons per year; version 1.0-July 2016. European Chemicals Agency.

144. Mathiassen, S. K., Boutin, C., Strandberg, B., Carpenter, D., & Damgaard, C. (2021). Effects of low doses of herbicides on different endpoints in the life cycle of nontarget terrestrial plants. *Environmental Toxicology and Chemistry, 40*(5), 1389–1404.

145. Meesters, J. A. J., Peijnenburg, W. J. G. M., Hendriks, A. J., van de Meent, D., & Quik, J. T. K. (2019). A model sensitivity analysis to determine the most important physicochemical properties driving environmental fate and exposure of engineered nanoparticles. *Environmental Science: Nano, 6*(7), 2049–2060.

146. Migliore, L., Civitareale, C., Brambilla, G., & Dojmi Di Delupis, G. (1997). Toxicity of several important agricultural antibiotics to *Artemia*. *Water Research, 31*(7), 1801–1806.

147. Moinard, V., Redondi, C., Etiévant, V., Savoie, A., Duchene, D., Pelosi, C., Houot, S., & Capowiez, Y. (2021). Short- and long-term impacts of anaerobic digestate spreading on earthworms in cropped soils. *Applied Soil Ecology, 168*, 104149.

148. Moreton, M. L., & Marlatt, V. L. (2019). Toxicity of the aquatic herbicide, Reward®, to the northwestern salamander. *Environmental Science and Pollution Research International, 26*(32), 31077–31085.

149. Movia, D., Bruni-Favier, S., & Prina-Mello, A. (2020). In vitro alternatives to acute inhalation toxicity studies in animal models—A perspective. *Frontiers in Bioengineering and Biotechnology, 8*, 549.

150. Nagpal, M. A., & Tiwari, Q. (2025). QSAR analysis of substituted benzylideneacetophenones as lipid peroxidation inhibitors. *Asian Journal of Chemistry, 17*(3), 1669–1677.

151. Nallani, G. C., Liu, Z., & Chandrasekaran, A. (2020). Toxicokinetic testing strategies to demonstrate bone marrow exposure in in vivo micronucleus study for genotoxicity assessment of agrochemicals. *Regulatory Toxicology and Pharmacology, 110, 104552*.

152. Naqvi, S. M., & Rizvi, S. A. (2000). Accumulation of chromium and copper in three different soils and bioaccumulation in an aquatic plant, *Alternanthera philoxeroides*. *Bulletin of Environmental Contamination and Toxicology, 65*(1), 55–61.

153. National Research Council. (2007). *Toxicity Testing in the 21st Century: A Vision and a Strategy*. The National Academies Press.

154. Nishimura, Y., Murakami, S., Ashikawa, Y., Sasagawa, S., Umemoto, N., Shimada, Y., & Tanaka, T. (2015). Zebrafish as a systems toxicology model for developmental neurotoxicity testing. *Congenital Anomalies, 55*(1), 1–16.

155. OECD. (2004). Test No. 218: Sediment-water chironomid toxicity using spiked water. *OECD Guidelines for the Testing of Chemicals, Section 2*. OECD Publishing. https://doi.org/10.1787/9789264067476-en.

156. OECD. (2021). Test No. 405: Acute eye irritation/corrosion. OECD.

157. OECD. (2002). Test No. 423: Acute oral toxicity—Acute toxic class method. OECD. https://doi.org/10.1787/9789264067414-en.

158. Olguin, C. J. M., Sampaio, S. C., dos Reis, R. R., Remor, M. B., & Olguin, C. F. A. (2019). QSPR modelling of the soil sorption coefficient from training sets of different sizes. *SAR and QSAR in Environmental Research, 30*(4), 299–311.

159. Olivares-Ferretti, P., Chavez, V., Hernandez, K., Peredo-Parada, M., & Parodi, J. (2022). Polyphenols extracts from *Didymosphenia geminata* (Lyngbye) Schmidt altered the motility and viability of *Daphnia magna*. *Aquatic Ecology, 56*(1), 35–45.

160. Ortiz-Andrade, R., Araujo-León, J. A., Sánchez-Recillas, A., Navarrete-Vazquez, G., González-Sánchez, A. A., Hidalgo-Figueroa, S., & Coral-Martínez, T. I. (2020). Toxicological screening of

four bioactive citroflavonoids: In vitro, in vivo, and in silico approaches. *Molecules, 25*(24), 5959. https://doi.org/10.3390/molecules25245959.

161. Palharini, K. M. Z., Vitorino, L. C., Bessa, L. A., & de Carvalho Vasconcelos Filho, S. (2021). *Parmotrema tinctorum* as an indicator of edge effect and air quality in forested areas bordered by intensive agriculture. *Environmental Science and Pollution Research, 28*(53), 68997–69011. https://doi.org/10.1007/s11356-021-16154-6.
162. Palharini, K. M. Z., Vitorino, L. C., de Oliveira Menino, G. C., & Bessa, L. A. (2020). Edge effects reflect the impact of the agricultural matrix on the corticolous lichens found in fragments of cerrado savanna in central Brazil. *Sustainability, 12*(17), 7149. https://doi.org/10.3390/su12177149.
163. Pereira, M. I. A., Monteiro, C. A. P., de Oliveira, W. F., Santos, B. S., Fontes, A., & Cabral Filho, P. E. (2020). Resazurin-based assay to evaluate cell viability after quantum dot interaction. In P. E. Cabral Filho (Ed.), *Methods in Molecular Biology: Cell Viability Assays* (Vol. 2135, pp. 213–221). Humana.
164. Pi, N., Ng, J. Z., & Kelly, B. C. (2017). Bioaccumulation of pharmaceutically active compounds and endocrine disrupting chemicals in aquatic macrophytes: Results of hydroponic experiments with *Echinodorus horemanii* and *Eichhornia crassipes*. *Science of the Total Environment, 601–602*, 812–820. https://doi.org/10.1016/j.scitotenv.2017.05.271.
165. Pott, F., & Roller, M. (2005). Carcinogenicity study with nineteen granular dusts in rats. *European Journal of Oncology, 10*, 249–281.
166. Poveda, J. (2021). Cyanobacteria in plant health: Biological strategy against abiotic and biotic stresses. *Crop Protection, 141*, 105450. https://doi.org/10.1016/j.cropro.2020.105450.
167. Präbst, K., Engelhardt, H., Ringgeler, S., & Hübner, H. (2017). Basic colorimetric proliferation assays: MTT, WST, and resazurin. In H. Hübner (Ed.), *Cell Viability Assays* (Vol. 1601, pp. 1–17). Humana Press.
168. Qiu, W., Fang, M., Liu, J., Fu, C., Zheng, C., Chen, B., & Wang, K. J. (2019). In vivo actions of bisphenol F on the reproductive neuroendocrine system after long-term exposure in zebrafish. *Science of the Total Environment, 665*, 995–1002. https://doi.org/10.1016/j.scitotenv.2019.02.185.
169. Raimets, R., Naudi, S., Mänd, M., Bartkevičs, V., Smagghe, G., & Karise, R. (2021). Translocation of tebuconazole between bee matrices and its potential threat on honey bee (*Apis mellifera* Linnaeus) queens. *Insects, 13*(1), 45. https://doi.org/10.3390/insects13010045.
170. Raja, V., & Shanmugasundaram, S. (2020). Development of capacitance based nondestructive ripening indices measurement system for sapota (*Manilkara zapota*). *Journal of Food Process Engineering, 43*, e13307. https://doi.org/10.1111/jfpe.13307.
171. Ramírez-Morales, D., Fajardo-Romero, D., Rodríguez-Rodríguez, C. E., & Cedergreen, N. (2022). Single and mixture toxicity of selected pharmaceuticals to the aquatic macrophyte *Lemna minor*. *Ecotoxicology, 31*(5), 714–724. https://doi.org/10.1007/s10646-022-02522-4.
172. Rápó, E., & Tonk, S. (2021). Factors affecting synthetic dye adsorption; Desorption studies: A review of results from the last five years (2017–2021). *Molecules, 26*(18), 5419. https://doi.org/10.3390/molecules26185419.
173. Rehn, B., Seiler, F., Rehn, S., Bruch, J., & Maier, M. (2003). Investigations on the inflammatory

and genotoxic lung effects of two types of titanium dioxide: Untreated and surface treated. *Toxicology and Applied Pharmacology, 189*(2), 84–95. https://doi.org/10.1016/S0041-008X(03)00192-0.

174. Reiss, R., Lewis, G., & Griffin, J. (2009). An ecological risk assessment for triclosan in the terrestrial environment. *Environmental Toxicology and Chemistry, 28*(7), 1546–1556. https://doi.org/10.1897/08-557.1.
175. Renick, V. C., Anderson, T. W., Morgan, S. G., & Cherr, G. N. (2015). Interactive effects of pesticide exposure and habitat structure on behavior and predation of a marine larval fish. *Ecotoxicology, 24*(2), 391–400. https://doi.org/10.1007/s10646-015-1565-7.
176. Romero, C., Giner, B., Haro, M., Artigas, H., & Lafuente, C. (2006). Thermophysical study of 1,4-dioxane with cycloalkane mixtures. *Journal of Chemical Thermodynamics, 38*(7), 871–878. https://doi.org/10.1016/j.jct.2005.09.008.
177. Roy, K., Das, R. N., & Popelier, P. L. A. (2015). Predictive QSAR modelling of algal toxicity of ionic liquids and its interspecies correlation with *Daphnia* toxicity. *Environmental Science and Pollution Research, 22*(9), 6634–6641. https://doi.org/10.1007/s11356-014-3840-5.
178. Safitri, R. R., Sudirman, L. I., & Koesmaryono, Y. (2020). Exploration of *Parmotrema tinctorum* and *Leptogium* sp. lichens as bioindicator of air quality in Mekarsari Fruit Park. In *IOP Conference Series: Earth and Environmental Science* (Vol. 457). IOP Publishing. https://doi.org/10.1088/1755-1315/457/1/012050.
179. Saidani, W., Sellami, B., Khazri, A., Mezni, A., Dellali, M., Joubert, O., & Beyrem, H. (2019). Metal accumulation, biochemical and behavioral responses on the Mediterranean clams *Ruditapes decussatus* exposed to two photocatalyst nanocomposites (*TiO2 NPs* and *AuTiO2 NPs*). *Aquatic Toxicology, 208*, 71–79. https://doi.org/10.1016/j.aquatox.2019.01.019.
180. Sanchez-Bayo, F., & Hyne, R. V. (2011). Comparison of environmental risks of pesticides between tropical and nontropical regions. *Integrated Environmental Assessment and Management, 7*(4), 577–586. https://doi.org/10.1002/ieam.230.
181. Santos-Silva, T., de Azambuja Ribeiro, R. I. M., Alves, S. N., Thomé, R. G., & Santos, H. B. Dos. (2021). Assessment of the toxicological effects of pesticides and detergent mixtures on zebrafish gills: A histological study. *Brazilian Archives of Biology and Technology, 64*. https://doi.org/10.1590/1678-4324-2021210198.
182. Schenker, U., Scheringer, M., & Hungerbühler, K. (2008). Investigating the global fate of DDT: Model evaluation and estimation of future trends. *Environmental Science & Technology, 42*(4), 1178–1184. https://doi.org/10.1021/es070700b.
183. Schmolke, A., Galic, N., Feken, M., Thompson, H., Sgolastra, F., Pitts-Singer, T., & Hinarejos, S. (2021). Assessment of the vulnerability to pesticide exposures across bee species. *Environmental Toxicology and Chemistry, 40*(10), 2640–2651. https://doi.org/10.1002/etc.5113.
184. Seben, D., Salbego, J., da Silva, E. G., Gressler, L. T., Baldisserotto, B., Marchesan, E., & Golombieski, J. I. (2021). Acute silver catfish (*Rhamdia quelen*) exposure to chlorantraniliprole insecticide. *Bulletin of Environmental Contamination and Toxicology, 107*(6), 883–888. https://doi.org/10.1007/s00128-021-03236-3.
185. Shariatzadeh, S., Emadi, H., Jamili, S., & Mashinchian Moradi, A. (2022). Pathological

and genotoxic effects of the herbicide oxadiargyl on common carp (*Cyprinus carpio*) fingerlings. *Iranian Journal of Fisheries Sciences, 21*(2), 316–330. https://doi.org/10.22092/IJFS.2022.131538.

186. Simpson, S. L., & Batley, G. E. (2016). *Sediment Quality Assessment: A Practical Guide*. CSIRO Publishing.
187. Simpson, S. L., Campana, O., & Ho, K. T. (2016). Sediment toxicity testing. In O. Campana & K. T. Ho (Eds.), *Marine Ecotoxicology* (pp. 199–237). Academic Press.
188. Smith, G. R., Krishnamurthy, S. V., Burger, A. C., & Mills, L. B. (2011). Differential effects of malathion and nitrate exposure on American toad and wood frog tadpoles. *Archives of Environmental Contamination and Toxicology, 60*(2), 327–335. https://doi.org/10.1007/s00244-010-9580-5.
189. Snell, T. W., & Joaquim-Justo, C. (2007). Workshop on rotifers in ecotoxicology. *Hydrobiologia, 593*(1), 227–232. https://doi.org/10.1007/s10750-007-9026-1.
190. Spirhanzlova, P., Leemans, M., Demeneix, B. A., & Fini, J. B. (2019). Following endocrine-disrupting effects on gene expression in *Xenopus laevis*. *Cold Spring Harbor Protocols, 2019*(12), pdb. prot098301. https://doi.org/10.1101/pdb.prot098301.
191. Stanton, D. T., Dimitrov, S., Grancharov, V., & Mekenyan, O. G. (2002). Charged partial surface area (CPSA) descriptors QSAR applications. *SAR and QSAR in Environmental Research, 13*(3–4), 341–351. https://doi.org/10.1080/10629360290025691.
192. Su, Q., Zheng, J., Xi, J., Yang, J., Wang, L., & Xiong, D. (2022). Evaluation of the acute toxic response induced by triazophos to the non-target green algae *Chlorella pyrenoidosa*. *Pesticide Biochemistry and Physiology, 182*, 105036. https://doi.org/10.1016/j.pestbp.2022.105036.
193. Taylor, S. K., Williams, E. S., & Mills, K. W. (1999). Effects of malathion on disease susceptibility in Wood house's toads. *Journal of Wildlife Diseases, 35*(3), 536–541. https://doi.org/10.7589/0090-3558-35.3.536.
194. Tian, S., Zhang, Y., Song, C., Zhu, X., & Xing, B. (2015). Bioaccumulation and biotransformation of polybrominated diphenyl ethers in the marine bivalve (*Scapharca subcrenata*): Influence of titanium dioxide nanoparticles. *Marine Pollution Bulletin, 90*(1–2), 48–53. https://doi.org/10.1016/j.marpolbul.2014.11.033.
195. Tiepo, E. N., Corrêa, A. X. R., Resgalla, C., Cotelle, S., Férard, J. F., & Radetski, C. M. (2010). Terrestrial short-term ecotoxicity of a green formicide. *Ecotoxicology and Environmental Safety, 73*(5), 939–943. https://doi.org/10.1016/j.ecoenv.2010.02.020.
196. Tongur, S., & Yıldız, S. (2021). Toxicity tests using flurbiprofen, naproxen, propranolol, and carbamazepine on *Lepidium sativum*, *Daphnia magna*, and *Aliivibrio fischeri*. *Desalination and Water Treatment, 221*, 359–366. https://doi.org/10.5004/dwt.2021.26938.
197. Triques, M. C., Oliveira, D., Goulart, B. V., Montagner, C. C., Espíndola, E. L. G., & de Menezes-Oliveira, V. B. (2021). Assessing single effects of sugarcane pesticides fipronil and 2,4-D on plants and soil organisms. *Ecotoxicology and Environmental Safety, 208*, 111622. https://doi.org/10.1016/j.ecoenv.2020.111622.
198. Vali, S., Majidiyan, N., Yalsuyi, A. M., Vajargah, M. F., Prokić, M. D., & Faggio, C. (2022). Ecotoxicological effects of silver nanoparticles (Ag-NPs) on parturition time, survival rate, reproductive success and blood parameters of adult common molly (*Poecilia sphenops*) and their larvae. *Water, 14*(1), 144. https://doi.org/10.3390/w14010144.

199. Van Loon, S., Vicente, V. B., & van Gestel, C. A. M. (2022). Long-term effects of imidacloprid, thiacloprid, and clothianidin on the growth and development of *Eisenia andrei*. *Environmental Toxicology and Chemistry, 41*(7), 1686–1695. https://doi.org/10.1002/etc.5472.

200. van Ravenzwaay, B., Landsiedel, R., Fabian, E., Burkhardt, S., Strauss, V., & Ma-Hock, L. (2009). Comparing fate and effects of three particles of different surface properties: Nano-TiO_2, pigmentary TiO_2 and quartz. *Toxicology Letters, 186*(3), 152–159. https://doi.org/10.1016/j.toxlet.2009.01.017.

201. Vargas, R., & Ponce-Canchihuamán, J. (2017). Emerging various environmental threats to brain and overview of surveillance system with zebrafish model. *Toxicology Reports, 4*, 467–473. https://doi.org/10.1016/j.toxrep.2017.07.006.

202. Vargesson, N. (2015). Thalidomide-induced teratogenesis: History and mechanisms. *Birth Defects Research Part C: Embryo Today: Reviews, 105*(2), 140–156. https://doi.org/10.1002/bdrc.21096.

203. Wang, K., Wang, C., Wang, J., Dong, Y., Che, W., & Li, X. (2022). Acute toxicity of broflanilide on neurosecretory system and locomotory behavior of zebrafish (*Danio rerio*). *Chemosphere, 305*, 135426. https://doi.org/10.1016/j.chemosphere.2022.135426.

204. Wang, L., Chen, Y., Zhao, Y., Du, M., Wang, Y., Fan, J., Ren, N., & Lee, D. J. (2020). Toxicity of two tetracycline antibiotics on *Stentor coeruleus* and *Stylonychia lemnae*: Potential use as toxicity indicator. *Chemosphere, 255*, 127011. https://doi.org/10.1016/j.chemosphere.2020.127011.

205. Wang, S., Han, X., Yu, T., Liu, Y., Zhang, H., Mao, H., Hu, C., & Xu, X. (2022). Isoprocarb causes neurotoxicity of zebrafish embryos through oxidative stress-induced apoptosis. *Ecotoxicology and Environmental Safety, 242*, 113870. https://doi.org/10.1016/j.ecoenv.2021.113870.

206. Wang, X., Zhang, C., Liu, Z., & Chen, L. (2015). Development of predicted no effect concentration (PNEC) for TCS to terrestrial species. *Chemosphere, 139*, 428–433. https://doi.org/10.1016/j.chemosphere.2015.07.009.

207. Warheit, D. B., Reed, K. L., & Webb, T. R. (2003). Pulmonary toxicity studies in rats with triethoxyoctylsilane (OTES)-coated, pigment-grade titanium dioxide particles: Bridging studies to predict inhalation hazard. *Experimental Lung Research, 29*(7), 593–606. https://doi.org/10.1080/01902140303771.

208. Webber, N. R., Boone, M. D., & Distel, C. A. (2010). Effects of aquatic and terrestrial carbaryl exposure on feeding ability, growth, and survival of American toads. *Environmental Toxicology and Chemistry, 29*(10), 2323–2327. https://doi.org/10.1002/etc.315.

209. Weitekamp, C. A., Koethe, R. W., & Lehmann, D. M. (2022). A comparison of pollen and syrup exposure routes in *Bombus impatiens* (Hymenoptera: Apidae) microcolonies: Implications for pesticide risk assessment. *Environmental Entomology, 51*(3), 613–620. https://doi.org/10.1093/ee/nvab208.

210. Wu, X., Nguyen, H., Kim, D., & Peng, H. (2022). Chronic toxicity of PFAS-free AFFF alternatives in terrestrial plant *Brassica rapa*. *Science of The Total Environment, 850*, 158100. https://doi.org/10.1016/j.scitotenv.2021.158100.

211. Xu, X. P., Xi, Y. L., Huang, L., & Xiang, X. L. (2015). Effects of multi-metal (Cu, Zn, Cd, Cr, and Mn) mixtures on the reproduction of freshwater rotifer *Brachionus calyciflorus*. *Bulletin of Environmental Contamination and Toxicology, 95*(6), 714–720. https://doi.org/10.1007/s00128-015-1585-5.

212. Yalçin, M., Kapiz, I., Kösoglu, M., Koca, Y. O., Turgut, N., Topal, E., & Özkaleli Akçetin, M. (2021). Translocation of clothianidin to guttation fluid and its potential impact on honey bee, *Apis mellifera anatoliaca* Maa, 1953 (Hymenoptera: Apidae). *Türkiye Entomoloji Dergisi, 45*(4), 511–522. https://doi.org/10.16970/ted.783894.

213. Yang, Y., Li, S., Wang, Z., Ren, Y., Mu, Y., Zhang, X., & Cheng, B. (2022). Acute toxicity, bioaccumulation and elimination of prometryn in tilapia (*Oreochromis niloticus*). *Chemosphere, 300*, 134565. https://doi.org/10.1016/j.chemosphere.2022.134565.

214. Yu, S., Wages, M. R., Cai, Q., Maul, J. D., & Cobb, G. P. (2013). Lethal and sublethal effects of three insecticides on two developmental stages of *Xenopus laevis* and comparison with other amphibians. *Environmental Toxicology and Chemistry, 32*(9), 2056–2064. https://doi.org/10.1002/etc.2315.

215. Yu, Y., Luan, Y., & Dai, W. (2022). Time evolution of protein corona formed by polystyrene nanoplastics and urease. *International Journal of Biological Macromolecules, 218*, 72–81. https://doi.org/10.1016/j.ijbiomac.2022.01.065.

216. Zhi, D., Yang, D., Zheng, Y., Yang, Y., He, Y., Luo, L., & Zhou, Y. (2019). Current progress in the adsorption, transport and biodegradation of antibiotics in soil. *Journal of Environmental Management, 251*, 109598. https://doi.org/10.1016/j.jenvman.2019.109598.

217. Zhu, F. P., Duan, J. L., Yuan, X. Z., Shi, X. S., Han, Z. L., & Wang, S. G. (2018). Hydrolysis, adsorption, and biodegradation of bensulfuron methyl under methanogenic conditions. *Chemosphere, 199*, 138–146. https://doi.org/10.1016/j.chemosphere.2018.01.163.

218. Zhu, Y. C., Wang, Y., Portilla, M., Parys, K., & Li, W. (2019). Risk and toxicity assessment of a potential natural insecticide, methyl benzoate, in honey bees (*Apis mellifera* L.). *Insects, 10*(11), 382. https://doi.org/10.3390/insects10110382.

219. Zuriaga, E., Giner, B., Ribate, M. P., García, C. B., & Lomba, L. (2018). Exploring the usefulness of key green physicochemical properties: Quantitative structure–activity relationship for solvents from biomass. *Environmental Toxicology and Chemistry, 37*(4), 1014–1023. https://doi.org/10.1002/etc.4067.

220. Zuriaga, E., Giner, B., Valero, M. S., Gómez, M., García, C. B., & Lomba, L. (2019). QSAR modelling for predicting the toxic effects of traditional and derived biomass solvents on a *Danio rerio* biomodel. *Chemosphere, 227*, 480–488. https://doi.org/10.1016/j.chemosphere.2019.04.158.

221. Zuriaga, E., Lomba, L., Royo, F. M., Lafuente, C., & Giner, B. (2014). Aggregation behavior of betablocker drugs in aqueous media. *New Journal of Chemistry, 38*(9), 4141–4148. https://doi.org/10.1039/C4NJ00580K.

Chapter 3

REPRODUCTIVE TOXICOLOGY

Contents

Introduction

The possibility of interference with normal reproductive function or proper development is one of the potential health effects of chemical exposure that is of most concern. The increasing number of women in the workplace and subsequent pregnancies associated with occupational exposure to various chemicals makes the general population particularly sensitive to the potential for this type of toxicity. Our environment is also often perceived as potentially toxic to reproduction, as awareness of the prevalence and persistence of some man-made (or human-related) chemicals grows. To what extent do these perceptions of increased reproductive risk correspond to currently available scientific information, and how can future scientific investigations be directed to address important questions? These questions can be answered by considering the interactions between reproductive processes and chemical (and non-chemical) exposures in the workplace or environment. Our knowledge of reproductive toxicity has expanded rapidly in recent decades, and we now have much more information available to critically assess potential reproductive risk.

This chapter examines the known toxic responses of the male and female reproductive systems and human fetal development. The focus is on the potential human health effects arising from occupational and/or environmental exposures and examples are given from this area. However, there is much additional mechanistic information from experimental systems and many other chemicals for which there is experimental evidence of potential reproductive toxicity. In evaluating the significance of such chemicals or mechanisms in terms of human exposure, two basic principles of toxicology must be considered: 1) what are the characteristics of a likely exposure, and 2) what might be a relevant dose. The key to answering these questions is to understand how reproductive processes respond to chemical challenges.

The topics to be covered include

- Male reproduction and the susceptibility of rapidly dividing gametes.
- Female reproduction and the regulation of endocrine status as a potential target for toxic reactions.

Many of the toxicological principles relating to reproduction can be made clear by examples relating to the male. Furthermore, many of the best characterized examples of toxic responses to human reproduction from occupational exposures are related to males. This state of knowledge may reflect a historical bias toward male effects due to the past predominance of men in industrial settings. However, male reproductive physiology and function provides certain vulnerabilities to toxicants that are useful to illustrate how toxicologic responses relate to reproductive biology in general. Understanding the underlying mechanisms will help to understand the more complex and less well understood issues of female and developmental toxicology. The interest continues to shift toward non-industrial occupational exposures and general environmental exposures, many new discoveries about the mechanisms of toxic injury to the female reproductive system and developing offspring can be expected.

Most of the best-described examples of reproductive toxicity rely on experimental results obtained in laboratory animals to explain them. While inferring the actual human potential for an adverse event from the results of animal studies must always be done critically and cautiously, there are certain factors related to reproductive endpoints that add unique uncertainties. The relevance of the experimental dose to the potential human exposure is always an important factor in the interpretation of animal studies. For reproductive endpoints, not only the dose level is an issue, but also the duration and interval of administration, as sequential, precisely timed sequences of physiological events are a hallmark of reproductive processes. Experimental testing for a given chemical must cover the time frame that is likely to be relevant to the toxicity mechanisms involved. Concurrent maternal toxicity can be a problematic complication when assessing developmental toxicity. When attempting to demonstrate effects, doses are often set so high that they lead to generalized emaciation, feeding problems or other distress in the animal. Therefore, it can be difficult to distinguish between direct toxicity to the developing offspring and females that are simply too impaired to maintain a normal pregnancy. In light of such complications, animal studies remain an important and valuable tool for characterizing reproductive toxicity. It is imperative to use test systems that can be easily manipulated to identify potential mechanisms of toxicity. The challenge is to interpret the implications of certain animal test results and determine how they relate to potential problems for humans.

Orientation and Directional Terms

Term	Definition	Illustration
Sertoli Cells	Sertoli cells are specialized cells located in the seminiferous tubules of the testes. They support and nourish developing sperm cells, regulate spermatogenesis, and provide a barrier between blood and germ cells.	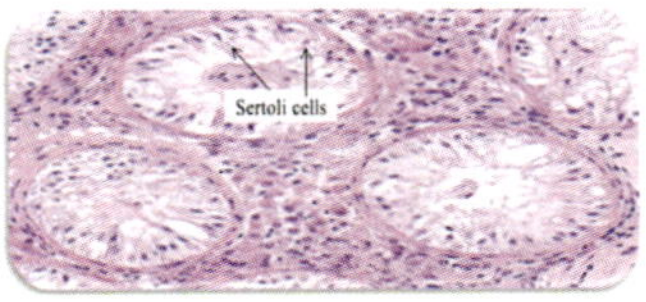
Leydig Cells	Leydig cells are located in the interstitial tissue of the testes and are responsible for producing testosterone and other androgens. They play a crucial role in male sexual development and spermatogenesis.	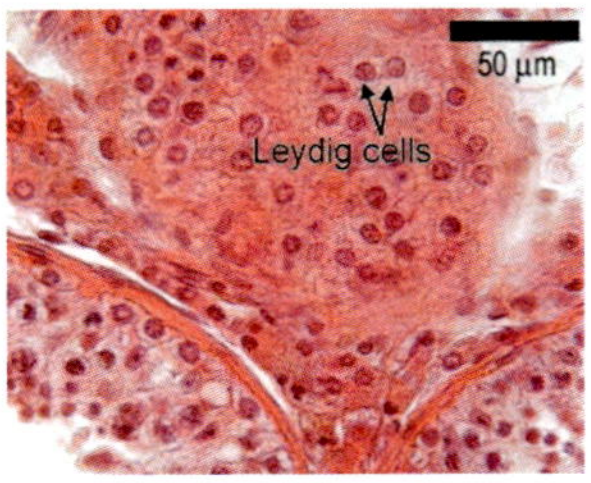
Oocyte Toxicity	Oocyte toxicity refers to damage or dysfunction of oocytes (egg cells) due to exposure to harmful substances or conditions, which can impact fertility and reproductive health.	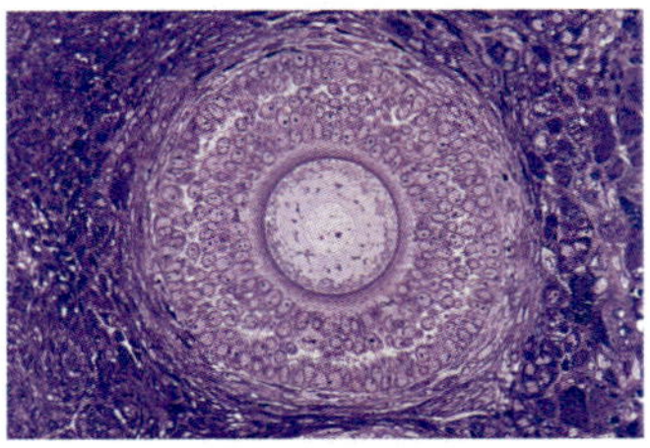
Fetal Hydantoin Syndrome	Fetal Hydantoin Syndrome is a condition caused by maternal use of hydantoin (a type of anticonvulsant medication) during pregnancy. It is characterized by physical and developmental abnormalities in the infant.	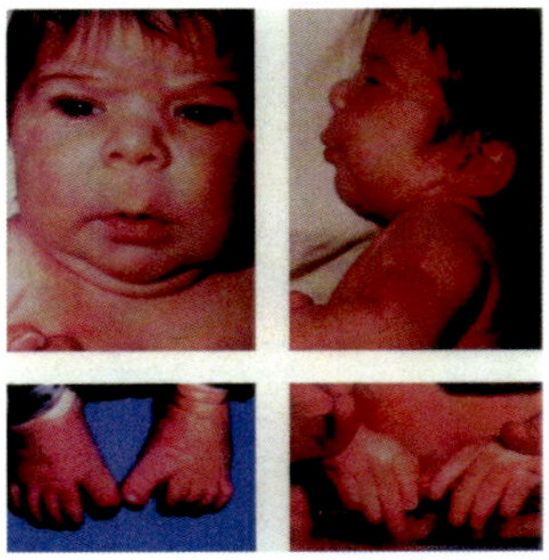
Methylmercury Poisoning	Methylmercury poisoning is a form of mercury poisoning caused by the ingestion of methylmercury, a toxic compound found in contaminated fish and seafood. It can lead to neurological and developmental damage.	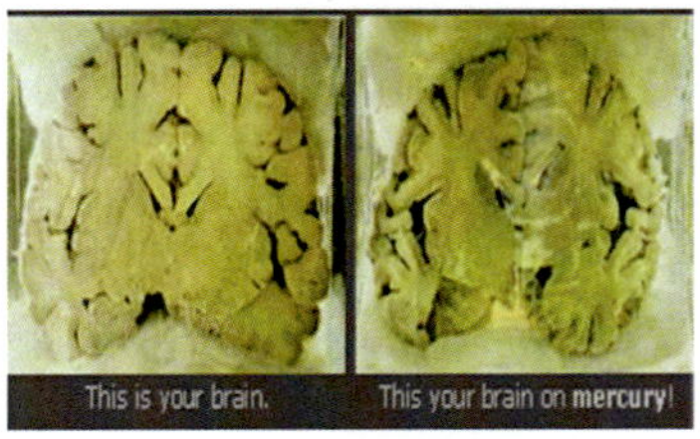

3.1. Male Reproductive Toxicology

Basically, the function of the male reproductive system is to produce the male germ cells, the spermatozoa and put them in a state that allows them to unite with a female germ cell and subsequently develop. Toxic reactions must either disrupt germ cell production or transmission. The reproductive organs are obvious targets for such reactions, but damage to the nervous and endocrine systems may also be important because of their role in controlling reproductive function. This section describes some of the toxic chemicals that affect germ cell production and their mechanisms of action. In addition, information is presented on some of the toxic reactions that can lead to problems with sperm release.

3.1.1. Susceptibility of Spermatogenesis

The process of germ cell formation in men, spermatogenesis, provides clear examples of how cells can exhibit increased sensitivity to certain classes of chemicals at certain times. In spermatogenesis, germ cells are generated from a pool of progenitor cells, the stem cells, through a series of mitotic and meiotic divisions that eventually give rise to large numbers of sperm from each original stem cell and provide replacement stem cells. Spermatogenesis takes place in specialized, thick-walled tubes in the testicles, the so-called seminiferous tubules. The germ cells are initially located at the outer edge of the tubule (Figure 3.1) and gradually migrate to the center of the tubule. From here, the sperm migrate along the tubules and into the ductal system that transports them out of the body.

In humans, it takes about 64 days for a mature sperm to emerge through this process, which continues throughout adult life. The rate of spermatogenesis increases dramatically after puberty until eventually a 100 million or more sperm are produced per day. Spermatogenesis can be equated with a mass production process that focuses on constantly high production rates and a high production volume. In a biological system, this requires an extremely active, rapidly dividing cellular environment in the testes.

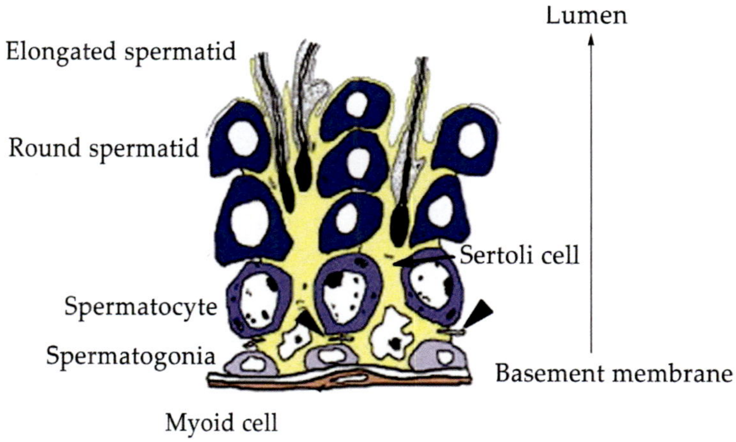

Figure 3.1. *Illustration of seminiferous tubule: An overview.*

Source: https://ars.els-cdn.com/.

The high rate of cell division and high metabolic activity associated with spermatogenesis are the basis for susceptibility to certain types of damage. During the duplication of genetic material and cell division, DNA is particularly susceptible to damage. In addition, many specialized cellular proteins and enzymes are required, and a high level of cellular respiration is needed. Therefore, chemicals that can cause DNA damage or impair the function of cell proteins or cellular respiration are particularly problematic in rapidly dividing tissues. Examples include reactive electrophilic chemicals such as alkylating agents and ionizing radiation. Many chemicals or their metabolites, which are considered to be relatively toxic, are capable of undergoing chemical reactions with DNA or important cell proteins. Depending on the chemical, DNA damage can result from direct interaction with the strands or with other cellular macromolecules involved in stabilizing DNA. Reactions with DNA can affect base pairing and strand linkage. Protein damage can alter enzymes and carrier molecules in such a way that they can no longer participate in biochemical reactions.

Antineoplastic drugs used in chemotherapy, such as methotrexate, adriamycin, cyclophosphamide, vincristine, and vinblastine, are good examples of reactive compounds that can lead to disruption of germ cell production. Some examples of reactive chemicals commonly encountered in the workplace or environment that are of particular concern with regard to rapidly dividing spermatogenic tissue are:

- Acrylamide and ethylene oxide – widespread industrial use.
- Polynuclear aromatic hydrocarbons (PAHs) – combustion products.
- Ethylene dibromide and dibromochloropropane fumigants/ pesticides.

An understanding of the general mechanisms of action can help categorize chemicals in terms of potential effects. It is important to remember that while there is a mechanism for cellular damage to spermatogenic cells for reactive chemicals in general, not every alkylating agent or reactive metabolite actually acts as a specific reproductive toxicant. Other factors determine the susceptibility of spermatogenic tissue to certain chemicals. Critical factors include the level of the ingested dose, the extent of distribution in the target tissue and how or where the metabolism of the chemical takes place. Individual and species-specific differences in these factors explain the variation in susceptibility and highlight the need for caution in predicting whether a chemical is toxic to human reproduction.

The energy associated with ionizing radiation, including X-rays, can also cause chemical changes to DNA that affect its potential to be copied correctly and control cell function. Although germ cells can be damaged at all stages of spermatogenesis, some of the early stages appear to be most susceptible to radiation-induced DNA strand breaks. Such breaks can lead to chromosomal malformations in germ cells. In addition, the death of damaged somatic cells (non-germ cells) can lead to the accumulation of cell debris in the ductal system that transports the germ cells.

In addition to DNA damage, which can lead to cell death, there is also the possibility that DNA modifications are incorrectly repaired, and a mutation occurs. There are cellular mechanisms to remove and replace damaged DNA segments, but this type of repair is associated with a certain, albeit small, error rate. If such repair errors occur in a germ cell, there is a possibility that the resulting mutation will be passed on to offspring and be heritable. Although this is theoretically possible and can be demonstrated in some experimental systems, the emergence of a heritable human mutation following chemically induced DNA damage has not been documented (Yamashita & Markert, 2021; Bicker, 2022).

3.1.2. Direct and Indirect Modes of Toxicity

Another important toxicological concept, which is well illustrated by the example of the male reproductive system, is the distinction between direct and indirect toxicants. Direct-acting toxicants may be reactive chemicals or chemicals that are structurally similar to molecules used in cellular communication in such a way that they can interfere with signaling pathways. Indirectly acting toxins may be able to cause damage in the same way, but must first be modified or bioactivated by metabolic reactions. Ironically, reactive metabolites often arise from the chemical reactions that are also used to degrade and eliminate foreign chemicals. Metabolism may take place in the cells or tissues that are ultimately damaged, or in other organs, such as the liver. In the latter case, the toxic metabolites must be transported to the target tissue.

Some of the best-known reproductive toxicants have a direct effect on male reproductive tissue. Lead and cadmium are two examples of metals in this category. Lead can damage genetic material, disrupt cell division and lead to cell death. While many different cell types can be damaged by lead, this process is particularly vulnerable due to the importance of continuous division during spermatogenesis.

Cadmium has an interesting direct effect on the vasculature surrounding the testes and epididymis, the adjacent tubular organ where sperm are stored and mature. Sperm must be kept at temperatures just below the body's core temperature. An extensive and specialized vascular system is present to dissipate the heat from the testicles. This vascular system is extremely susceptible to direct damage from cadmium. If such damage occurs, the remaining vessels can no longer remove as much blood and therefore as much heat. The combination of reduced blood flow with oxygen-rich blood and higher temperatures can subsequently destroy the spermatogenic cells.

Many of the alkylating chemotherapeutic agents have a direct mode of action that leads to toxicity to male reproduction, including busulfan and cyclophosphamide. Ethylene oxide, used extensively as a chemical intermediate in industry and for gas sterilization of medical devices and even food, also acts directly on cellular biomolecules, and experimental studies suggest that germ cells are particularly susceptible to its damage in later stages.

DNA is stabilized by extensive interactions with structural elements called protamines during later stages of spermatogenesis and protamines are particularly vulnerable to reactions with ethylene oxide.

These examples from medicine illustrate the delicate balance between therapeutic or beneficial uses and potential reproductive toxicity. The strong alkylating properties of chemotherapeutic agents allow them to act against rapidly dividing cancer cells, and the risk of side effects on other cells, even overt reproductive toxicity, may be an acceptable trade-off for the cancer patient. The safety and benefits of dry gas sterilization with ethylene oxide are also clearly important. While we can experimentally document the mechanisms of action leading to male reproductive toxicity, there is no evidence that ethylene oxide exposure associated with sterilization has led to reproductive toxicity in males. Again, the toxicology shows what could happen if the right conditions were present, not what happens in the typical situations in which the chemicals are found. Many of the compounds of interest in occupational or environmental toxicology require metabolic activation to cause reproductive effects. The testis has the enzymatic capabilities for oxidative metabolism, a metabolic pathway that frequently generates reactive intermediates. Although this activity is low compared to the liver, it is high enough to produce toxic levels of metabolites of some compounds.

The metabolism of common industrial chemicals, including the solvents n-hexane and glycol ether, appears to contribute to their reproductive toxicity. Some of the phthalates, a chemical class used extensively as plasticizers and widely distributed in the environment, may also affect male reproductive tissue after metabolism. All of these examples are discussed further in terms of the specific cells they affect and are at least claimed to affect in humans. There are many other examples of indirectly acting male reproductive toxicants for which there is at least experimental or mechanistic information on toxic potential, including the intermediate acrylamide and vinyl chloride, another common industrial intermediate that is also found in the environment, often as a degradation product of dry cleaning products.

3.1.3. Cell-Type Specific Toxicity

Another principle that becomes clear in the study of male reproductive toxicology is the specificity of the effect on certain cell types based on the characteristics of the cells or their metabolic potential. For some reproductive toxicants, there is a difference in sensitivity between somatic and germ cells. While in some cases this can be explained by the high cell division and activity of germ cells, in other cases more specific factors seem to be involved. In addition to germ cells, there are two important types of somatic cells in the testis that are required for spermatogenesis: Sertoli and Leydig cells. These two cell types can also be specific targets for some toxins. In addition, the testicular microvasculature may be a specific target, and the functional consequences of impaired blood flow to the testis have already been described.

Developing spermatozoa As the germ cells undergo spermatogenesis, different terms are used to distinguish the different stages of maturation. The earliest stages are the spermatogonia, followed by the spermatocytes, the spermatids and finally the spermatozoa (Figure 3.1). These distinctions not only describe the developmental stage of the germ cells but also correspond to a certain degree of toxicological specificity, as certain stages are attacked by certain compounds. This specificity generally refers to which stages are most sensitive to a particular compound. In most cases, more than one stage can be affected with increasing doses or changing exposure conditions.

One of the workplace events that sparked interest in the effects on male reproductive function was the reported sterility in workers handling the pesticide dibromochloropropane (DBCP). Subsequent investigations suggested a toxic effect that would certainly explain the sterility. The most important cell type damaged by DBCP is probably the spermatogonia. Since these precursor germ cells form the basis for the cellular expansion of spermatogenesis, their destruction precludes future cycles of spermatogenesis. Thus, the expected observation would be a depletion of all the later stages and an inability to recover spermatogenic potential after the toxicant was removed. This fits the observed effects on occupationally exposed humans.

Spermatocytes, especially in the pachytene stages, are susceptible to damage by ethylene glycol monoethyl ether (EGME), one of the glycol ethers with significant exposure potential for humans. A metabolite of EGME, 2-methoxyacetic acid (MAA), can indirectly damage spermatocytes by reducing lactate production in Sertoli cells. Lactate is an important metabolic substrate for developing spermatocytes.

Spermatids can be a particular target for ethylene dibromide (EDB) toxicity. This is another compound used as a fumigant for which there is at least some evidence that occupational exposure may have adverse effects on male reproduction. Effects on the later stages of spermatogenesis, the spermatids, would be consistent with the abnormalities and deficits observed in some occupationally exposed workers. Experimentally, however, EDB proves to be an example where stage specificity breaks down with increasing doses.

Spermatozoa can be damaged by various toxic mechanisms. Epichlorohydrin (a widely used intermediate in plastics/rubbers) is an example of a compound that appears to impair sperm motility by interfering with metabolism. Motility is required for fertilization and the energy required is generated by specialized metabolic pathways within the sperm. Chlorpromazine, a drug used to treat psychosis, appears to have metabolic effects on sperm by making their membranes permeable. Agents such as mercury and lead may have a combined effect on both sperm membrane dynamics and the epididymis. Sperm complete their maturation in the epididymis, and the secretory and absorptive functions of the epididymal epithelium are necessary for the maintenance of viable sperm.

Another important mechanism of toxicity may also be important for mature sperm. Many biochemical reactions lead to the formation of highly reactive radical groups. Cellular phospholipids, which are important for the structure of cell membranes, are particularly sensitive targets for reactions with these radicals. The resulting damage, known as lipid peroxidation, can impair the integrity of cell membranes. Free radicals can be generated during the oxidative metabolism of many different compounds. Some of these that can be toxic to male reproduction are adriamycin, ethylene dibromide and the herbicides paraquat and diquat.

Free radical-induced lipid peroxidation may be important to sperm for two reasons: 1) the detoxification pathways that normally keep free radicals in check are altered in reproductive tissues and appear to be particularly limited in sperm, and 2) sperm contain highly specialized membranes that can be easily damaged. The study of lipid peroxidation in sperm has only recently begun, and currently, the only clear occurrence of such damage in human sperm is found in frozen sperm samples. Freezing appears to destroy one of the key antioxidant defense enzymes, making sperm particularly vulnerable. Further investigation of chemically induced lipid peroxidation may better explain some of the membrane disruption associated with spermatotoxicity.

3.1.4. Sertoli Cells

The Sertoli cells are in direct contact with the germ cells and support them both structurally and functionally (Figure 3.1). Through specialized connections between the Sertoli cells that isolate the germ cells from all other somatic cells outside the testicular canal, the Sertoli cells form a barrier that provides a degree of insulation and protection from chemicals that are distributed through the circulatory system. Thus, when the Sertoli cells are attacked by toxins, not only is their support of germ cell production compromised, but the blood-testis barrier may also be disrupted, exposing the germ cells to greater potential damage.

Because of their close relationship with germ cells, it is not surprising that toxins that specifically affect Sertoli cells also affect germ cell production. One of the characteristics of Sertoli cell damage is that all stages of developing germ cells are affected and the damage is often irreversible. This is since Sertoli cells can only be replaced to a limited extent; they divide relatively little in mature men. Also, part of the function of Sertoli cells is to initiate the sequence of germ cell development. Without Sertoli cells, the remaining progenitor germ cells are unable to start the spermatogenic cycle.

The solvent n-hexane is a proven reproductive toxicant. Its testicular toxicity is related to the disruption of microtubule formation in Sertoli cells by the metabolite 2,5-hexanedione. The susceptibility of Sertoli cells to microtubule toxin is understandable because Sertoli cells form a scaffold that supports multiple layers of germ cells, and this function relies on microtubule assembly. This process involves extensive remodeling of the Sertoli cell architecture as the germ cells are moved through the seminiferous tubule, and such remodeling is highly dependent on microtubule formation.

Some of the phthalate plasticizers also appear to affect Sertoli cells. The toxicity appears to occur in the Sertoli cells, destroying the connections between Sertoli cells and germ cells. Thus, all spermatogenic cells may be impaired in the developmental sequence at the time of intoxication.

Bioactivation of triocresyl phosphate (TOCP) is required before it acts on Sertoli cells. Interestingly, the metabolism takes place in the Leydig cells but does not appear to affect their function. The reactive metabolite subsequently reaches the Sertoli cells, which are damaged so that spermatogenesis is impaired.

Another Sertoli cytotoxin of interest in occupational toxicology is dinitrobenzene (DNB). This compound and structurally related analogs appear to interfere with Sertoli cell function, possibly by participating in a metabolic reaction cycle that deprives the cells of important reducing equivalents, thereby impairing their functional support of spermatogenic cells. As a consequence, all stages of germ cell development may be impaired.

The tight junctions of Sertoli cells can also be impaired by toxic agents, which disrupts the blood-testis barrier. Platinum-based antineoplastic drugs, such as cisplatin, appear to act in this way. However, it is not clear whether this is directly due to exposure through the disrupted barrier or whether the Sertoli cells are unable to properly control germ cell development (Yamashita & Markert, 2021; Bicker, 2022).

3.1.5. Leydig Cells

The Leydig cells are located outside the seminiferous tubules but surround them. Their main function is the production of testosterone, a key to the regulation of spermatogenesis and the development and behavior of male reproduction. There are several toxins that have been shown experimentally to attack Leydig cells. However, it is not clear whether detectable reproductive toxicity in humans is primarily due to the effect on Leydig cells. This is partly because androgen regulation is so complex that it is difficult to determine which observations are primary toxic responses and which are secondary to hormonal dysregulation. In addition, several of the toxicants with specific effects on Leydig cells may also induce responses in other cell types, depending on the dose.

One well-described experimental Leydig cell toxicant that does not appear to have direct effects on other testicular cell types is ethane 1,2-dimethanesulfonate (EDS). This compound interferes with androgen production by Leydig cells and appears to interfere with certain early steps in the synthesis of steroid hormones. The mechanism leading to cell death is not clear, but EDS kills the Leydig cells. The ultimate result of EDS toxicity is, somewhat predictably, impaired spermatogenesis. In addition, Sertoli cells, which are to some extent dependent on Leydig cell secretions, may also be damaged.

Among the toxicants with significant human exposure that primarily affect the testes, diethylhexyl phthalate and its metabolites are the only examples with specific effects on Leydig cells. In addition to their effects on Sertoli cells, phthalates also appear to affect steroid synthesis and Leydig cell function. It is not yet clear what relative contribution the damage to Leydig cells makes to the resulting spermatotoxicity.

3.1.6. Hormonal Regulation and the Hypothalamic-Pituitary-Gonadal Axis

Disorders of male reproductive function can also occur secondary to toxic reactions in the endocrine system. Androgen production in the testes is regulated primarily by luteinizing hormone (LH), a gonadotropin released by the pituitary gland. Gonadotropin secretion is in turn regulated by the gonadotropin-releasing hormone (GnRH), which is secreted by the hypothalamic part of the brain. This hierarchical arrangement, in which the hypothalamus regulates the pituitary gland, which in turn regulates the gonads, is known as the hypothalamic-pituitary-gonadal axis. The hypothalamic-pituitary-gonadal axis is illustrated in Figure 3.2 for both the male and female organism. From a toxicological point of view, this arrangement creates even more sites where toxic reactions can affect reproduction. With this in mind, it is not surprising that some compounds generally thought to affect the central nervous system can also affect Leydig cell function and male reproduction.

The toxic effects of ethanol are far-reaching and complex. Experimental evidence of direct testicular toxicity is inconclusive, but it is clear that alcoholics suffer from reduced testosterone levels and subsequently reduced gonadal function. The ability to stimulate testosterone production appears to be impaired in alcoholics. Experiments have shown that ethanol influences the release of LH. It is clear that alcohol impairs male reproduction by affecting endocrine regulation and ultimately partially affecting testosterone production in Leydig cells, but the relative contributions of direct testicular effects and toxic responses elsewhere in the regulatory axis are not known.

A number of other drugs and industrial compounds also affect male reproduction via endocrine-related mechanisms. These include the antihypertensive drug propanolol, opiates, and tetrahydrocannabinol (THC). The use of such drugs is relevant to occupational toxicology as their effects may confound observations of reproductive impairment associated with direct occupational exposure. Carbon disulfide, the pesticide chlordecone, and phthalates are examples of industrial chemicals that can disrupt the endocrine axis.

In addition to the potential effects on spermatogenesis, there is another aspect of toxicity to the hypothalamic-pituitary-gonadal axis that affects male reproductive function. Both libido, i.e., the behavioral drive, and the physical aspects, such as penile erection and ejaculation, are controlled by the central nervous system. Libido is controlled primarily by androgens and any of the drugs or industrial compounds that can dysregulate the endocrine axis and affect androgen production can affect libido. Alcohol and THC are common examples of compounds that decrease libido. Workers exposed to carbon disulfide and chlordecone also reported a reduced libido. However, it should be borne in mind that neurological and psychological factors play a huge role in libido and the relative importance of chemical-related mechanisms in reducing libido is probably small. If there are demonstrable effects on endocrine balance, it is not surprising that effects on libido are reported. However, if the claimed effect is simply a report of reduced libido, it is unlikely that a clear toxicological basis can be demonstrated.

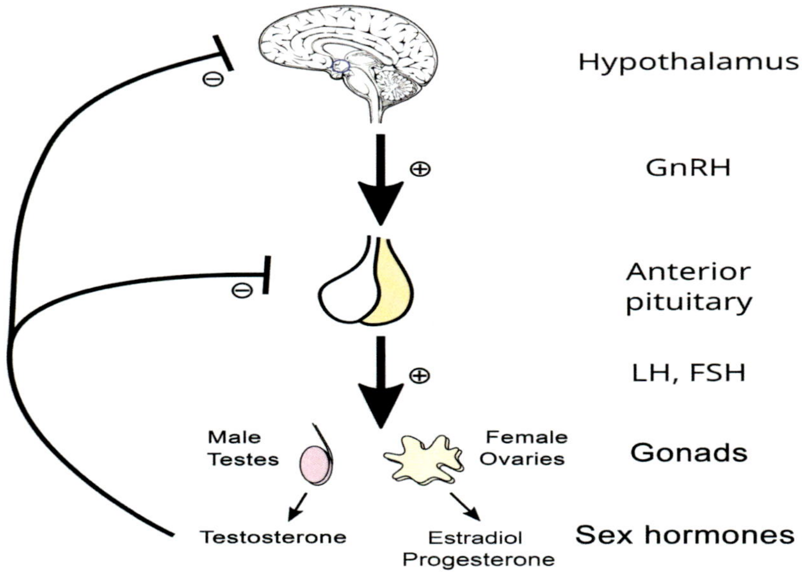

Figure 3.2. *The hypothalamic-pituitary-gonadal axis for human males and females.*

Source: By Artoria2e5 – Own work, CC BY 3.0; https://commons.wikimedia.org/w/index.php?curid=81460023.

Other factors that may prevent sperm release include impotence and the inability to ejaculate. These aspects of reproductive function are centrally controlled, but the autonomic nervous system also plays an important role in coordinating bodily processes. The most common examples of chemically induced impotence are some of the adrenergic antihypertensives, methyl-DOPA, clonidine, and guanethidine, as well as opiates and ethanol. Psychotropic drugs such as chlorpromazine and diazepam can also lead to impotence. As with the effects on libido, psychological factors also contribute significantly to impotence. Clinical findings in humans indicate that the majority of reported impotence problems are psychological and not due to toxic reactions (Yamashita & Markert, 2021; Bicker, 2022).

3.1.7. Endocrine Feedback and Potential Dysregulation

Some of the key signaling molecules that are important for endocrine feedback loops are the steroid hormones and other proteinaceous hormones. Since both the absolute levels and the ratio between androgens and estrogens serve as signals to the hypothalamic-pituitary-gonadal axis, changes in this balance can subsequently disrupt endocrine function and lead to reproductive effects.

A high-profile case of occupational exposure leading to reproductive dysfunction involves the pesticide chlordecone. Occupationally exposed men appeared to have reduced fertility. Subsequent analyses revealed a possible mechanism for these effects, as chlordecone was found to have an estrogenic effect. The endocrine dysregulation caused by increased estrogenic feedback could explain the neurotoxic and reproductive effects attributed to chlordecone.

The role of exogenous compounds with estrogenic, anti-estrogenic, and anti-androgenic effects is currently the subject of considerable controversy. The extremely potent toxin dioxin can disrupt the endocrine balance and the contribution of this activity to its toxicity is controversial. A number of pesticides, including DDT, the carbamates and Mirex, are thought to have endocrine activity, as are some polychlorinated biphenyls (PCBs). It is not yet clear whether exposure to such compounds in the environment can actually cause endocrine-mediated toxic effects. Most synthetic steroid-like molecules can only displace the actual endogenous compounds in molecular interactions to a very limited extent. In addition, the typical exposure levels of exogenous compounds are extremely low, and metabolic deactivation before they reach the target tissue further limits potential activity. On the other hand, the endocrine system functions with very low effective concentrations of signaling molecules at the target cells. The significance of endocrine-mediated toxicity in the male reproductive system is not yet clear, but it is a topic of great interest with potentially far-reaching implications for the future.

3.1.8. Male Reproduction Summary

There are many industrial and pharmaceutical compounds that are potentially toxic to reproduction in men (Table 3.1). Such chemicals can directly or indirectly affect germ cell development by interfering with the cellular and endocrine factors involved in supporting and regulating spermatogenesis. The regulatory functions of the neuroendocrine system are also important for sperm delivery. However, the potential of various compounds to act via a specific toxic mechanism does not necessarily mean that there is a relevant risk to human reproduction associated with that mechanism or even with the compound itself. Mechanistic possibilities and experimental results must be carefully evaluated with respect to those effects that are actually observed in exposed humans.

Table 3.1. *Suspected Human Male Reproductive Toxicants*

Industrial/ Environmental	Pharmaceutical Agents and Drugs
Cadmium	Adriamycin
Carbon disulfide	Busulfan
Chlordecone	Chlorambucil
Dibromochloropropane (DBCP)	Chlorpromazine
DDT	Clonidine
Diethylhexyl phthalate	Cyclophosphamide
Dinitrobenzene	Diazepam
Epichlorohydrin	Ethanol
Ethylene dibromide	Guanethidine
Ethylene oxide	Methotrexate
n-Hexane	Methyl DOPA
2-Hexanedione	Opiates
Ionizing radiation	Propanolol
Lead	Tetrahydrocannabinol
Mercury	Vincristine
2-Methoxyethanol	Vinblastine
Tri-o-cresylphosphate	–

Source: (Wu, 2022)

There have been relatively few instances of occupational exposure leading to demonstrable decreases in male fertility.

The susceptibility of cell types to toxic damage can be broadly generalized, with germ cells being the most sensitive, followed by Sertoli and then Leydig cells. This is due to the hierarchical regulation of spermatogenesis, as germ cell development is often impaired by toxins acting on the Sertoli and Leydig cells. Sertoli cells, in turn, are often affected by both Sertoli and Leydig cell-specific toxins. Furthermore, there does not have to be a specific site in the testis to be affected by a reproductive toxicant. Reproductive function is susceptible to agents that affect the central nervous system and autonomic nervous function because neuroendocrine regulation is so important.

3.2. Female Reproductive Toxicology

Female reproductive toxicology includes only toxic reactions in mature females that do not directly affect the fertilized egg or subsequent development. All post-fertilization toxicity related to the developing offspring is considered developmental toxicology. With this limitation, the female reproductive function can be described with the same characteristics described for the male — the main characteristics being the production of female gametes, eggs, and the transport of the gametes, in this case sperm and eggs, to the site of fertilization.

With regard to occupational and environmental human exposure, much less is known about female-specific toxicology than about male or developmental toxicology. One of the reasons for this is that reproductive impairment in females is difficult to detect and analyze. Unless a persistent inability to maintain a pregnancy is observed, there is often little reason to investigate whether toxic reactions may have impaired female reproductive function. While this may also be true for occupationally exposed men, there are rapid and quite sensitive means of testing male reproductive function. Semen samples can be easily obtained and analyzed, and although such analysis cannot definitively determine fertility, abnormalities are obviously a sign of a potential problem. On the other hand, germ cell production by women is very difficult to monitor and potential indicators, such as failure to menstruate or irregular menstruation, occur frequently enough and for such a variety of reasons that associating these occurrences with a particular exposure is difficult. In addition, pregnancy losses are also common, which may be due to problems with the woman or the developing embryo.

There are also some fundamental differences in female germ cell production that are related to the possible mechanisms of toxic damage. In contrast to the constant cell division required to produce millions of new sperm each day, the ovary at the time of birth contains all the eggs that will ever be ovulated and then some. All mitotic divisions and the initial stages of meiosis are completed by the middle of fetal development, leading to the formation of approximately 10 million primary oocytes arrested in meiotic progression. This is followed by a rapid degeneration process (atresia), leaving around 1 million primary oocytes at birth. Atresia continues somewhat more slowly over the course of a woman's life, and the mature woman has around half a million oocytes that have the potential to develop into mature oocytes.

In humans, a handful of primary oocytes begin the process of folliculogenesis in each menstrual cycle, but usually, only one of them forms a fully mature follicle and is brought to ovulation. Estimating the number of menstrual cycles in a typical reproductive life, only about 500 germ cells will ever complete their development. There is no further division of germ cells before they leave the ovary, and while there are somatic cells that divide and develop to support the maturing egg, this occurs for about two weeks. It is clear that female germ cell production is not based on mass production and rapidly dividing cell populations. Accordingly, the overall process is less susceptible to cytotoxic substances that act against dividing cells.

3.2.1. Oocyte Toxicity

However, some of the strong antineoplastic drugs such as cyclophosphamide, chlorambucil, busulfan, and vinblastine are still able to interfere with oocyte development. Experimental results suggest that busulfan may be able to destroy the arrested primordial oocytes and thus prevent further maturation and ovulation. Other alkylating agents appear to act only on the follicles that are developing at the time of exposure. This is beneficial for the reproductive process as a whole, as more primordial oocytes are available for future cycles of folliculogenesis.

Although there is experimental evidence that ovarian-derived metabolites of some polycyclic aromatic hydrocarbons (PAHs – combustion by-products) are also capable of destroying primordial oocytes, there is little information on ovotoxicity associated with occupational or environmental exposures. There are no good examples of reproductive toxicants in humans that appear to affect egg production in such circumstances. This is certainly due in part to the difficulties in analyzing ovarian toxicity, which have slowed the identification of toxicants that may affect the ovaries.

3.2.2. Somatic Ovarian and Reproductive Tract Toxicity

There are some experimental examples of toxic compounds that may have a direct effect on somatic ovarian cells or the reproductive tract. In the ovaries, this toxicity relates to successful germ cell production as ovarian cells differentiate into layers known as granulosa and theca, both of which are essential for the development of mature follicles. 4-Vinylcyclohexene, an industrial compound used in the manufacture of epoxy resins, appears to be capable of inducing generalized ovarian atrophy. A similar atrophy can be induced by the antibiotic nitrofurantoin, which also has a certain specific toxicity towards the cells lining the follicles. In particular, the granulosa layer can be attacked by metabolites of some phthalates. It is not clear how this toxicity is related to other effects of these compounds.

The female reproductive tract is responsible for the transport of eggs and sperm to the site of fertilization and the subsequent transport of the fertilized embryo to the site of implantation in the uterus. Fertilization takes place in the uterus, which is also known as the fallopian tube or oviduct (Figure 3.3).

The early stages of embryonic development occur in the uterine tube, and then the embryo moves down to the uterus to implant. This transportation requires an open lumen in the fallopian tube, and movement is achieved by a combination of ciliary beat and muscle movement. In other words, the tract is more than just a transport tube, and adequate biological function is required to support the early embryo in particular.

Atrophy of the fallopian tube or the uterus can clearly prevent the transportation of the germ cells and the embryo. Cadmium can cause such atrophy, and presumably, so can other metals that cause general tissue degeneration. In the case of cadmium, the response is a general metabolic inhibition of cells in the reproductive tract, leading to cell death and decreased organ weight. Not surprisingly, the cyclicity of both the uterus and the ovaries is impaired. Lead is another example of a metal that can directly affect the cells lining the uterus, which in turn affects the proper cyclicity of the uterus.

The functions responsible for the movement of germ cells and the early embryo appear to be a potential target for some components of cigarette smoke. Experimental exposures have resulted in both an increase in muscle-induced tubal and uterine motility and immobility of the cilia lining the fallopian tube. The relevance of these observations to human exposure and the observed effects of smoking are not clear. However, the possible consequences – insufficient migration of germ cells preventing fertilization or an early embryo that cannot implant properly – are consistent with the overall decreased fertility and increase in irregular cycles observed in smokers (Yamashita & Markert, 2021; Bicker, 2022).

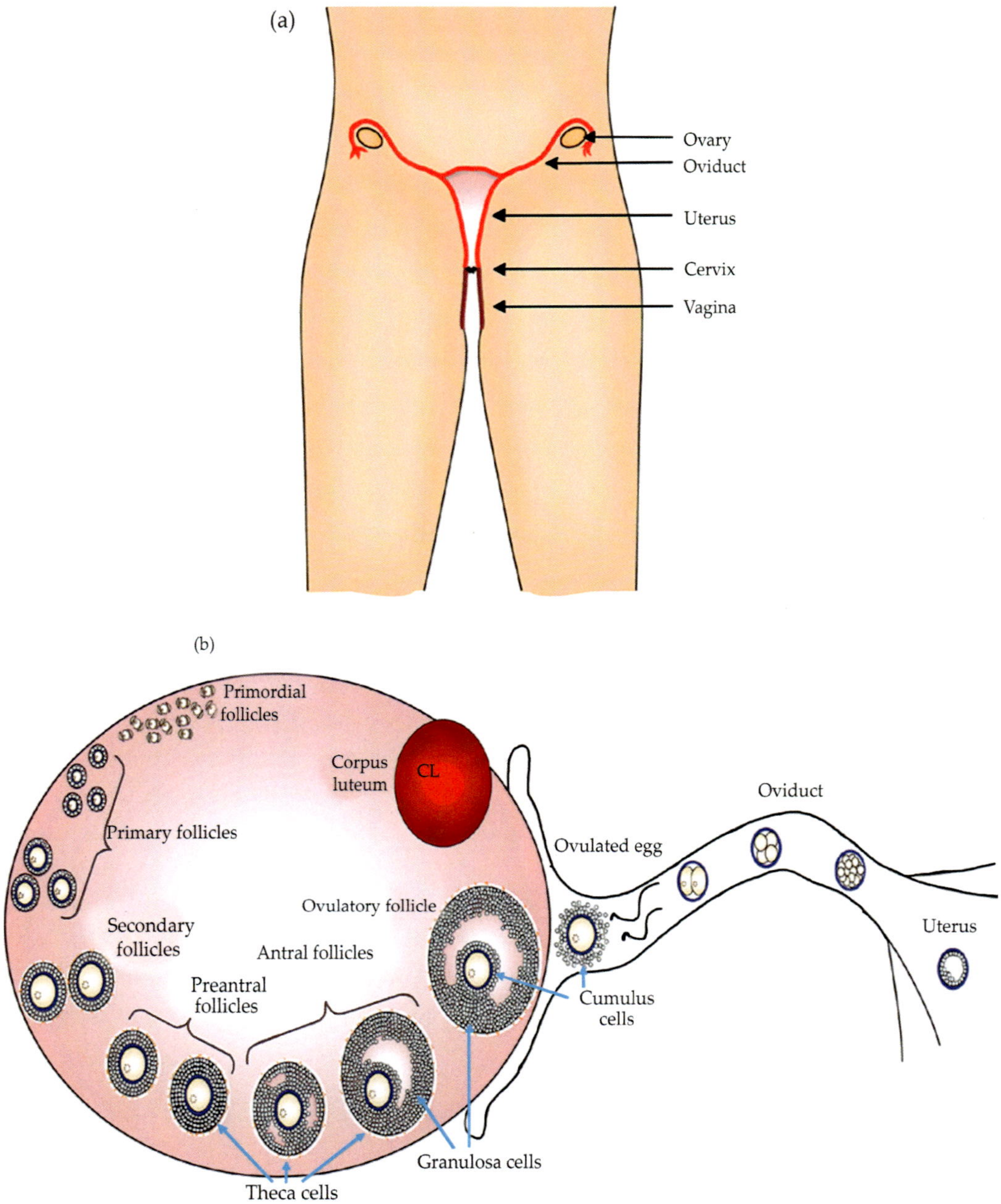

Figure 3.3. *Follicular development cycle and the course of the human female reproductive tract.*

Source: https://static.cambridge.org/.

3.2.3. Hormonal Regulation of Reproductive Function and Associated Toxicity

The endocrine regulation of female reproduction is actually extremely complex. In females, the hypothalamic-pituitary-gonadal axis is present, and the release of GnRH and the temporal changes in the relative levels of the two major gonadotropins, LH and follicle-stimulating hormone (FSH), are linked to the ovarian follicular cycle (Figure 3.2). This is achieved through endocrine feedback loops involving the steroid hormones estrogen and progesterone, as well as some protein hormones.

In simple terms, the female hormonal cycle begins with increased FSH production by the pituitary gland in the early stages of follicular maturation. As the follicles develop, the granulosa cells surrounding the oocyte are an important source of estrogen. As estrogen levels rise, FSH production is decreased and production of the other gonadotropin LH is increased. When the follicle is fully mature, there is a strong release of LH, which triggers ovulation and the subsequent formation of a progesterone-producing tissue, the corpus luteum, at the site of the follicle. The progesterone level rises and supports the development of a pregnancy. Progesterone also causes the levels of both gonadotropins to fall. If pregnancy does not occur, the corpus luteum regresses and the progesterone level falls, which removes the inhibition of gonadotropin secretion. FSH can rise again and the cycle begins anew. In humans, this is the time when menstruation begins, which lasts until the start of the next follicular cycle.

Disorders in the gonads, the pituitary gland or the hypothalamus during the pre-ovulatory phases can lead to a failure of folliculogenesis, so that ovulation does not occur in the affected cycle. Later disorders can lead to failure of corpus luteum maintenance, preventing pregnancy if the egg has been fertilized, or causing a shortened cycle. Alternatively, a disorder of corpus luteum degeneration can lead to a prolonged cycle, which may result in delayed menstruation. It is clear that there are many ways in which endocrine-disrupting toxins can affect both the follicular cycle and the ability to maintain a pregnancy.

There are examples of toxins that can interfere with female hormone regulation. Lead toxicity, for example, has been linked to decreased progesterone production. This may partly explain its historical use as an abortifacient, as progesterone is the most important hormone for the establishment and maintenance of pregnancy. The actual mechanism of lead-induced progesterone inhibition is not clear. However, it can be assumed that the proven effects of lead on the neuroendocrine system impair the hypothalamic or pituitary secretory patterns required for the luteal phase of the cycle.

Both cigarette smoking, probably nicotine, and alcohol can impair GnRH release. Alcoholics have been observed to be unable to produce the LH surge required for ovulation, and tobacco use is associated with reduced estrogen levels. These observations are consistent with the cycle irregularities that have been associated with alcohol and tobacco use. The decreased libido and lack of cyclicity associated with the abuse of narcotics may be related to the hypothalamic depression that these substances cause. It is clear that drug abuse and smoking have wide-ranging physiological effects, and that their toxicity is not specifically associated with female reproductive function. However, the endocrine effects of such substances clearly represent a mechanism by which the associated reproductive impairments could be explained.

Clomiphene citrate is an example of a compound that is used therapeutically to the female endocrine balance. This anti-estrogen is used to stimulate ovulation in infertile women. It appears to increase the release of gonadotropin so that more follicles can develop. The anti-oestrogenic properties prevent the estrogen-mediated shutdown of FSH production. However, the anti-oestrogenic effect has other consequences, such as reduced luteal function and a reduced ability of the uterus to induce pregnancy. The mixture of desired and undesired effects is a good example of the complex consequences of endocrine interventions.

Occupational and environmental exposures that could disrupt the female hormone system are an important topic of current research. Dioxins, other polycyclic chlorinated compounds, and organochlorine and organophosphorus pesticides are all compounds of potential concern. As described in the section on male reproductive toxicology, there is concern that many of these compounds have some type of estrogenic or androgenic activity due to their ability to substitute for endogenous compounds in cellular interactions. The theoretical potential of such compounds to impair female reproductive function is obvious. However, demonstrating such an effect is extremely difficult and there are still no convincing examples of endocrine-disrupting compounds causing reproductive impairment in women through typical occupational or environmental exposures.

The endpoints that can generally be observed in women are the menstrual interval, fertility as measured by time to pregnancy, and the ability to carry a pregnancy to term. The latter potential effect is discussed in the Developmental Toxicology section. There are such extreme interpersonal differences in menstrual interval and regularity, and so many proven causes for the absence or delay of menstruation, that it is difficult to link any variation to a particular chemical exposure. Many cultural and occupational factors clearly play a role in influencing the time to pregnancy, and difficulty achieving pregnancy at the desired time can at times affect up to 25% of couples in the United States. It is clear that this is not always due to female reproductive problems, but this "natural" background masks possible toxicologically mediated effects.

The great interest in endocrine disruption as a possible mechanism for female reproductive toxicity is leading to extensive investigations of this hypothesis. In the future, it should become clearer whether estrogens and other endocrine-disrupting compounds in the environment can actually reach levels at which they can cause significant endocrine disruption and thus reproductive impairment. Currently, we have a potential mechanism for reproductive effects and candidates that could act via this mechanism, but no clear evidence that any of the candidates pose an actual risk to humans via such a mechanism following occupational or environmental exposure.

The potential exposure to chemicals that could alter endocrine processes and the need to use pharmacologic agents known to have reproductive toxicity lead to controversial occupational and societal questions about limiting women's exposure to chemicals. What types of data or experimental results should be sufficient to support the need for occupational exposure controls? When considering whether women should be excluded from certain activities during certain periods of their reproductive lives, the need to go beyond the uncertainties of extrapolating doses and mechanisms of toxicity from animal studies suddenly becomes apparent. The issues involved are as varied as the economic impact of potentially requiring workers to change certain jobs or requiring specialized equipment to control exposure, to potential claims of discrimination if women are excluded from opportunities based on concerns they feel are not relevant to them.

Or what is adequate information to the patient about the risks to herself or the developing fetus if she chooses a particular therapy? It is clear that we cannot always reject effective treatments. The recent return of thalidomide, discussed below as the cause of one of the most notorious cases of human developmental toxicity, is a shining example. Thalidomide is proving to be a particularly effective treatment for patients suffering from complications of leprosy or certain complications of AIDS. It can also be an effective sedative for cancer patients and patients with autoimmune diseases. These uses expand the range of patients for whom reproductive effects are a potential problem. Effective patient education and a carefully planned distribution policy may be relatively easy with thalidomide since the timing and dosage of toxic effects are known and the results can be easily documented, but what is the appropriate balance between protection and restriction with other drugs?

3.2.4. Female Reproduction Summary

Compared to men, there are relatively few female-specific reproductive toxicants that are not related to developmental toxicity (Table 3.2). (Developmental toxicants are discussed in the following section) In part, this is due to the difficulties in analyzing oocyte production and determining when there is a reproductive impairment.

Table 3.2. *Suspected Human Female Reproductive Toxicants*

Category	Industrial/Environmental Toxicants	Pharmaceutical Agents and Drugs
Metals	Arsenic	–
–	Cadmium	–
–	Lead	–
	Mercury	–
Organic Compounds	Dioxins	–
–	Diethylhexyl phthalate	–
Polychlorinated biphenyls	PCBs—coplanar forms	–
Radiation	Ionizing radiation	–
Pharmaceuticals	–	Androgens, estrogens, and progestins
–	–	Busulfan
–	–	Chlorambucil
–	–	Cyclophosphamide
–	–	Ethanol
–	–	Opiates
–	–	Vinblastine

Source: (Chelimsky, 2000)

The relatively small proliferative cell population in the ovary and the intermittent nature of the proliferative phase also make the ovary less susceptible to cell division disorders. The compartmentalization of the active germ cell and its supporting follicle is also important for ovarian toxicology, as it means that only a few germ cells are susceptible during a given cycle. This reduces the likelihood that toxic damage will lead to permanent impairment of oogenesis. Although there are occasional toxins, such as busulfan, that can wipe out the arrested population of primordial oocytes and prevent future follicular development, in general, the arrested cells are quite resistant to damage.

Probably the most significant type of toxins for female reproductive function are those that disrupt the dynamic endocrine balance required for follicle formation and ovulation. A wide range of toxins have at least the potential to disrupt female hormonal patterns, including heavy metals, drugs of abuse and some chlorinated biphenyls. Chemicals that may structurally mimic steroid hormones or have competing functional activity are found among a variety of therapeutic drugs, pesticides, and environmental pollutants. Although a mechanism for impairment of female reproductive function is suspected, the effects of endocrine disrupting chemicals, particularly through environmental exposure, on human reproduction are not yet clear.

3.3. Developmental Toxicology

The realization that environmental factors can cause congenital defects grew after the 1941 report by Gregg, who found a link between exposure to rubella virus (German measles) during pregnancy and the occurrence of blindness and deafness in the offspring. Further analysis following the rubella epidemic and the thalidomide case made people more aware of the potential of prenatal exposure to cause developmental disorders. The fact that this realization came so late, even in the scientific community, was partly due to the belief that the placenta served as a barrier to prevent potentially harmful substances from reaching the fetus. Since the 1960s, it has become clear that the placenta is quite permeable to chemicals with a molecular size that includes all but the largest drugs and industrial compounds. Developmental toxicity testing has become commonplace, and many chemical and biological agents and physical phenomena that can affect development have been identified.

As we have seen in the field of male and female reproductive toxicology, the experimental evidence of toxic potential is far more numerous than the proven cases of developmental toxicity in humans. This may be due in part to species differences and the high doses used in experimental protocols; however, in the case of developmental disorders, it is also not always clear whether the experimentally demonstrated differences in structure or behavior can be extrapolated to humans and considered abnormal. Overall, the class of chemicals with proven effects on humans is less significant in the population than biologically infectious agents such as rubella, syphilis, and cytomegalovirus and maternal metabolic disorders, such as diabetes and phenylketonuria. Genetically determined developmental disorders, in turn, continue to surpass all environmental phenomena that can impair development in terms of proportional importance within the population.

This section deals with toxicology relevant to all stages of development from fertilization onwards. This includes the effect of toxicants on the mother, affecting the ability to establish and maintain a pregnancy, as well as the direct effect on the fetus. The developmental stages can be divided into 1) the preimplantation stage, where toxicity generally affects the entire organism and there is typically an all-or-nothing response (i.e., repair occurs or the developing organism is aborted), and 2) the later embryonic and fetal stages, where specific structural defects may occur. The most sensitive period for teratogenesis, i.e., the development of congenital defects, is organogenesis at the embryonic stage.

Mammalian development can be visualized as a comprehensive flow chart (Figure 3.5). After fertilization, there is a very specific sequence of events that is controlled by the expression of specific genes at specific times. From a toxicological point of view, disturbances in this relatively linear phase usually derail the entire developmental sequence. Certain developmental steps serve as branching points, and once certain branches are followed, the occurrence of events on that branch does not necessarily affect other branches. As development progresses, many smaller branches are reached, each of which may relate to the development of specific tissues, cell types or regions of a structure. When specific sequences are affected, the response may be limited to the features that develop from that particular sequence. This illustrates the extent to which specific defects can occur in response to toxins or other environmental factors and have a clear time dependence.

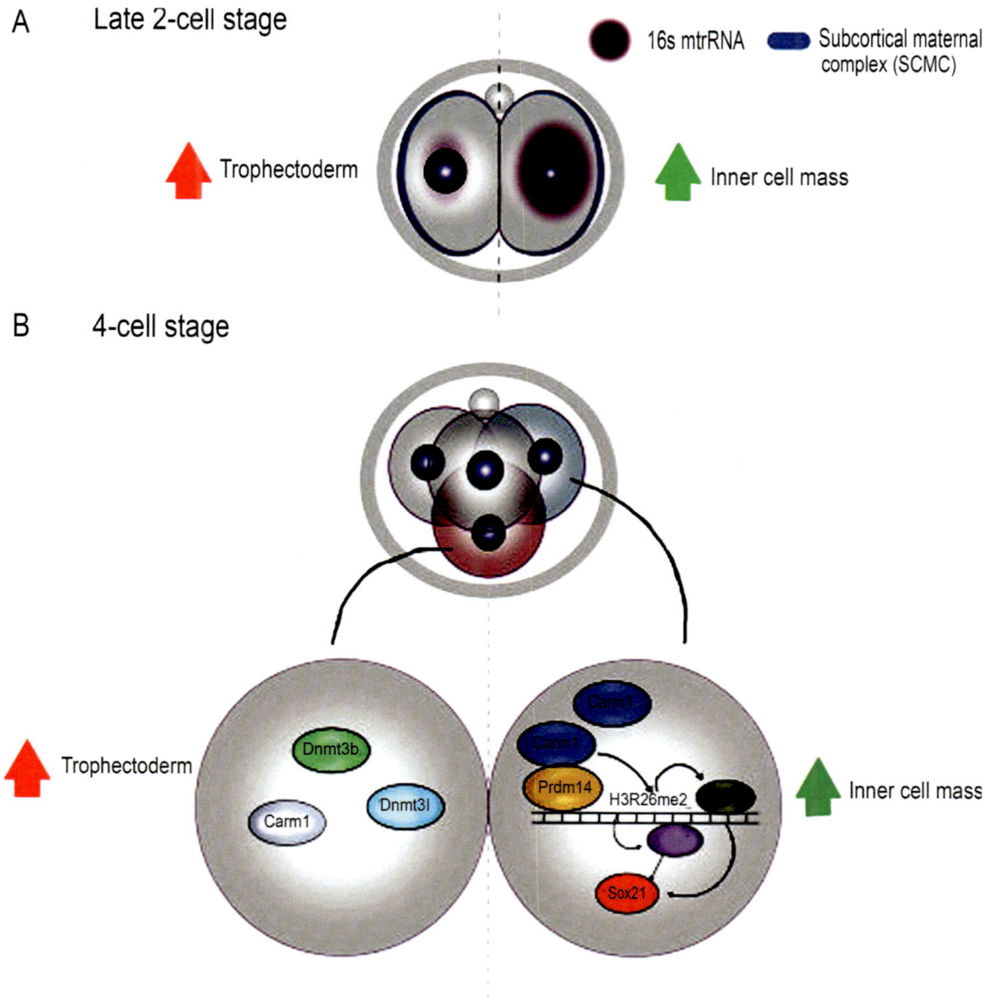

Figure 3.4. *Mammalian development stages.*

Source: https://ars.els-cdn.com/.

3.3.1. Spontaneous Abortion and Embryonic Loss

Recent improvements in the measurement of human chorionic gonadotropin, a very early indicator of the presence of an embryo, have allowed reasonable estimates of early pregnancy loss. Overall, more than 50% of fertilized eggs/embryos are lost through spontaneous abortion. About 30% are lost after implantation but before the first menstrual period. A further 20 to 25% are lost after they have been clinically recognized as a pregnancy. There are probably also considerable losses before implantation, but these are much more difficult to estimate accurately. In other words, the chance of achieving pregnancy in a menstrual cycle in which fertilization is likely to have occurred (based on non-contraceptive intercourse with ovulation) is around 25.

The majority of embryo losses occur in the so-called linear development phase. On the basis of chromosome analyses of spontaneously aborted embryos, around two-thirds of this loss can be explained by gross genetic abnormalities. About 10% can be attributed to a known environmental cause, and for the remainder, no cause can be determined. While some of the genetic loss could be due to environmental DNA damage, it is clear that the majority is due to major chromosomal aberrations associated with germ cell production and fusion. Again, the potentially chemically induced responses are hidden in an extremely high background rate of embryo loss.

In general, the response to toxicological impairment at the early embryonic stage is considered an all-or-nothing event, where damage up to minor cell death is fully reparable, whereas major cellular disruption or death leads to termination of the pregnancy. This is due to the flexibility of cells in the early embryo, which allows them to functionally replace some lost cells. As development progresses, most cell lineages become committed to a specific fate, making such compensation less likely.

The limited response options during early embryogenesis mean that the endpoint for toxic exposures is usually a spontaneous miscarriage. While this criterion has held true for most toxicants over the years, there are recent experimental results suggesting that very early exposure to ethylene oxide and some other mutagens can induce responses that do not occur until much later in development. This implies that the exposure may result in a sublethal injury that is not repaired, nor are all of the affected cells replaced. It is not clear how many toxins could cause developmental defects in this way, as they should probably be able to induce specific, minor changes in DNA, nor is it clear whether the experimental conditions are relevant to humans.

Spontaneous abortions remain the most useful indicator of early embryonic toxicity, and there are both experimental and occupational examples that chemical exposures appear to affect spontaneous abortion rates. One of the best-studied and most controversial occupational examples involves anesthetic gasses. Large and small studies have reported both positive and negative results when it comes to increased rates of spontaneous abortions in healthcare professionals using anesthetic gasses such as nitrous oxide and halothane. The potential effect does not appear to be related to paternal exposure, as no increase in spontaneous abortion rates is observed in the wives of occupationally exposed men. Methodological flaws have called some of the positive results into question. At this stage, the most reasonable conclusion is that there is an increased incidence of spontaneous abortion in women in such occupations based on the available data; however, the association between anesthesia exposure and spontaneous abortion rates cannot be reliably established. This suggests that other unidentified factors may play an important role in the study populations. Carbon disulfide, dimethylformamide, and some phthalates are other examples where studies of spontaneous abort rates have found differences that may be due to occupational exposures of women. The data for carbon disulfide are the most convincing in documenting an association, but even this conclusion is weakened by the fact that the proportional increases are small and not clearly outside the expected background range.

Chloroprene, an industrial chemical used in the manufacture of polymers, is an example of how male exposure can have an impact on spontaneous abortion. In this case, the wives of occupationally exposed men showed increased spontaneous abortion rates.

This could be classified as an effect on male reproduction if it is due to an effect on sperm that necessarily occurs prior to fertilization and suggests that some types of sperm damage may still be compatible with the ability to fertilize an egg. While such a mechanism of toxicity could explain the observations, it is not recognized as a common type of toxic effect, so it is difficult to rule out another explanation that is not directly related to male exposure to chloroprene.

There are many compounds that have been experimentally shown to induce spontaneous abortion. Some of these substances, such as antineoplastic drugs and heavy metals could be expected due to their general toxic effects. Their cytotoxicity is well known, so the impairment of the embryo is hardly surprising. In addition, solvents such as benzene and toluene, many chlorinated pesticides and herbicides, PAHs, and aldehydes such as formaldehyde can experimentally prevent early pregnancy. In short, most cytotoxic chemicals are capable of interfering with early development under experimental conditions. The relevance to human exposure conditions and potential doses, especially in occupational settings, is not clear.

A common occupational chemical exposure that illustrates the difficulties in detecting embryotoxicity in humans is the use of ethylene oxide. This chemical is used in large quantities in manufacturing, particularly in the production of ethylene glycol antifreeze.

Female workers are clearly potentially exposed industrially. In terms of the number of workers exposed, the use of ethylene oxide as a sterilizing agent for medical devices is even more significant.

Exposure to ethylene oxide during unloading of sterilizers and in the area where the sterilized packages are ventilated can be high enough to cause toxic reactions in other organ systems. This was particularly true before interest in the possible long-term effects increased in the 1980s. In addition, ethylene oxide clearly causes embryotoxicity and death in animal studies, as well as structural abnormalities during the fetal stages. These factors suggest that ethylene oxide may pose a problem for development in occupational exposure.

Epidemiologic studies of workers exposed to ethylene oxide are inconclusive. Although increased spontaneous abort rates have occasionally been reported in potentially exposed workers, this finding has not been consistently observed. In addition, the largest studies, which are best designed to account for exposure levels and potential bias, have routinely been negative.

So, the database stacks up as follows: 1) the toxic potential from animal tests is clear, 2) the potential for human exposure is clear, 3) suggestive associations have been reported in relatively few worker studies that have been criticized for inability to clearly establish exposure levels and for sensitivity to possible biases, and 4) no association is supported by the biggest and best-controlled studies.

3.3.2. Toxic Responses of the Embryo and Fetus

For many people, the possibility of congenital defects is the most alarming aspect of reproductive toxicology. Congenital defects are any morphological, biochemical or functional abnormalities that are due to an event before birth. The defect may not be discovered until later, as in some learning disabilities, but the biological basis for the defect arises during uterine development. Most congenital defects are not due to chemical exposure, but it is clear that some defects are caused by drugs and environmental exposures.

The rate of major congenital structural malformations is about 2% to 3% of live births. If other, more subtle congenital defects are added, the rate reaches about 7% of live births. About 15 of these defects are associated with a hereditary disorder at a known gene locus, such as Tay-Sachs disease or hemophilia. A further 10% are associated with major chromosomal abnormalities such as monosomies or trisomies. Overall, genetic factors can be responsible for up to 35 of congenital defects. Recognizable external factors (physical, biological, and chemical) are responsible for about 10 of congenital defects. It is estimated that additional, uncharacterized chemical and drug-induced defects account for between 1% and 5%. This leaves a large proportion of defects for which there is no clear cause.

Teratogens are chemical or other substances that can cause congenital defects. It is generally assumed that they cause specific defects during organogenesis, which in humans begins around five weeks after fertilization and lasts for almost the entire second trimester of pregnancy in various organs. For many teratogens with specific structural targets, the fetus shows a sensitivity period that corresponds to the development of the target structure. This is important for humans as it means that exposure generally has to occur in a specific time window during pregnancy to cause a defect.

3.3.3. Disruptions of Tissue Organization

The prototypical example of a teratogen with a narrow window of toxic potential is thalidomide. This drug was used in the late 1950s and 1960s to treat morning sickness and as a sedative. A sudden increase in children with limb malformations was noted in mothers who had taken thalidomide. The critical window of sensitivity was determined based on the severity of the malformations and the length of time the mother had been taking the drug. A relatively narrow window was identified at 6 to 7 weeks gestation, during which exposure to thalidomide resulted in malformations in almost all infants. Exposures after this time were associated with fewer and less common defects. In addition to the conspicuous limb malformations, thalidomide-exposed infants also exhibited congenital heart and kidney defects and ear malformations.

Despite extensive animal experiments following the thalidomide incident, the mechanism of action is still not clearly understood. The probable reactive metabolites have been identified and mechanisms of action such as disruption of vitamin or amino acid metabolism in the developing limb bud and direct disruption of DNA in this region have been proposed. Unfortunately, it seems ironic that while so many chemicals have a clear potential mechanism of action but no clearly observable effects in humans, perhaps the best example of an actual human teratogen has defied studies that could identify the mechanisms that actually disrupt human development.

Since thalidomide can no longer be used by pregnant women, the most significant teratogenic drug is isotretinoin or Accutane, a highly effective cystic acne drug. This drug is particularly important in terms of teratogenicity precisely because it is so effective and there is no suitable substitute. Therefore, it continues to be used despite its ability to cause severe fetal malformations. Despite aggressive warnings by physicians and many exclusionary policies that attempt to prevent patients at risk for becoming pregnant from taking the drug, developmental deformities related to isotretinoin exposure continue to be reported.

The defects associated with isotretinoin are wide-ranging and include craniofacial deformities, including cleft palate, and abnormalities of the heart and central nervous system. This can be understood on the basis of the role of retinoids in normal development. Isotretinoin is a synthetic retinoid, a chemical relative of vitamin A. The distribution of certain retinoids in tissues appears to play an important role in the organization and direction of tissue growth. For example, the direction of cell growth required for the elongation of a limb is controlled by retinoid signaling. Disruption of this roadmap by exogenous retinoids could clearly be a basis for maldevelopment. Exogenous exposure to most retinoids can, at least experimentally, lead to developmental defects. Isotretinoin is a good example of a teratogen that acts by disrupting the chemical signals that control development.

3.3.4. Fetal Hydantoin Syndrome

Another class of teratogenic drugs is still taken by pregnant women because the developmental risks are less than the risks associated with removing the drug. Diphenylhydantoin–phenytoin, valproic acid and other anticonvulsants are used in epileptics to prevent seizures. They are also teratogenic. In these cases, however, the treatment regimens are not associated with a significant number of congenital defects, and the risk of harm to the fetus and mother in the event of a seizure is more of a concern. A number of characteristic developmental features associated with anticonvulsant treatment have been classified as fetal hydantoin syndrome. There are craniofacial features, limb changes and growth and learning deficits. While the structural effects may be mild, the growth and learning delays are usually permanent. However, the syndrome is not particularly common and many studies conclude that the risk is low, especially when the potential for epileptic seizures is taken into account. In experimental protocols, phenytoin leads to more severe, specific craniofacial defects, including cleft palate, when administered in the time window associated with palatogenesis. Subsequent administrations have effects on the limbs.

Valproic acid is also clearly teratogenic in experimental protocols. The primary effects appear to be on the central nervous system, but skeletal and cranial defects may also occur. There are reports of neural tube defects and spina bifida in humans exposed to valproic acid through maternal treatment, and the incidence appears to be higher than expected in some studies. However, most of these studies have examined selected cases and it is not clear what the true incidence rate of valproic acid-related defects in humans is. Again, the situation is complicated by concomitant epilepsy.

3.3.5. DES: A Teratogen Associated with Cancer Endpoints

Another type of teratogen is exemplified by another human tragedy. Diethylstilbestrol (DES) is a synthetic steroid hormone that was used to prevent miscarriages in women who had difficulty maintaining a pregnancy. In this case, it took not just half a decade for the effects of thalidomide to become apparent, but about a quarter of a century between the mid-1940s and 1970 before the teratogenicity of DES became clear. A number of women whose mothers had taken DES during the first trimester of pregnancy were found to have an extremely rare form of cancer of the reproductive tract, clear cell adenocarcinoma. Although the risk of cancer was first detected in some girls in their early teens, it peaked between the ages of 19 and 22. This explains the delay in detecting the effects of DES and illustrates an example where the congenital defect was not immediately obvious. DES is also an interesting example of a teratogen that causes cancer as a congenital defect. It is currently the only proven carcinogen in humans that has a transplacental effect.

In addition to the cancer risk associated with DES, a number of other reproductive abnormalities were observed as the exposed children grew up. In female children, there was an increased risk of ectopic pregnancy, spontaneous miscarriage, menstrual disorders and infertility. In male children, abnormalities of the genitals, reduced sperm production, cryptorchidism, and a possible increase in testicular cancer were observed. All of these reproductive tract defects indicate the likely effects of DES on developing children. The development of the internal and external genitalia is coordinated by the production of steroid hormones, primarily by the fetal gonads. The hyperestrogen environment produced by DES is consistent with improper formation of the male internal and external genitalia and may have disrupted the development of the steroid feedback loops in the hypothalamic-pituitary-gonadal axis of the females.

3.3.6. Additional Human Teratogens

Other drugs that have been shown to be teratogenic include lithium, tetracyclines, aminopterin, and the coumarin anticoagulants. Antineoplastic agents such as busulfan and cyclophosphamide are teratogenic in addition to their numerous other reproductive toxicities. Androgenic hormones used to maintain pregnancies are also teratogenic and impair the reproductive development of the fetus, similar to estrogenic DES. For all of these therapeutic agents, the dose that leads to teratogenicity, the problems that arise if the underlying disease is left untreated, and the actual likelihood of teratogenic effects must be considered when characterizing their toxicological potential.

3.3.7. Drugs of Abuse and Maternal Nutrition

Some of the abused drugs are teratogenic, but their effects are usually related to general metabolic disturbances rather than impairment of specific developmental characteristics. Fetal alcohol syndrome (FAS) is the best example of this class of teratogens. The main features of FAS include growth retardation, psychomotor disturbances and craniofacial anomalies. Growth retardation is the most sensitive and widespread consequence of alcohol consumption during pregnancy. This can be demonstrated at relatively low doses, about 1 drink per day, but the effects of a low dose are controversial. At higher doses, i.e., 5 or more drinks at the same time and at least 2 drinks per day, the risk of a child being classified as too small for gestational age increases threefold. One third of children of chronic alcoholics have been classified as FAS in some studies. Later development is characterized by reduced height and the inability to catch up in postnatal development. In children classified as FAS, the rate of mental retardation is 85%. Impulsivity, attention deficit disorder and language deficits are frequently observed.

The mechanism by which FAS develops has not yet been clarified. In chronic alcoholics in particular, it seems most likely that it is primarily related to the mother's general nutritional status, metabolism, and endocrine imbalance. Nutrient deficiencies and disturbances of metabolism and transport in the placenta are clearly mechanisms that can affect fetal growth and neuronal function. Children of heroin addicts also exhibit growth retardation, which is probably related to the overall maternal nutritional and metabolic status.

Maternal cigarette smoking has also been linked to general developmental deficits. The growth retardation in the fetuses of smokers is clear. However, the large number of chemicals contained in tobacco smoke makes it difficult to determine the decisive pathway. It has been suggested that nicotine, carbon monoxide and cyanide interfere with the transport of amino acids across the placenta. In addition, cadmium is capable of causing placental necrosis and could impair placental exchange. Furthermore, PAHs induce metabolic enzymes in the placenta that can produce toxic reactive metabolites. It is unclear which of these mechanisms actually operate in humans and which are the main cause of growth retardation.

Maternal deficiencies of certain nutrient factors have been reported to be associated with teratogenicity. Zinc, folic acid and retinoic acid deficiencies have negative effects on development. It is clear that these nutrients are all needed by the fetus, just like any other human, but the degree of deficiency that must be reached to cause developmental problems is not clear. A severe deficiency of any of the vitamins, minerals or amino acids can be expected to impair development. A deficiency of zinc, folic acid and retinoic acid may not be very well tolerated, as the growth processes in development are heavily dependent on them. Zinc and folic acid are consumed to a high degree in the metabolism of rapidly growing tissue. The role of retinoic acid as an important signaling molecule during fetal growth has already been described.

3.3.8. Methylmercury Poisoning

In the 1950s, Minamata disease was described and linked to the pollution of Minamata Bay in Japan by industrial plants. Fish from these coastal waters, which are an important food source for women in the region, were found to have elevated levels of methylmercury. Mercury levels realized by the women were not high enough to produce obvious signs of mercury toxicity. However, the accumulation of methylmercury was sufficient to cause CNS abnormalities in developing fetuses, with cerebral palsy being the most common problem. It was later found that mercury levels increased in the placenta and fetal membranes of pregnant women exposed to metallic mercury at work. However, this exposure was apparently not sufficient to cause developmental toxicity, as the spontaneous abortion rate did not increase and no defects were found in the offspring.

3.3.9. Developmental Toxicity Summary

Developmental toxicity can be divided into two categories. In early pregnancy, the predominant effect of chemical and other exposures is spontaneous abortion. Later, when the specific differentiation of the various organs and structures takes place, some toxins react with congenital structural or functional disorders. Determining whether a spontaneous abortion was caused by a specific chemical exposure is extremely difficult, especially because the background rate is so high and there are so many non-toxicologic causes. Detecting a difference in spontaneous abortion rates within a population is difficult for similar reasons.

Most congenital defects are due to inherited or developmental genetic factors rather than teratogenic chemicals. Although in many cases there is a desire to determine whether a defect is due to external factors, it is often impossible to clearly identify the relevant factors and isolate the ultimate cause. From a population perspective, it is difficult to find a relevant, common factor that can be blamed for a particular set of defects, and even more difficult to determine the causal role of such a factor. It should be borne in mind that the best examples of chemically induced teratogenesis involve therapeutic doses of chemicals administered with the knowledge and documentation of a health professional.

Table 3.3. *Suspected Human Developmental Toxicants and Teratogens*

Category	Industrial/ Environmental	Pharmaceutical Agents and Drugs
Anesthetic gases	Halothane	–
Organic solvents and compounds	Benzene	Aminopterin
–	Cadmium	Busulfan
–	Carbon disulfide	Coumarin anticoagulants
–	Chloroprene	Cyclophosphamide
–	Chlorobiphenyls	Diethylstilbestrol (DES)
–	Dimethylformamide	Ethanol
–	Diethylhexyl phthalate	Isotretinoin and other retinoids
–	Dioxins	Lithium
–	Ethylene oxide	Phenytoin
–	Lead	Opiates
–	Methylmercury	Tetracyclines
–	Toluene	Thalidomide
–		Valproic acid
Miscellaneous nonchemical agents	–	–
–	Cytomegalovirus	Rubella
–	Diabetes	Syphilis
–	Ionizing radiation	Toxoplasmosis
–	Phenylketonuria	–

Source: (Council et al., 2000)

Experimental results have clearly demonstrated mechanisms by which both early and later development can be influenced by exogenous chemicals. This information is useful in prioritizing investigations of potential human health effects and judging whether reported effects could reasonably be expected to occur from certain candidate chemicals. However, development is a very finely regulated process that depends on small pools of cells that serve as the starting point for various structures, and it is not surprising that many experimental protocols can interfere with this process. The challenge is to decide which of these experimental sources of developmental effects should be of concern to humans. Table 3.3 summarizes the suspected developmental toxicants (Yamashita & Markert, 2021; Bicker, 2022).

3.4. Current Research Concerns

This section describes some areas of reproductive toxicology that are currently of great interest to researchers. Some of these areas of research are likely to cross over into applied toxicology and become topics that will impact the future regulatory framework in the United States and consequently influence industry and environmental decisions and concerns. The goal is to both highlight exciting areas of research and suggest areas of toxicology that may be of importance to both regulators and industry in the future.

3.4.1. Endocrine Disruption

Since the passage of the Food Quality Protection Act of 1996, a law requiring the EPA to screen pesticides for estrogenic effects in humans, endocrine disruption has become the focus of toxicology research and legislative controversy. The potential for some chemicals to cause adverse effects through interactions with the endocrine system has already been discussed in earlier sections of this chapter for male and female toxicology and developmental toxicology. Although scientific and regulatory attention is recent, ecologists, agricultural scientists and farmers have been aware of the practical effects of endocrine disruptors for many years. A large number of chemicals produced by one organism can affect the hormonal status of other organisms. On an ecological level, this type of chemical signaling between species is critical to the functioning of certain communities. Farmers have long known that grazing sheep or cattle on rich, newly growing clover reduces the number of pregnancies. This effect is due to compounds produced by clover that can mimic estrogens, known as phytoestrogens. Many different classes of chemicals produced by plants or fungi can affect reproduction. One question that is attracting a lot of attention in toxicology and from regulatory authorities is whether exposure to synthetic chemicals at levels relevant to the environment or the workplace can also have hormonal effects. A second question is whether synthetic chemicals with weak hormonal potency could impair endocrine function, given that the human diet already contains large amounts of naturally derived endocrine disruptors. A third critical question is whether it is practicable to regulate chemicals on the basis of suspected mechanisms of action—i.e., on the basis of a potential endocrine mechanism — rather than on the basis of producing adverse effects such as reproductive or developmental disorders.

There is little doubt that exposure of certain wildlife exposures to high concentrations of synthetic chemicalshave produced has reproductive and developmental effects. However, scientists disagree as to which chemicals or environmental factors may be are responsible, and whether the effects are caused by hormonal mechanisms or by other types of toxicity. There Even more controversial is even greater controversy regarding the question of whether adverse effects are also occur in humans and other wildlife at lower exposure levels (the so-called endocrine disruptor hypothesis). Proponents of this hypothesis claim support rely on three main hypotheses: the effects observed in wildlife inhabiting in highly contaminated environments;, the chemical similarities between endogenous hormones, naturally occurring hormonally active agents, endocrine disruptors and certain synthetic chemicals;, and, the fact that the endocrine system is responds to minute very low levels of hormones. Those who consider the hypothesis untenable point to several principles: that synthetic chemicals are much less effective than natural hormones; that the human diet already contains many naturally occurring hormonally active substances that can actually improve health; that there is a tendency for weak hormonal chemical signals to cancel each other out through antagonistic effects; and that the reproductive health of people in industrialized societies has increased rather than decreased in recent decades.

The basis for the assumption that exposure to endocrine disruptors can lead to significant risks is mechanistically sound and clearly works in certain high-dose situations, such as birth control pills and other therapeutic uses of synthetic hormones like DES. However, there are well-understood biological reasons for expecting endocrine response characteristics to differ at dramatically different levels of stimulation (i.e., doses). Since the dose of DES prescribed in the first three months of pregnancy is equivalent to a woman's natural estrogen production for more than 150 years, this example is probably not relevant to the potential risks posed by low levels of weakly estrogenic environmental pollutants. It is important to note that the effect of "environmental estrogens" is typically hundreds to millions of times less than that of estradiol itself. Although there are factors that could reduce these differences in potency, such as binding to serum proteins, these factors are not sufficient to answer the serious questions that arise as to whether synthetic chemicals could affect endocrine signaling in humans at realistic exposure levels.

Other putative developmental effects of endocrine disruptors in humans are due to environmental exposures, some of which occurred at high doses in accidental poisonings. Prenatal and postnatal exposure to PCBs and polychlorinated dibenzofurans (PCDFs) in accidental poisonings with high doses of contaminated rice oil in Yusho, Japan, and Yucheng, Taiwan, has resulted in various developmental disorders. The effect syndrome includes low birth weight, dark pigmentation of the skin and mucous membranes, gingival hyperplasia, exophthalmic ocular edema, edentulism at birth, abnormal calcification of the skull, rocker-bottom heel, and low birth weight. Most of the affected infants were smaller and had a lower total lean mass and soft tissue mass. Follow-up studies of poisoned individuals suggest effects on neurobehavior and cognitive deficits. However, proponents of the endocrine disruptor hypothesis point out that typical body burdens of PCBs and dioxins are relatively close to the levels measured in epidemiologic study groups that have found adverse effects on IQ and neuromuscular development. Nevertheless, these PCB exposures have not been shown to cause any specific adverse effects in the body, and the overall epidemiologic evidence is equivocal and does not support a causal relationship between typical PCB exposures in the body and adverse developmental outcomes.

Another highly publicized suspected consequence of endocrine disruption in humans is reduced sperm counts in men in industrialized countries. Increasing background levels of a number of persistent estrogenic environmental chemicals have been identified as a possible cause. This theory is somewhat mechanistically plausible, as sperm production is controlled by androgen levels and some effects of androgens can be reversed by estrogens. This theory also has some precedent in the form of DES, a potent estrogenic compound that may have reduced sperm counts in men exposed to therapeutic levels in utero. However, several of the studies reporting declining sperm counts have been criticized for methodological flaws, failure to account for alternative factors, and bias in data collection. The statistical tests used and the correct interpretation of the tests have also been questioned. Due to these difficulties and criticisms, many scientists doubt that sperm counts in men from industrialized countries have actually declined.

It is important to recognize that the presumed decrease in sperm count is not the type of readily apparent pathological condition that has been observed in DBCP manufacturers (see above under Toxicology of Male Reproduction). The decrease in sperm count suggested by some authors (up to about 50%) is unlikely to be associated with an overall decrease in fertility due to the large excess of sperm produced by most men.

Numerous methodological difficulties arise when evaluating sperm counts from different laboratories over a long period of time, so the degree of change supposedly related to environmental exposures may be too subtle to be easily measured. Collection and processing methods have changed over the years, and different criteria have been used to categorize typical or "normal" sperm counts. Different studies have handled samples from potentially infertile patients differently, with some studies including them and others excluding them according to different criteria. These differences in methodology have complicated attempts to summarize the results for integrated analysis in a larger database. For these reasons, many scientists are convinced that reported sperm count declines are an artifact of methodological and analytical flaws of the studies. Many synthetic chemicals have been suggested as potential endocrine disruptors due to widespread human exposure and their hormone-like effects in certain laboratory tests. Various lists of suspected endocrine disruptors have been published or otherwise publicized in the media or on the Internet. It is important to note that the quality of the data supporting the inclusion of chemicals on these lists varies widely and that there is currently no universally recognized scientific source that provides an authoritative list. Most lists contain chemicals from different chemical classes, many of which have tested positive in at least one of the various bioassays and receptor binding methods developed to determine a chemical's potential interaction with the endocrine system. Despite positive results in laboratory tests, only a few chemicals - such as the drugs and chemicals discussed earlier in this section — have been shown to cause adverse developmental outcomes in exposed humans. Some prominent examples of chemicals listed as endocrine disruptors are organochlorine pesticides (e.g., toxaphan, methoxychlor, chlordecone, DDT, and metabolites), alkylphenol ethoxylates (detergents or dispersants in household cleaners), PAHs (combustion products), dioxins (TCDD), coplanar PCBs, phthalates, and phenolic plasticizers (e.g., benzyl butyl phthalate, di-n-butyl phthalate, bisphenol A). However, more definitive laboratory studies and risk assessments developed for a number of these chemicals (e.g., alkylphenol ethoxylates, phthalates, and phenolic plasticizers) indicate that there is little or no potential for adverse effects on humans at environmentally relevant exposure levels. In the controversy over endocrine disruption, two particular issues have arisen that deserve special mention. In 1996, just months before Congress passed the Food Quality Protection Act, Arnold and his associates published an article in the journal Science that brought national attention to the issue of endocrine disruption. The report claimed that a combination of synthetic chlorinated pesticides was one thousand times more potent in stimulating an estrogenic response than either chemical alone. This so-called evidence of estrogenic synergism was later shown to be in error, and the publication was retracted more than a year later. Despite the lack of evidence of synergy, this study sparked a debate among the scientific community, authorities, and regulators about the frequency of occurrence of synergistic interactions and their significance for human and environmental health. Although interest in synergistic effects has waned considerably since the Arnold publication was withdrawn, intensive work is still underway to determine whether such chemical interactions are relevant to risk assessment.

The second question at issue concerns the dose-response function for endocrine disruptors. First, is there a threshold for endocrine-mediated adverse effects, and second, do toxic effects of high doses of endocrine disruptors mask more subtle adverse effects that can only be detected at low doses using specialized test systems? These questions arise from two publications suggesting that very low doses of plasticizers may have subtle effects on the developing male reproductive tract that are not seen at higher doses, possibly because subtle effects are masked by more overt toxicity at higher doses. Neither study could be replicated, although attempts were made with more comprehensive study designs. Nonetheless, the issue has led to an outcry from consumer and environmental activist groups who want to ban the use of certain plastics in baby bottles and children's toys. The former Surgeon General of the United States, Dr. C. Everett Koop, has responded by calling this reaction irresponsible.

In summary, a number of critical questions have been raised about the identification of endocrine disruptors in general and laboratory studies purporting to show potential endocrine activity in particular.

- Are positive results in short-term in vivo and in vitro laboratory tests an indication of adverse health effects in humans?
- Can measurements of hormonal potency in laboratory tests at environmentally relevant exposure levels be extrapolated to human populations?
- Given that the human diet contains large amounts of naturally occurring endocrine disruptors, is it conceivable that synthetic chemicals with weak hormonal potency could interfere with human hormonal function?
- Is there no threshold for adverse effects in the dose-response curves of endocrine disruptors?
- Do the toxic effects of high doses of endocrine disruptors conceal more subtle adverse effects that can only be detected at low doses using specialized test systems?
- Are endocrine disruptors more susceptible to interactive effects (synergism or antagonism) than chemicals that act via other mechanisms?
- Does it make sense to regulate chemicals on the basis of suspected mechanisms of action—i.e., on the basis of a potential endocrine mechanism — rather than on the basis of producing adverse

effects such as reproductive or developmental disorders?

The way science and regulators answer these questions could have profound implications for the risk assessment of endocrine disruptors in the workplace and in the environment (Yamashita & Markert, 2021; Bicker, 2022).

3.4.2. Lead Poisoning and the Lowering of the Threshold

A current focus of research is the sensitivity of the developing nervous system to low-dose lead exposure. Lead toxicity is evident in a variety of organ systems. As mentioned above, the effects of lead on male and female reproduction have been studied, and the use of lead salts to induce abortions dates back to ancient times. The neurological system is considered one of the most important targets for toxic reactions to lead. Some recent reports have suggested that lead exposure to large populations, particularly in urban areas, may be sufficient to cause adverse cognitive effects. This has led to extensive research into both the mechanisms of lead toxicity in animals and the occurrence of cognitive deficits in children. Although reports of the effects of low doses of lead in parents and in society have raised eyebrows, the research findings on intelligence and cognitive performance do not show a consistent relationship with current levels of lead exposure in the environment.

Instead of the traditional applied dose, lead exposure is usually considered on the basis of a measured blood level. It is undisputed that lead poisoning can occur in children when chronic blood levels reach 30–50 μg/dl or more. A standard criterion for concern is 10 μg/dl. However, there is evidence that cognitive effects can occur at this threshold, perhaps as low as 10-fold lower. Unfortunately, the endpoints of intelligence and language ability, which have been proposed as the most sensitive indicators, are extremely difficult to measure in a repeatable, reliable, and objective way. A further complication is the considerable plasticity of learning processes and the ability of children to 'catch up' " as they develop.

Scientists argue about the language abilities of two-year-olds and the significance of IQ differences of less than one or two points on the typical scale. Research suggests that language development is a brain function that is particularly vulnerable to lead. Despite the statistical significance claimed in some studies, the uncertainty associated with the assessment of these endpoints, which is not captured statistically, makes it impossible to draw firm conclusions. The test methods used to assess cognitive development and language abilities in infants and young children are generally not considered sensitive enough to reliably distinguish between interindividual variability and exposure-related effects at the required levels.

However, information from animal studies has begun to shed light on the mechanisms by which lead may affect brain development. The brain cells of fetuses and newborns appear to be more sensitive to lead effects compared to those of adults. This could be related to the much more active process of forming connections between nerve cells and the expansion of blood vessels and blood-carrying elements in the fetal and neonatal period. However, it is not clear to what extent this process needs to be altered to represent a negative response to lead, as there is considerable variation and plasticity in this process anyway.

Two important areas for further investigation are: 1) the development of better tools to study human cognitive function and ability, and 2) the characterization of the relationship between the dose-response characteristics of experimental animals and humans for lead. These issues are important for both public health and industry. In general, the scientific and regulatory communities have viewed the marked and dramatic decline in children's blood lead levels since the 1970s as a real public health improvement achieved through the control of lead in gasoline and paint. If neurocognitive development turns out to be as sensitive to the effects of lead as some suspect, far more difficult questions will arise about whether and how to address exposures down to the range associated with naturally occurring lead. Without obvious and easily replaceable major sources of exposure, such as gasoline or paint, the costs associated with additional incremental reductions in lead exposure to the population at large may be dramatic (Yamashita & Markert, 2021; Bicker, 2022).

A Closer Look

Oocyte Toxicity

Oocyte toxicity is the detrimental impact of toxic substances on female germ cells that poses significant threats to reproductive health. Oocytes, or female egg cells, are crucial for reproduction, and their vulnerability to toxic agents can lead to infertility, developmental defects, and transgenerational effects. Understanding oocyte toxicity is imperative for safeguarding reproductive health, especially given the increasing exposure to environmental pollutants, pharmaceuticals, and lifestyle-related toxins.

At the core of oocyte toxicity is the susceptibility of oocytes to various toxicants during different stages of development. Oocytes are formed during fetal development and remain dormant until puberty, when they undergo maturation during each menstrual cycle. This prolonged dormancy period renders them particularly vulnerable to the accumulation of toxic substances. Environmental pollutants like heavy metals, pesticides, and industrial chemicals can permeate ovarian tissue, causing oxidative stress, DNA damage, and disrupted cellular processes. These toxicants can impair oocyte quality and viability, leading to reduced fertility and increased risk of miscarriages and birth defects.

Pharmaceuticals, including chemotherapeutic agents, also contribute significantly to oocyte toxicity. Chemotherapy targets rapidly dividing cells, but it can inadvertently affect oocytes, leading to premature ovarian failure and infertility. The delicate balance of hormonal regulation necessary for oocyte maturation is disrupted, further compromising reproductive potential. Similarly, lifestyle factors such as smoking and excessive alcohol consumption introduce toxins that can adversely affect oocyte health. Nicotine and alcohol metabolites induce oxidative stress and DNA damage in oocytes, reducing their developmental competence and increasing the risk of genetic abnormalities in offspring.

The molecular mechanisms underlying oocyte toxicity involve oxidative stress, mitochondrial dysfunction, and apoptosis. Oxidative stress, a condition characterized by an imbalance between reactive oxygen species (ROS) and antioxidants, plays a pivotal role in oocyte damage. Excessive ROS levels lead to lipid peroxidation, protein oxidation, and DNA damage, compromising oocyte integrity. Mitochondria, the energy powerhouses of cells, are particularly susceptible to oxidative damage, leading to impaired energy production and increased apoptosis. Apoptosis, or programmed cell death, is triggered by severe cellular damage and further depletes the ovarian reserve.

Research into oocyte toxicity has revealed potential protective strategies. Antioxidants, such as vitamins C and E, have shown promise in mitigating oxidative stress and preserving oocyte quality. Dietary interventions rich in antioxidants, coupled with lifestyle modifications to reduce toxin exposure, can enhance reproductive health. Additionally, advancements in assisted reproductive technologies (ART) offer hope for individuals facing oocyte toxicity-induced infertility. Techniques like in vitro maturation (IVM) and oocyte cryopreservation provide alternative pathways to parenthood, circumventing the impact of toxicants on natural conception.

Addressing oocyte toxicity requires a multifaceted approach involving regulatory measures, public awareness, and scientific advancements. Stricter regulations on environmental pollutants and safer pharmaceutical alternatives can minimize exposure risks. Public awareness campaigns can educate individuals about the impact of lifestyle choices on reproductive health, promoting healthier behaviors. Continued research into the molecular mechanisms of oocyte toxicity and the development of novel protective agents are essential for mitigating its impact.

A comprehensive approach involving regulation, education, and scientific innovation is crucial for addressing oocyte toxicity and safeguarding future generations.

Summary

- This chapter examines the complex interactions and toxic responses of the male and female reproductive systems, as well as the developing fetus, to various toxicants. It is particularly insightful in highlighting the differential sensitivity of tissue and cell types within these systems to specific toxicants, underscoring the nuanced nature of toxicological impacts.
- One of the key takeaways is the varied sensitivity of male and female reproductive tissues to different toxicants. This differential sensitivity can significantly affect reproductive health and function, emphasizing the need for a tailored approach when assessing reproductive toxicology. The chapter effectively illustrates how certain toxicants selectively affect specific cell types, which can lead to disparate outcomes in reproductive capabilities and overall health in males and females.
- Moreover, the chapter explores the functional and toxicological implications associated with the distinct patterns of cellular division and germ cell maturation observed in males and females. This aspect is crucial as it underpins the foundational biological processes that govern reproductive function and are susceptible to disruption by toxic substances. The discussion provides a clear explanation of how toxicants can interfere at various stages of germ cell development, potentially leading to long-term reproductive issues.
- An additional focal point is the interaction between the reproductive and endocrine systems, particularly how these systems are interconnected with broader hormonal regulations. The balance of endocrine regulation plays a vital role in maintaining normal reproductive functions, and its disruption by toxicants can lead to significant health repercussions. This section of the chapter illustrates the complex network of hormonal pathways that are vulnerable during toxic exposures and how these disruptions can affect not only reproductive health but also overall physiological well-being.
- The sequential nature of developmental processes and their relationship to toxic responses is another critical topic covered. This discussion is particularly important in understanding how timing and exposure levels during development can influence the severity and type of toxic response. The chapter provides examples of how toxicants can have varied impacts during different stages of development, such as between the embryonic and fetal periods. This distinction is vital for developing strategies to mitigate risks and protect developmental health.
- Importantly, the chapter addresses the challenges in translating findings from experimental toxicants used in research to actual human health outcomes. It acknowledges the considerable gap that often exists between the demonstrated toxic potential in experimental models and the established effects in human occupational or environmental exposures. This gap underscores the complexities of extrapolating from laboratory studies to real-world scenarios, which is crucial for formulating effective public health policies and safety regulations.
- By highlighting examples of known human reproductive and developmental toxicants, the chapter serves as a resource for identifying chemicals that currently pose a risk to human health. These examples not only enrich the reader's understanding but also guide future research and policy-making in the area of reproductive and developmental toxicology.

- This chapter provides a thorough overview of the mechanisms through which toxicants affect the reproductive and developmental systems, offering valuable insights into the critical factors that must be considered in toxicological assessments and interventions.

References

1. Abbott, L. C., & Nigussie, F. (2021). Mercury toxicity and neurogenesis in the mammalian brain. *International Journal of Molecular Sciences, 22*(14), 7520. https://doi.org/10.3390/ijms22147520.
2. Albarano, L., Zupo, V., Guida, M., Libralato, G., Caramiello, D., Ruocco, N., & Costantini, M. (2021). PAHs and PCBs affect functionally intercorrelated genes in the sea urchin *Paracentrotus lividus* embryos. *International Journal of Molecular Sciences, 22*(22), 12498. https://doi.org/10.3390/ijms222212498.
3. Beamish, C. R., Love, T. M., & Rand, M. D. (2021). Developmental toxicology of metal mixtures in *Drosophila*: Unique properties of potency and interaction of mercury isoforms. *International Journal of Molecular Sciences, 22*(22), 12131. https://doi.org/10.3390/ijms222212131.
4. Bicker, G. (2022). Looking at developmental neurotoxicity testing from the perspective of an invertebrate embryo. *International Journal of Molecular Sciences, 23*(4), 1871. https://doi.org/10.3390/ijms23041871.
5. Chung, D. D., Pinson, M. R., Bhenderu, L. S., Lai, M. S., Patel, R. A., & Miranda, R. C. (2021). Toxic and teratogenic effects of prenatal alcohol exposure on fetal development, adolescence, and adulthood. *International Journal of Molecular Sciences, 22*(16), 8785. https://doi.org/10.3390/ijms22168785.
6. Closset, M., Cailliau, K., Slaby, S., & Marin, M. (2022). Effects of aluminum contamination on the nervous system of freshwater aquatic vertebrates: A review. *International Journal of Molecular Sciences, 23*(1), 31. https://doi.org/10.3390/ijms23010031.
7. Erhirhie, E. O., Ihekwereme, C. P., & Ilodigwe, E. E. (2018). Advances in acute toxicity testing: Strengths, weaknesses and regulatory acceptance. *Interdisciplinary Toxicology, 11*, 5–12. https://doi.org/10.2478/intox-2018-0001.
8. Galanjuk, S., Zühr, E., Dönmez, A., Bartsch, D., Kurian, L., Tigges, J., & Fritsche, E. (2022). The human induced pluripotent stem cell test as an alternative method for embryotoxicity testing. *International Journal of Molecular Sciences, 23*(6), 3295. https://doi.org/10.3390/ijms23063295.
9. Saputra, F., Uapipatanakul, B., Lee, J. S., Hung, S. M., Huang, J. C., Pang, Y. C., & Hsiao, C. D. (2021). Co-treatment of copper oxide nanoparticle and carbofuran enhances cardiotoxicity in zebrafish embryos. *International Journal of Molecular Sciences, 22*(15), 8259. https://doi.org/10.3390/ijms22158259.
10. Stuart, S. D. F., & Villalobos, A. R. (2021). GSH and zinc supplementation attenuate cadmium-induced cellular stress and stimulation of choline uptake in cultured neonatal rat choroid plexus epithelia. *International Journal of Molecular Sciences, 22*(16), 8857. https://doi.org/10.3390/ijms22168857.
11. Yamashita, M., & Markert, U. R. (2021). Overview of drug transporters in human placenta. International Journal of Molecular Sciences, 22(24), 13149. https://doi.org/10.3390/ijms222413149.

Chapter

PROPERTIES AND EFFECTS OF TOXICITY OF PESTICIDES

4

Contents

Introduction

The term "pesticide" refers to a category of chemical compounds specifically designed to eliminate or manage pests. These substances play a critical role in agriculture, disease control, and household maintenance by targeting various types of pests through their unique chemical properties. Pesticides are categorized into different classes based on their intended targets, including insecticides for insects, fungicides for fungi, herbicides for unwanted plants, rodenticides for rodents, and molluscicides for mollusks. Each type is tailored to address specific challenges in pest management, making pesticides a fundamental tool in maintaining agricultural productivity and public health.

Pesticides have been instrumental in controlling vector-borne diseases, such as malaria and Rocky Mountain Spotted oxicity Fever. These diseases pose significant health risks, and the effective use of pesticides has reduced their prevalence dramatically, saving countless lives. In agriculture, pesticides contribute to the stability and increase of food production, enabling farmers in the United States and worldwide to protect crops from pests and diseases and yield more produce. Homeowners also benefit from pesticides to manage household and garden pests, enhancing living conditions and maintaining hygiene.

Exposure to pesticides can occur in various settings. Occupationally, individuals working in industries related to pesticide formulation or commercial pesticide application are at higher risk. These workers might come into contact with pesticides at manufacturing plants or during the application of these chemicals in agricultural settings. For the general public, exposure typically occurs through environmental routes, such as consuming fruits and vegetables treated with pesticides. Additionally, residential use of pesticides in home gardens and indoor spaces can lead to direct exposure. The management and regulation of pesticide use are meticulously overseen in the United States by several regulatory bodies to ensure safety and effectiveness. The primary legislation governing pesticide regulation is the Federal Insecticide, Fungicide, and Rodenticide Act (FIFRA), which oversees the registration, distribution, sale, and use of pesticides. Under FIFRA, the Environmental Protection Agency (EPA) plays a crucial role in assessing and approving pesticides before they can be marketed. The agency ensures that these substances do not pose unreasonable risks to human health or the environment when used as directed.

Specific regulations targeting the protection of workers who handle pesticides are outlined in the 40 Code of Federal Regulations Parts 156 and 170, which were enhanced by the EPA in 1992. These regulations include safety protocols like proper labeling, the use of personal protective equipment, and safety training requirements to minimize health risks to workers. Additionally, guidelines for occupational exposure to airborne pesticides have been published by the Occupational Safety and Health Administration (OSHA) and the American Conference of Governmental Industrial Hygienists (ACGIH), providing further safeguards for those in the industry.

Despite their benefits, the use of pesticides is not without controversy. Concerns over potential health risks to humans, impacts on non-target species, and environmental pollution drive continuous evaluation and discussion about the safety and sustainability of pesticide use. As a result, there is a growing interest in developing and implementing integrated pest management (IPM) strategies, which use a combination of biological, cultural, and chemical practices to control pests in a more environmentally friendly and sustainable manner.

Orientation and Directional Terms

Term	Definition	Illustration
Carcinogenicity	The ability or tendency of a substance to cause cancer or increase the risk of developing cancer.	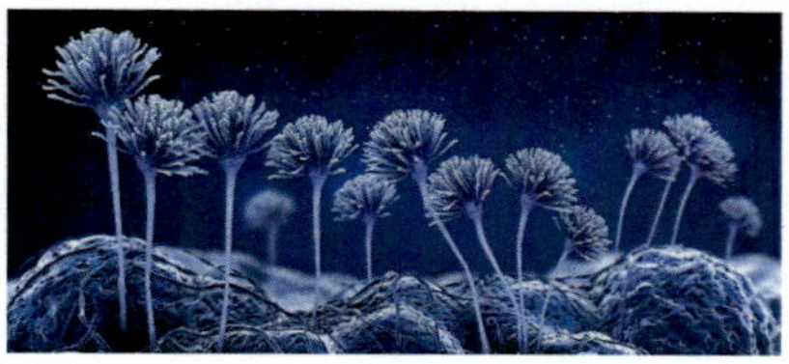
Pharmacokinetics	The branch of pharmacology concerned with the movement of drugs within the body, including absorption, distribution, metabolism, and excretion.	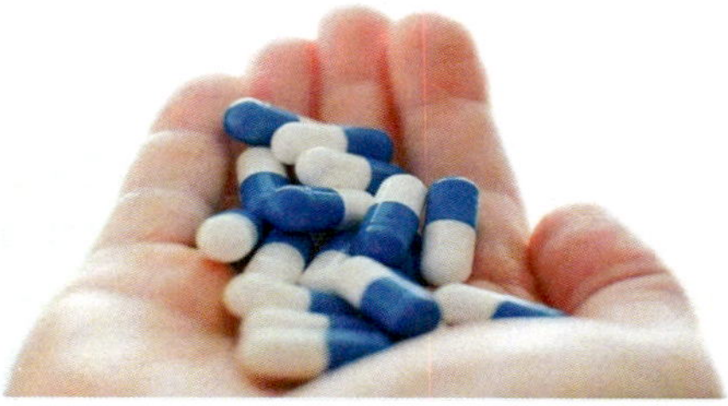
Synthetic Pyrethroids	A class of synthetic chemicals modeled after natural pyrethrins, used as insecticides for their effectiveness in pest control.	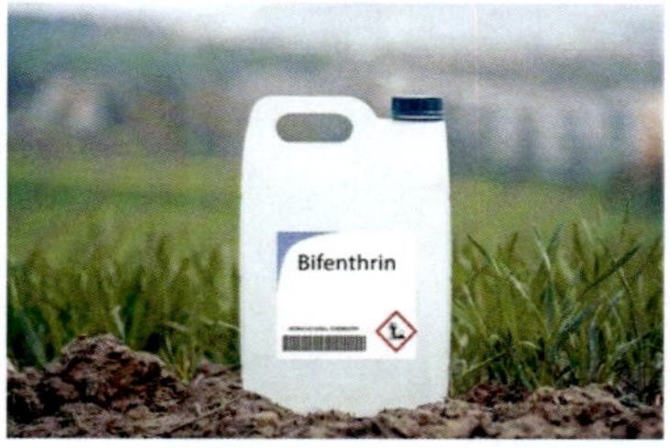
Triazines	A group of herbicides containing a triazine ring structure, commonly used to control weeds in crops like corn and wheat.	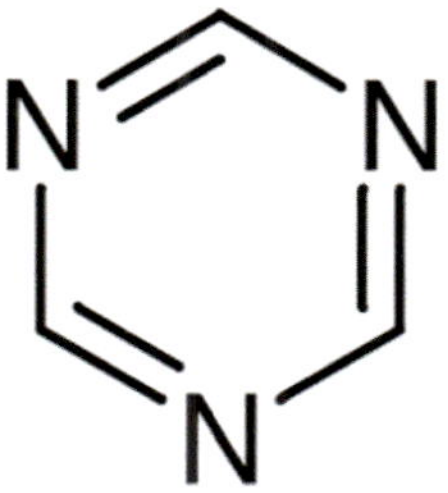
Sodium Fluoroacetate	A highly toxic chemical compound used as a rodenticide and for pest control, also known as 1080.	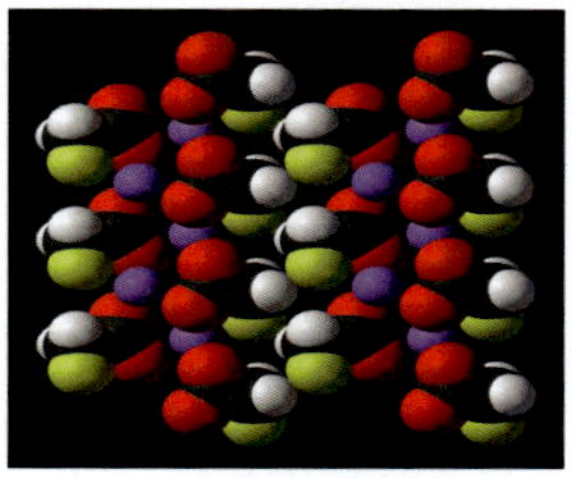

4.1. Organophosphate and Carbamate Insecticides

Organophosphorus compounds have become widely used pesticides, replacing the more persistent organochlorine insecticides (see section 4.2). Organophosphorus insecticides do not accumulate in tissues and organisms or accumulate in the environment, as is the case with organochlorines. In fact, chlorpyrifos, an organophosphate compound, has become a widely used termiticide and serves as a replacement for the more persistent organochlorines used in the past. However, due to the acute toxicity of some organophosphate compounds, another class of pesticides — pyrethrins (see section 4.3)—is becoming more widely used. Examples of commonly used organophosphates include Dursban (chlorpyrifos), Knox Out 2FM (diazinon) and Vapona (dichlorvos) (*see* Figure 4.1 for examples of organophosphate insecticides). Examples of commonly used carbamate pesticide products are Sevin (carbaryl) and Temik (aldicarb) (*see* Figure 4.2 for examples of carbamate insecticides). It should be noted that organophosphate compounds are not only used as pesticides; chemicals in this class are also used as therapeutic agents to treat glaucoma and myasthenia gravis in humans. For example, the organophosphate echothiophate iodide is used to treat glaucoma.

The first organophosphate insecticide developed was tetraethyl pyrophosphate (TEPP), which was developed in Germany during the Second World War as a substitute for nicotine. As TEPP was an effective but unstable compound in the environment, efforts were made to develop more stable compounds. These efforts led to the development of the organophosphate insecticide parathion in 1944.

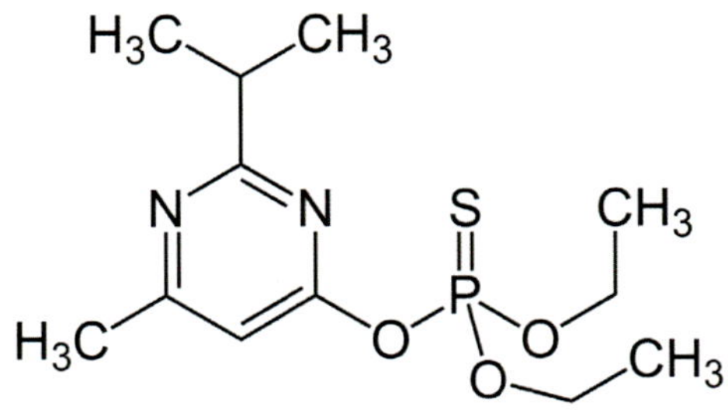

Figure 4.1. *Examples of organophosphate insecticides.*

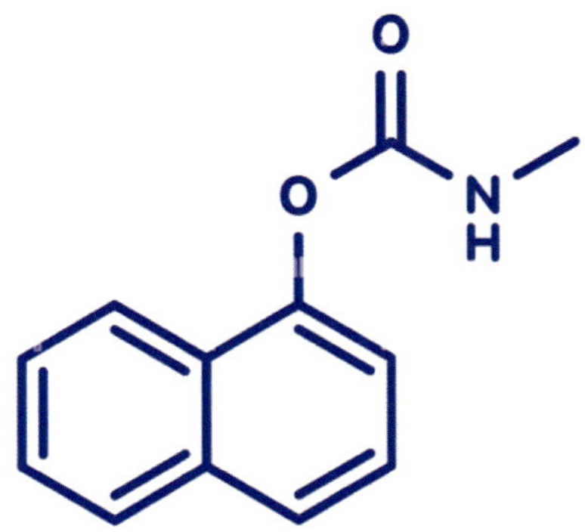

Carbaryl

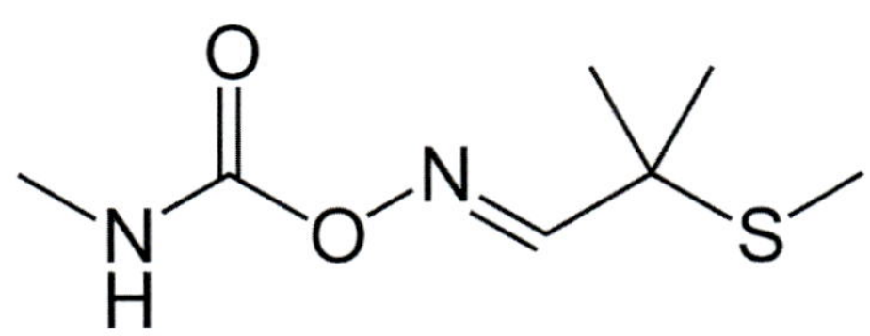

Aldicarb

Figure 4.2. *Examples of carbamate insecticides.*

Source: Wikipedia

4.1.1. Mechanism of Action

The two compound classes of organophosphates and carbamates have the same mechanism of action in both insects and mammals (including humans): inhibition of the enzyme acetylcholinesterase. Inhibition of acetylcholinesterase by organophosphates and carbamates is the mechanism of action responsible for the acute symptomatology associated with these compounds. Acetylcholinesterase is an enzyme located in the synaptic cleft whose function is to break down acetylcholine, the neurotransmitter present in postganglionic parasympathetic nerves, somatic motor nerve endings in skeletal muscle, preganglionic fibers in the parasympathetic and sympathetic nerves, and in some synapses in the central nervous system. Organophosphate and carbamate insecticides act by inhibiting the enzyme acetylcholinesterase at its ester site, which leads to an accumulation of the neurotransmitter acetylcholine in the nervous tissue and at the effector organ. This accumulation then leads to persistent stimulation of cholinergic synapses and, at sufficient levels, to the signs and symptoms associated with overexposure to these compounds (see later in this section) (Bernhardt et al., 2017; Mesnage et al., 2021; Brühl et al., 2022).

4.1.2. Absorption and Metabolism

Organophosphates and carbamates can be easily absorbed by ingestion, skin contact and inhalation due to their lipophilic nature. Organophosphate insecticides, which do not require metabolic activation (see below) and are also referred to as direct inhibitors, may cause local toxic effects at the site of exposure, such as sweating (dermal exposure), miosis or stinging pupils (eye contact) and/or bronchospasm (inhalation exposure). Both organophosphate and carbamate insecticides have a relatively short biological half-life and are metabolized and excreted relatively quickly.

Within the class of organophosphate insecticides, there are direct organophosphate inhibitors (those containing O) and indirect organophosphate inhibitors (those containing S), depending on whether or not they require metabolic activation before they can inhibit acetylcholinesterase. In other words, the indirect organophosphate compounds (containing S) must be bioactivated to become biologically active (containing O). The indirect inhibitory compounds, including organophosphates such as parathion, diazinon, malathion, and chlorpyrifos, become more toxic than the parent compound during metabolism. With these indirect inhibitors, oxidative desulphurization (replacement of the sulfur atom by an oxygen atom as described above) leads to the formation of the oxon of the parent compound (e.g., parathion → paraoxon, diazinon → diazoxon, malathion → maloxon and chlorpyrifos → chlorpyrifos–oxon).

This metabolism takes place via the liver's mixed-function oxidase system. Once the cholinesterase activity in the body has been inhibited by an organophosphate compound, the recovery of this compound depends on the reversal of inhibition, aging, and the regeneration rate of a new enzyme. A chemical reaction that organophosphate insecticides can undergo in the body once they are bound to the cholinesterase enzyme is called "aging." During aging, the compound is dealkylated as soon as it is bound to the enzyme cholinesterase. In this "aged" form, the organophosphate compound is firmly bound to the enzyme and can no longer be released from the enzyme. Once the aging reaction has occurred, treatment with drugs (such as pralidoxime, which will be discussed later) is no longer effective with these aged complexes. Once a cholinesterase molecule has been irreversibly inhibited (by the aging process), enzyme activity can only be restored by synthesizing a new enzyme.

In addition to the aging reaction, organophosphates can also undergo various phase I and II biotransformation pathways, including oxidative, hydrolytic, GSH-mediated transfer and conjugation reactions.

Carbamate compounds do not require metabolic activation to inhibit cholinesterase. Furthermore, carbamate insecticides are not considered irreversible inhibitors like some organophosphate insecticides. Inhibition of cholinesterase by carbamate compounds is readily reversible, with reversal of inhibition usually occurring within a few hours of exposure. This rapid reversal of cholinesterase enzyme activity results in a much shorter duration of action and therefore a shorter duration of intoxication than overexposure to organophosphates. Furthermore, carbamates are not subject to "aging" like organophosphates. Like organophosphates, carbamates can also undergo various phase I and phase II metabolic reactions.

4.1.3. Acute Effects of Organophosphate and Carbamate Insecticides

The effects of organophosphate and carbamate insecticides can be either local (e.g., sweating from localized skin exposure) or systemic. Signs and symptoms of overexposure to organophosphate and carbamate compounds occur relatively quickly after exposure, with effects typically 5 minutes to 12 hours after exposure. Diagnosis of organophosphate poisoning is usually based on a duration of exposure of 6 hours or less before the onset of signs and symptoms. If symptoms appear more than 12 hours after exposure, another etiology should be considered, and if symptoms begin 24 hours after exposure, organophosphate intoxication should be considered doubtful.

Symptoms of carbamate overexposure usually occur within 15 minutes to 2 hours of exposure and usually last only a few hours, much shorter than typical overexposure to organophosphate pesticides. Symptoms occurring 24 hours after exposure are unlikely to be due to overexposure to carbamate insecticides.

The acute signs and symptoms associated with overexposure to organophosphate and carbamate pesticides are related to the degree of inhibition of acetylcholinesterase in the individual. The clinical manifestation of overexposure to organophosphate and carbamate compounds is the result of muscarinic, nicotinic, and CNS symptoms. In systemic intoxications with organophosphate and carbamate compounds, muscarinic effects are generally the first to occur.

Muscarinic symptoms (parasympathetic nervous system) include sweating, increased salivation, increased lacrimation, bronchospasm, dyspnea, gastrointestinal effects (nausea, vomiting, abdominal cramps and diarrhea), miosis (pinpoint pupils), blurred vision, frequent urination and incontinence, wheezing, and bradycardia (decreased heart rate). Nicotinic effects (sympathetic and motor nervous system) include pallor, hypertension, muscle fasciculations, muscle cramps, motor weakness, tachycardia (increased heart rate) and paralysis. Central nervous system signs include dizziness, tension, anxiety, restlessness, insomnia, nightmares, headaches, tremors, drowsiness, confusion, slurred speech, ataxia, coma, Cheyne–Stokes respiration and convulsions.

The diagnosis of organophosphate poisoning is based on the possibility of exposure to the compound, signs, and symptoms suggestive of organophosphate overexposure, and significant inhibition (i.e., 50 inhibition) of the enzyme cholinesterase as measured in plasma and red blood cells (discussed later). The signs and symptoms of overexposure to these organophosphate and carbamate compounds are best described using the mnemonic DUMBELS: Diarrhea, Urination, Miosis (pinpoint pupils), Bronchospasm, Emesis (vomiting), Lacrimation (tear-ing), and Salivation. Signs and symptoms associated with overexposure to organophosphates and carbamate compounds generally do not occur unless acetylcholinesterase activity is approximately 50% or less of normal activity. Signs and symptoms of mild to moderate organophosphate poisoning usually subside within days to weeks after exposure. In severe organophosphate poisoning, it takes 3 months for the cholinesterase levels in the red blood cells to return to normal. Death from organophosphate poisoning is usually due to respiratory failure due to depression of the respiratory center in the brain, paralysis of the respiratory muscles and excessive bronchial secretion, pulmonary edema and bronchial constriction. Death in persons with acute organophosphate poisoning who are not treated usually occurs within the first 24 hours, and within 10 days in treated persons. In the absence of anoxia, full recovery generally occurs within about 10 days of the exposure event.

Carbamate poisoning is similar to organophosphate poisoning. Cases of carbamate intoxication resolve much faster than cases of organophosphate overexposure due to rapid reversal of the acetylcholinesterase enzyme and rapid biotransformation in vivo.

4.1.3.1. Chronic Effects of Organophosphate and Carbamate Insecticides

In general, the main reported chronic effect that may result from exposure to organophosphate insecticides is delayed neuropathy. Organophosphate-induced delayed neuropathy has been associated with exposure to only a few organophosphate compounds, with cases occurring almost exclusively at near-lethal exposure levels. Studies of individuals handling or formulating organophosphate compounds (e.g., chlorpyrifos) have not shown permanent health effects. Carbamate poisoning generally has no lasting effects; delayed neuropathy does not occur with carbamate poisoning (see below) (Bernhardt et al., 2017; Mesnage et al., 2021; Brühl et al., 2022).

4.1.3.2. Organophosphate-Induced Delayed Neuropathy

Some of the organophosphates have been associated with the development of a delayed, predominantly motor peripheral neuropathy called organophosphate-induced delayed neuropathy (OPIDN). In the United States, OPIDN, also known as " ginger jake" paralysis, developed in the 1930s following the consumption of ginger liquor contaminated with triorthyl cresyl phosphate (TOCP). Other outbreaks of OPIDN have occurred in connection with the consumption of cooking oil contaminated with TOCP. Organophosphates that have been associated with OPIDN include TOCP, mipafox, trichlorophos, leptophos, and methamidophos. It should be noted that only a few of the organophosphate compounds are actually capable of causing OPIDN.

The development of OPIDN is not physiologically related to the inhibition of cholinesterase. OPIDN is a distally symmetrical, predominantly motor polyneuropathy of the long, large-diameter axons (the short, small-diameter nerves appear to be spared) in the peripheral nerves. OPIDN, as the name implies, occurs approximately 1–3 weeks after an acute life-threatening exposure to an organophosphate that can cause delayed neuropathy. The initial symptoms of OPIDN include calf cramps with numbness and tingling in the feet and later in the hands. This is followed by weakness in the lower limbs. There may be bilateral drooping of the feet and wrist, and reflexes are usually absent or normal. A high-stepping gait has also been described in individuals with OPIDN. Motor weakness of the limbs may also occur, and motor nerve conduction studies may show abnormalities.

The current theory of the cause of OPIDN is based on a two-stage process in the nervous system. First, it is assumed that phosphorylation of a target protein in the nervous system is required. This enzyme is known as neuropathy target esterase (NTE), formerly also referred to as neurotoxic esterase. The biological effect of NTE in the body is not known. The second and essential step leading to OPIDN is probably the conversion or "aging" of the enzyme. This "aging" process involves the cleavage of an R group from the phosphorus, leaving a negatively charged residue bound to the active site of the enzyme. It appears that compounds that are able to inhibit NTE and aging can only lead to OPIDN if an inhibition threshold is reached. A high inhibition threshold — 70 to 80 inhibition of NDEs in the brain, spinal cord or peripheral nerve of the experimental animal—shortly after administration of an organophosphate that can trigger OPIDN is required for this condition to develop. Thus, the critical factor for the development of OPIDN is the formation of a critical mass of aged, inhibited NDEs.

A term used to express the concentration of a substrate (e.g., an organophosphate compound) required to inhibit 50% of an enzyme is IC_{50}. One way to predict whether a compound will cause OPIDN compared to the concentrations that cause acute cholinergic symptoms is to compare the AChE and NTE IC_{50} values for a given compound. In vitro and in vivo IC_{50} values for NTE and AChE in humans and chickens (the test species used to evaluate the delayed neuropathic potential of organophosphate insecticides) were compared for several organophosphate compounds, and it was found that for organophosphate compounds with an IC_{50}-AChE/IC_{50}-NTE ratio of less than 1, OPIDN may occur only after recovery and treatment from an acute, otherwise fatal, cholinergic crisis.

The scientific literature indicates that, at least for the few compounds studied that are known to cause OPIDN, the ratio of AChE-IC_{50} to NTE-IC_{50} is generally less than one. This means that the concentration of a chemical that inhibits 50% of the AChE molecules is less than the concentration of the same chemical required to inhibit 50% of the NTE molecules. Therefore, at a certain concentration, AChE is inhibited more strongly than NTE. As mentioned above, it is currently believed that more than 50% of the NTE (i.e., 70% to 80%) must be inhibited to develop OPIDN. Similarly, 50–80 inhibition of AChE leads to clinical manifestations. Human case reports indicate that virtually all patients who develop OPIDN were initially treated for a cholinergic crisis.

It is important to note that carbamates do not cause delayed neuropathy. While some carbamates are capable of inhibiting the NDE, aging does not occur. In fact, experiments have shown that some carbamates that inhibit NTE protect chickens from developing OPIDN (Bernhardt et al., 2017; Mesnage et al., 2021; Brühl et al., 2022).

4.1.3.3. Neurobehavioral Sequelae

Several studies have been conducted on individuals exposed to organophosphates occupationally or through accidental or intentional poisoning to investigate the late effects of organophosphate poisoning. In most of these studies, no changes in permanent memory impairment or other psychological problems were found in individuals exposed to organophosphate insecticides or poisoned. Most of the papers reporting neuropsychological changes in people exposed to organophosphates had serious methodological flaws, including failure to control for exposure level, age, education, and alcohol consumption. One study examined 117 individuals who had suffered acute organophosphate poisoning and found no neuropsychiatric symptoms attributable to organophosphate poisoning. While certain neuropsychiatric symptoms (e.g., headache, tension, dizziness, confusion, insomnia) may occur in the acute phase of organophosphate poisoning, there is no objective evidence of permanent neuropsychiatric sequelae associated with organophosphate poisoning.

4.1.3.4. Biological Monitoring for Organophosphates and Carbamates

Organophosphates and carbamates are able to inhibit pseudocholinesterase, red blood cell cholinesterase and nervous system cholinesterase, although the biological effects are only due to the actual inhibition of nervous system cholinesterase. The level of cholinesterase in the blood, particularly in the red blood cells, can be used to estimate the extent to which the nervous system is affected by anticholinesterases. As mentioned above, a 50 drop in cholinesterase levels in plasma and red blood cells is usually required before clinical manifestations are observed. Acute overexposure to organophosphates can be categorized as mild (20–50 of baseline cholinesterase level), moderate (10–20 of baseline cholinesterase level) or severe (10 or less of baseline cholinesterase level).

Plasma cholinesterase is susceptible to the inhibitory effects of organophosphate insecticides but has no known biological function in the body. Plasma cholinesterase levels may vary in an individual due to various disease states or conditions (e.g., decreased plasma cholinesterase levels in liver diseases such as cirrhosis and hepatitis, in multiple metastases, and during pregnancy). Plasma cholinesterase is produced by the liver, and this enzyme is found in nerve tissue, the heart, the pancreas and the white matter of the brain. The level of cholinesterase in plasma usually decreases and regenerates faster than the level of cholinesterase in red blood cells. In the first 7–10 days, the cholinesterase level in the plasma usually regenerates by 25. After organophosphate intoxication, the cholinesterase level in the plasma can remain low for a period of 1 to 3 weeks. The cholinesterase enzyme in the red blood cells is the same enzyme that is also found in the nervous system. Red blood cell cholinesterase regenerates in the body at a rate of about 1 per day and is dependent on the synthesis of new red blood cells in the body. As already mentioned, it can take up to three months for the cholinesterase in the red blood cells to regenerate in cases of severe poisoning by organophosphate pesticides.

The measurement of cholinesterase activity in carbamate poisoning is not useful due to the rapid reactivation of cholinesterase after carbamate overexposure.

4.1.3.5. Treatment for Organophosphate and Carbamate Symptomatology

There are two effective treatments for organophosphate poisoning: Atropine and pralidoxime. Atropine competes with muscarinic sites, and treatment relieves the symptoms of nausea, vomiting, abdominal cramps, sweating, salivation, and miosis. Treatment with atropine has no effect on nicotinic symptoms, such as muscle fasciculations and muscle weakness. Atropine has no effect on muscle weakness in respiratory insufficiency. Furthermore, atropine does not reactivate cholinesterase.

The second therapeutic agent, pralidoxime (also known as 2-PAM), is a drug that reactivates the cholinesterase enzyme inhibited by organophosphates by removing the phosphate group attached to the ester site. However, 2-PAM should be administered quite soon after exposure, as the aged enzyme can no longer be reactivated. 2-PAM is effective in improving symptoms of respiratory depression and muscle weakness. Individuals suffering from carbamate intoxication should possibly not be treated with 2-PAM, as reversal of the carbamate inhibitor could exacerbate the damage. Decontamination of the individual should include removal of all contaminated clothing (rubber gloves should be worn to avoid contact with contaminated clothing and materials) and thorough washing of contaminated skin with soap and water.

4.1.3.6. Regulatory Information on Organophosphates and Carbamates

OSHA PELs and ACGIH TLVs exist for some of the organophosphate and carbamate insecticides. Biological Exposure Indices (BEI) also exist for exposure to parathion (*see* Table 4.1). There is an ACGIH BEI for urinary p-nitrophenol (a metabolite of parathion) levels and a BEI for cholinesterase activity for workers exposed to organophosphate cholinesterase inhibitors (Bernhardt et al., 2017; Mesnage et al., 2021; Brühl et al., 2022).

Table 4.1. *1999 ACGIH Biological Exposure Indices (BEI)*

Pesticide Determinant	Sampling Time	BEI
Organophosphorus Cholinesterase Inhibitors		
Cholinesterase activity in red cells	Discretionary	70% of individual's baseline
Parathion		
Total p-nitrophenol in urine	End of shift	0.5 mg/g creatinine
Cholinesterase activity in red cells	Discretionary	70% of individual's baseline

Source: (Lauwerys & Hoet, 2001)

4.2. Organochlorine Insecticides

While organochlorine insecticides were widely used in agriculture and malaria control programs from the 1940s to the mid-1960s, their use was almost completely phased out due to their environmental impact. Examples of organochlorine insecticides that were commonly used in the past include toxaphene (Toxakil), endrin (Hexadrin), aldrin (Aldrite), endosulfan (Thiodan), BHC (Hexachlorocyclohexane), dienoclor (Pentac), heptachlor (Heptagran), dicofol, mirex (De-cloran), chlordane, and DDT. One organochlorine compound that is still used today is lindane, which is used in the drug Kwell against ectoparasite infestation in humans (as well as in products for home and garden and for animals, e.g., Acitox, Gammex). In addition to their use as insecticides in agriculture and forestry, organochlorine compounds were also frequently used in the past as structural protection against termites. Some of these compounds are still widely used in some developing countries.

4.2.1. Physical and Chemical Properties

The physical and chemical properties of organochlorine compounds — their lipophilicity, low vapor pressure and slow degradation rate — not only made them effective pesticides, but also led to their persistence in the environment and their bioaccumulation in the food chain, which eventually led to their discontinuation of use.

4.2.2. Mechanisms of Action

Organochlorine chemicals act on the nervous system and have harmful effects there. This class of chemicals is thought to act by disrupting cation exchange at nerve cell membranes, resulting in nerve hyperactivity.

Benzene hexachloride (BHC) compounds (lindane and related compounds) are examples of isomers that have different effects on the nervous system.

The γ-isomer, also known as lindane, causes severe, rapid-onset convulsions, while other BHC isomers generally cause central nervous system depression. The relative contribution of each isomer may explain the toxicological differences between the formulations of these products. The cyclodiene organochlorine compounds (e.g., dieldrin) affect the central nervous system.

4.2.3. Pharmacokinetics

Organochlorine compounds are lipophilic and can be absorbed not only through the intestine but also through the lungs and skin. Some of these compounds (e.g., lindane, endrin, and chlordane) are more readily absorbed through the skin than other compounds in this class, such as DDT or toxaphene.

This class of insecticides (e.g., DDT) can also be stored in the body's fatty tissue. Organochlorine compounds can be detected in fatty tissue, serum, and milk. Some compounds (e.g., DDT) are mainly stored unchanged in adipose tissue (part of DDE is stored in adipose tissue), while others (e.g., endrin) are stored in a metabolized form, where aldrin is metabolized to endrin (this conversion also occurs in the environment) or heptachlor is metabolized to heptachlor epoxide. Organochlorine insecticides are primarily excreted in the feces.

4.2.4. Acute and Chronic Health Effects of Organochlorine Insecticides

The main adverse effect associated with overexposure to organochlorine insecticides is hyperactivity of the nervous system (e.g., headache, dizziness, paraesthesia, tremor, incoordination or convulsions). Early symptoms seen in chlorinated insecticide intoxications, such as with DDT, include hyperesthesias and paresthesias of the face and limbs, dizziness, nausea, and vomiting, headache, tremor, and mental disturbances. Myoclonic movements and convulsions are sometimes observed in severe cases of intoxication. It should be noted that the first sign of overexposure to toxaphene and cyclodiene compounds (e.g., aldrin, endrin, chlordane, and heptachlor) is convulsions, even if the early symptoms mentioned above are absent. In these cases, cramps may not occur until 2 days after exposure. A group of factory workers overexposed to chlordecone (Kepone) showed signs and symptoms such as gait disturbances, opsoclonus, headache, tremors, hepatomegaly/splenomegaly and neurological behavioral changes.

Studies on the carcinogenicity of organochlorine compounds have shown positive effects at high doses in mice, but generally not in rats, but there is generally no evidence of cancer in humans, even in the most highly exposed individuals (e.g., workers involved in the manufacture and formulation of organochlorine insecticides) (Bernhardt et al., 2017; Mesnage et al., 2021; Brühl et al., 2022).

4.2.5. Biological Monitoring for Organochlorine Insecticides

Organochlorine insecticides can be detected at background concentrations in the biological tissues of individuals not occupationally exposed to these compounds. Serum and adipose tissue tests have been performed to detect organochlorine pesticides in the general population. The NHAT (National Human Adipose Tissue) study was conducted in 1982. In this study, 763 individual adipose tissue samples from the general population were analyzed for various compounds, including several organochlorine compounds (β-BHC, p,p -DDE, dieldrin, heptachlor epoxide and DDT).

These results are presented in the NHATS Broad Scan Analysis. The results for organochlorine insecticides detected in the serum of the general population are presented in the Health and Nutrition Examination Survey II (HANES II).

4.2.6. Treatment of Organochlorine Intoxication

The treatment of organochlorine poisoning is supportive (e.g., control of convulsions with benzodiazepines or barbiturates). A chlorinated insecticide that can be effectively removed from the body is chlordecone (Kepone, the compound used in the factory worker poisoning described above).

In this case, cholestyramine was used therapeutically to treat the workers who had been poisoned with chlordecone. In nine patients, the administration of 24 g cholestyramine per day led to a 3.3–17.8-fold increase in the fecal excretion of chlordecone. The treatment also led to a reduction in the half-life of chlordecone in the blood from 165 to 80 days (Bernhardt et al., 2017; Mesnage et al., 2021; Brühl et al., 2022).

4.3. Insecticides of Biological Origin

Many compounds in nature have insecticidal properties, including extracts from the chrysanthemum flower and from the Legumionocae genera (e.g., rotenone). Trade names for insecticides in this classification are Pyrocide (Pyrethrum) and Prentox (Rotenone).

4.3.1. Pyrethrum and Pyrethrins

Pyrethrum is an extract from the chrysanthemum flower, *Pyrethrum cinerariaefollium* ("Dalmatian insect flower") and other species. This extract contains about 50% natural pyrethrins—the insecticidal component of the extract. The pyrethrins Jasmoline I and II, Cinerine I and II as well as Pyrethrins I and II are extracted from the powder and processed into commercially available aerosols and sprays. These compounds are often formulated with a synergist such as piperonyl butoxide or n-octylbicycloheptene dicarboximide. These synergists are added to slow down the degradation of the pyrethrin compounds. This class of compounds is commonly used in household insecticides and pet products (e.g., flea and tick repellents and sprays).

Pyrethrins and pyrethrum are very rapidly metabolized and excreted from humans and have very low toxicity to mammals. Crude pyrethrum has been associated with allergic reactions in humans, although this effect is most likely due to the non-insecticidal components of this compound. A study of 59 workers employed between 1 and 25 years in a pyrethrum factory found essentially no adverse health effects, except for inflammatory pleuritic changes in some individuals exposed to high airborne pyrethrum concentrations. Treatment of pyrethrin and pyrethrum exposure is primarily symptomatic.

4.3.2. Synthetic Pyrethroids

Pyrethrins and pyrethrum insecticides are unstable in light and heat. Because of this instability, synthetic pyrethroids have been developed that have better light and heat stability and are used in both agriculture and home pest control. Over the years, more than 1,000 synthetic pyrethroids have been developed, including compounds such as cyfluthrin, cypermethrin (Cymbush), deltamethrin, fenpropathrin (Danitol), fluvalinate (Mavrik), permethrin (Ambush), resmethrin (Chryson) and tralomethrin (Scout) (Figure 4.3).

The sites of action of pyrethroids are the voltage-dependent sodium channels in the nerves. The general basis for the generation and transmission of nerve impulses is the ionic permeability of the membrane in conjunction with the concentration gradients of sodium (high values outside the cell) and potassium (high values inside the cell). The resting cell membrane is maintained by the sodium–potassium pump, and the inside of the cell is negatively charged compared to the outside. A normal nerve impulse is triggered by a rapid, transient increase in the permeability of the membrane to sodium ions, resulting in an inward inflow of sodium, followed by an increase in potassium permeability, which causes an outflow of potassium. The ionic currents cause a temporary reversal of the membrane potential from negative to positive, which leads to the conduction of nerve impulses along the nerve fiber. Pyrethroids exert their effect by slowing the closing of the sodium activation gate. Type I pyrethroids prolong individual channel currents, prolonging sodium influx into the whole cell and increasing the afterpotential until the threshold potential is reached and repetitive discharges occur. Examples of type I pyrethroids are allethrin, cismethrin, permethrin, and resmethrin. Type I pyrethroids have caused increased sensitivity to external stimuli, tremors, increased body temperature and rigor immediately prior to death in animals at high concentrations. Type II pyrethroids cause an extremely prolonged sodium current, which leads to depolarization of the nerve and blockage of impulse conduction. Type II pyrethroids include cyfluthrin, cyhalothrin, cypermethrin, deltamethrin, and fenvalerate. Type II pyrethroids cause behavioral problems in the early stages of poisoning, leading to salivation, miosis, bradycardia, tremors, reduced startle response to sound and ataxia.

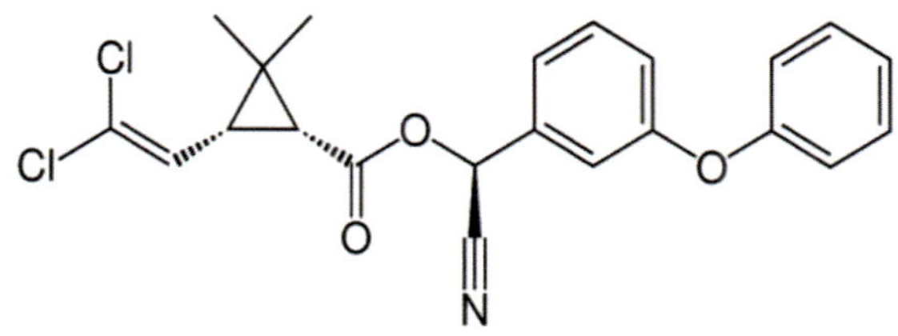

Alpha-Cypermethrin

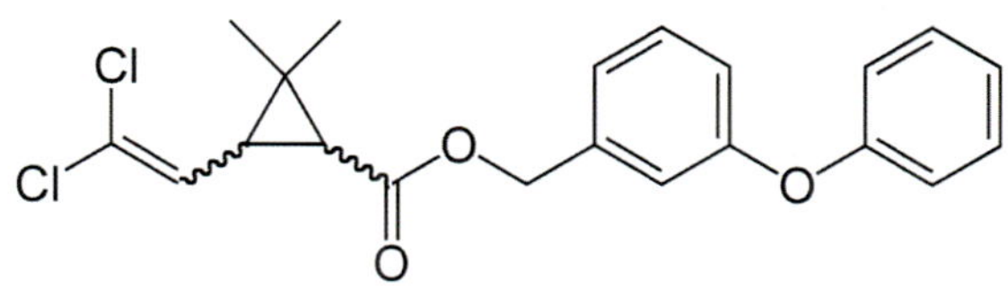

Permethrin

Figure 4.3. *Synthetic pyrethroids.*

Like pyrethrins and pyrethrum, synthetic pyrethroids are rapidly metabolized and excreted in humans and do not accumulate. The relative resistance of mammals, including humans, is due to the ability to metabolize these compounds rapidly and efficiently. Synthetic pyrethroids have a stronger insecticidal effect and lower toxicity to mammals than organophosphate, carbamate, and organochlorine insecticides. Experimental animals treated with high doses of pyrethroids show symptoms such as tremors, salivation, and/or convulsions. In general, animals that survive acute poisoning with pyrethroids recover within a few hours after exposure.

The most important reported reaction to exposure to synthetic pyrethroid insecticides in humans occurs with pyrethroids containing cyano groups (e.g., fenvalerate and cypermethrin). This reaction consists of paresthesias that typically occur in the mouth region in workers exposed to these compounds. This paresthesia is reversible and usually disappears within 24 hours of cessation of exposure. An occupational study of 199 workers involved in dividing and packaging pyrethroids (fenvalerate, deltamethrin, and cypermethrin) found that apart from transient facial paresthesia, sneezing, and increased nasal secretions, there were essentially no adverse health effects from pyrethroid exposure. The treatment of pyrethrin overexposure consists of decontamination and supportive treatment.

4.3.3. Rotenone

Rotenone (Noxfish) occurs naturally in several plant species (e.g., the Leguminocae genera) and is used mainly as an insecticide as well as to eliminate fish in lakes and ponds. The mechanism of action for rotenone is as a respiratory toxin, blocking electron transport at ubiquinone, and preventing oxidation of NADH. Rotenone seems to have low toxicity in humans, and few reports of serious injury appear to have been reported. Occupational exposure to the powder of the plant that contains rotenone has reportedly caused dermal and respiratory tract irritation and numbness in the mouths of workers. Treatment of rotenone overexposure consists mainly of decontamination and supportive therapy.

4.3.4. Bacillus thuringiensis

Microbial insecticides, such as various strains of *Bacillus thuringiensis* (e.g., Dipel, variety kurstaki), have been developed as effective insecticides. The endotoxin of *Bacillus thuringiensis* is insecticidal in certain sensitive species. *Bacillus thuringiensis* is not generally associated with mammalian or human toxicity; only a few cases of adverse effects in humans have been reported. A group of 18 volunteers who ingested 1 gram of a *B. thuringiensis* formulation for 5 days, with 5 of these 18 volunteers also inhaling 100 mg of the powder for 5 days, reported no adverse effects. A group of workers exposed to various processes in the formulation of a commercial product containing the biological insecticide also showed no adverse health effects (Bernhardt et al., 2017; Mesnage et al., 2021; Brühl et al., 2022).

4.4. Herbicides

4.4.1. Chlorophenoxy Herbicides

The chlorophenoxy herbicides 2,4-dichlorophenoxy acetic acid (2,4-D) and 2,4,5-trichlorophenoxy acetic acid (2,4,5-T) are probably the most commonly recognized of the chlorophenoxy herbicides. These compounds exert their action in plants by acting as growth hormones, but have no such hormonal action in animals or humans. Some of the commonly used chlorophenoxy herbicides include Banvel (dicamba), Weedone (2,4-D), and Basagran M (MCPA) (*see* Figure 4.4).

4.4.2. Acute Toxicity

2,4-Dichlorophenoxyacetic acid (2,4-D) is produced commercially by the reaction of 2,4-dichlorophenol and monochloroacetic acid. Other chlorophenoxy herbicide analogs are 2,4-DB, 2,4-DP, MCPA [(4-chloro-2-methylphenoxy)-acetic acid], MCPP and the herbicides 2,4,5-trichlorophe-noxyacetic acid (2,4,5-T) and 2-(2,4,5-trichlorophenoxy)-propionic acid (2,4,5-TP; Silvex), which are no longer used.

Dioxin (2,3,7,8-TCDD) was not detected in 2,4-D formulations (WHO, 1984). While contamination of 2,3,7,8-TCDD in 2,4-D may have occurred in the past, this was due to contamination during the manufacture of 2,4,5-T. The synthesis of 2,4-D does not produce 2,3,7,8-TCDD.

The most important routes of exposure to chlorophenoxy herbicides are the skin and inhalation. Chlorophenoxy compounds act by uncoupling oxidative phosphorylation and reducing oxygen consumption in tissues. These compounds are excreted relatively quickly and do not accumulate in the body. These compounds are primarily excreted in the urine, and apart from the conjugation of acids, there is little biotransformation in the body.

The acute toxicity of chlorophenoxy herbicides after ingestion includes irritation of the mucous membranes and gastrointestinal mucosa. Large deliberate overdoses with chlorophenoxy acids have led to symptoms such as coma, metabolic acidosis, myotonia, mucosal irritation and myalgias. Although sporadic cases of peripheral neuropathy following exposure to 2,4-D have been reported in the literature, no causal relationship between this compound and neuropathy has been established.

Treatment of cases of overexposure to chlorophenoxy herbicides is symptomatic and includes decontamination.

4.4.3. Carcinogenicity

2,4-D is currently classified by the USEPA as a "D" carcinogen (unclassifiable). A recent mortality study of chemical workers exposed to 2,4-D and its derivatives found no evidence of increased mortality from cancer, including non-Hodgkin's lymphoma. A recent review of available animal and human data for the chlorophenoxy herbicides 4-chloro-2-methylphenoxyacetic acid (MCPA),

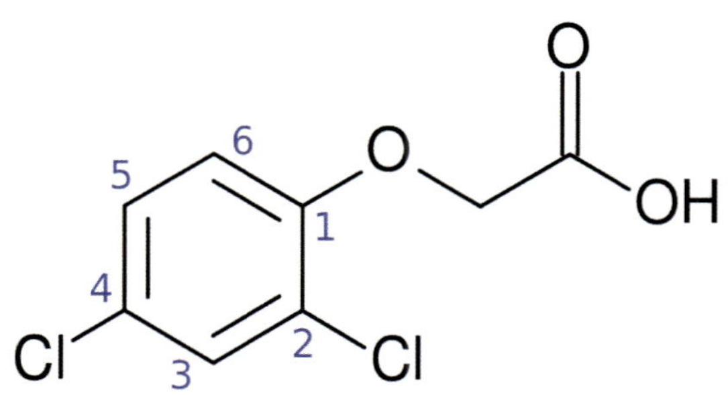

Figure 4.4. *2,4-Dichlorophenoxyacetic acid (2,4-D).*

Source: Wikipedia

2-(4-chloro-2-methylphenoxy)-propionic acid (MCPP) and 2-(2,4-dichlorophenoxy)-propionic acid (2,4-DP) concluded that there is no evidence that these compounds are carcinogenic to humans.

4.4.4. Bipyridyl Compounds – Paraquat and Diquat

Paraquat (1,1 -dimethyl-4,4 -d ipy r id y liu m) (*see* Figure 4.5) and diquat (1,1 -ethylene-2,2 -bipyridylium) are bipyridylium herbicides known under the trade names Gramoxone (paraquat) and Aquacide (diquat), among others. The majority of reported cases of toxicity associated with paraquat and diquat are observed with accidental or intentional (suicidal) ingestion, with paraquat having a higher toxicity than diquat. An emetic, valeric acid, is added to paraquat solutions.

Paraquat poisoning (e.g., by suicide attempts) can lead to multi-organ toxicity (e.g., gastrointestinal tract, kidneys, heart, and liver), including pulmonary fibrosis. Early deaths following intoxication with paraquat are due to acute pulmonary edema, oliguric renal failure and liver failure. Deaths occurring one to three weeks after intoxication are usually the result of pulmonary fibrosis. Paraquat is generally not readily absorbed through the skin, but reports of toxicity following sufficient dermal absorption have been observed in individuals with skin abrasions or in individuals with prolonged dermal exposure to paraquat. Sufficient dermal exposure to paraquat may also cause skin irritation, blistering, and ulceration. Similar irritant effects are observed in the esophagus and stomach of people who swallow paraquat. Paraquat accumulates in the lungs, where the proposed mechanism of action leading to pulmonary fibrosis is the formation of free radicals leading to lipid peroxidation. Pulmonary fibrosis, which can be fatal with sufficient exposure, begins within 2 days to 2 weeks of paraquat exposure. Inhalation is not thought to be a toxic route of exposure. Paraquat aerosol droplets larger than 5 μm in diameter have been measured, indicating that they do not reach the alveolar membrane to cause direct or systemic toxicity via inhalation. In two field trials in which the absorption of paraquat was measured by paraquat urine levels, systemic absorption did not appear to be significant. The authors of this study concluded that "ordinary care in personal hygiene is sufficient to avoid any risk from surface injury or systemic absorption." A recent study of a group of 85 paraquat sprayers also found no adverse health effects (other than irritant effects), including no effects on the lungs, attributable to long-term occupational use of this herbicide.

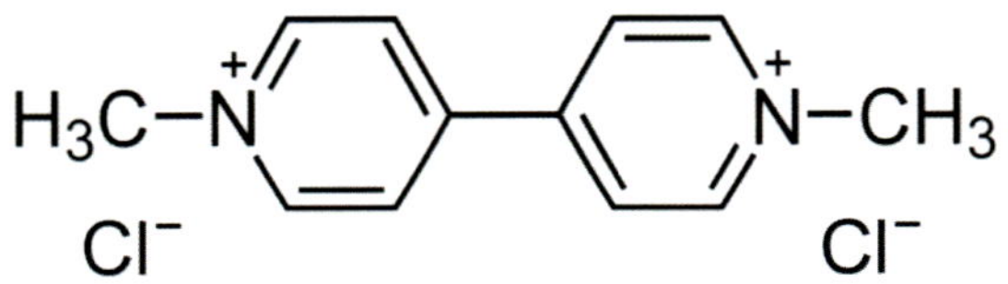

Figure 4.5. *Paraquat.*

Source: Wikipedia

Diquat causes less skin irritation and injury than paraquat, and diquat is not selectively concentrated in lung tissue like paraquat. Diquat, unlike paraquat, causes little or no damage to the lungs; however, diquat does have effects on the central nervous system, whereas paraquat does not. The mechanism of action of diquat is thought to be similar to that of paraquat and involves the formation of superoxide radicals that cause the destruction of lipid membranes. Exposure of the skin to sufficient quantities of diquat can lead to damage to the fingernails and irritation of the eyes and mucous membranes. Oral intoxication with diquat has been reported to cause signs and symptoms such as gastrointestinal irritation, nausea, vomiting, and diarrhea. Both paraquat and diquat have been reported to be associated with renal toxicity. There is no known specific antidote for paraquat or diquat poisoning.

Glyphosate (Round-Up) [N-(phosphonomethyl)glycine] (*see* Figure 4.6) is a widely used herbicide that interferes with amino acid metabolism in plants. In animals, it presumably acts as a weak uncoupler of oxidative phosphorylation. Glyphosate is moderately absorbed via the gastrointestinal tract, undergoes minimal biotransformation and is excreted via the kidneys. Several cases of poisoning have been reported in the literature, usually due to accidental or suicidal ingestion following overexposure to the glyphosate-containing product Round-Up. The various signs and symptoms include irritation and damage to the gastrointestinal tract and dysfunction in various organ systems (e.g., lung, liver, kidney, CNS, and cardiovascular system). It is suspected that the toxicity observed after poisoning with Round-Up is due to the surfactant in the commercial product. One study found that the irritation potential of the commercial preparation of Round-Up is comparable to that of baby shampoo.

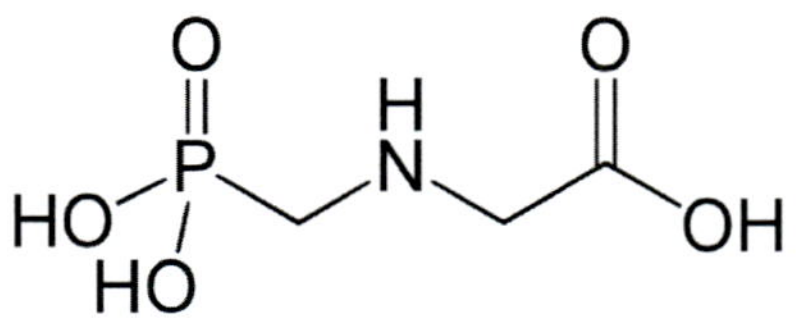

Figure 4.6. *Glyphosate.*

Source: Wikipedia

4.4.5. Triazines

Examples of triazine and triazole herbicides are atrazine (2-chloro-4-ethylamino-6-isopro-plyamine-s-triazine), propazine, simazine [2-chloro-4,6-bis(ethylamino)-s-triazine] and cy-anazine [2-chloro-4-(1-cyano-1-methylethylamino)-6-ethylamino-s-triazine]. Triazine herbicides have a relatively low toxicity and apparently, no cases of systemic poisoning have been reported. Occasionally, skin irritation following exposure to triazine herbicides has been reported in the literature.

4.5. Fungicides

Fungicides are compounds used to control fungal growth and are used in many different products, from their use to protect grain after harvest during storage to their use in paints.

Pentachlorophenol, also known as penta, is used as a wood preservative against fungal infestation and termites and as a molluscicide. The trade names of pentachlorophenol include Pentacon, Penwar, and Penchlorol (Figure 4.7).

Pentachlorophenol is readily absorbed through the skin, lungs, and gastrointestinal tract. Pentachlorophenol and its biotransformation products are mainly excreted via the kidneys. The biochemical mechanism of action of pentachlorophenol is an increase in oxidative metabolism by uncoupling oxidative phosphorylation.

This increase in oxidative metabolism can lead to an increase in body temperature in cases of poisoning. In fatal cases of poisoning with pentachlorophenol, the body temperatures of (almost) 41.8 °C (107.4 °F) were reported. Severe overexposure to pentachlorophenol may cause signs and symptoms such as delirium, flushing, pyrexia, diaphoresis, tachypnea, abdominal pain, nausea, and tachycardia.

Because pentachlorophenol volatilizes from treated wood and fabric, excessively treated indoor surfaces may cause irritation to the skin, eyes, and upper respiratory tract. Contact dermatitis has been reported in workers exposed to pentachlorophenol on the skin. Treatment of pentachlorophenol poisoning consists primarily of decontamination of clothing and skin and/or gastrointestinal tract and supportive treatment of symptoms associated with exposure (e.g., temperature control).

Pentachlorophenol can be detected in blood, urine, and adipose tissue. The ACGIH biological exposure index for pentachlorophenol is 2 mg/g creatinine total pentachlorophenol in urine before the last shift of the work week or 5 mg/L free pentachlorophenol in plasma at the end of the work shift.

4.5.1. Dithiocarbamates/ Thiocarbamates

The dithiocarbamates and thiocarbamates are used as fungicidal compounds and, in contrast to the N-methylcarbamates already mentioned (e.g., the acetylcholinesterase-inhibiting carbaryl), have only a low insecticidal toxicity. Examples of thiocarbamate fungicides are thiram (AAtack), metam sodium (Vapam), ziram (Ziram 76), ferbam, and the ethylene bisdithiocarbamate compounds (EBDC) — maneb, zineb, and mancozeb. In general, the thiocarbamate class of fungicides has low acute toxicity. Thiram dust has been reported to cause eye, skin, and mucous membrane irritation, with contact dermatitis and sensitization reported to have occurred in a few workers. Systemic intoxications associated with exposure to thiram have resulted in symptoms similar to reactions to disulfiram (Antabuse), a dithiocarbamate drug used to treat alcoholism.

Thiram, like disulfiram, is not a cholinesterase inhibitor but does inhibit the enzyme acetaldehyde dehydrogenase (responsible for converting acetaldehyde to acetic acid), and workers exposed to thiram have reportedly complained of "Antabuse" reactions after ingesting alcoholic beverages in rare cases.

Exposure to ziram, ferbam, and the EBDC compounds has been associated with skin, eye, and respiratory tract irritation in humans. Maneb and Zineb have been linked to cases of chronic skin disease, possibly due to the skin sensitization of workers to these compounds.

4.5.2. Chlorothalonil

Chlorothalonil (Bravo, Daconil) (2,4,5,6-tetrachloro-1,3-benzenedicarbonitrile) has been reported to cause skin and mucous membrane irritation in humans exposed to this compound. Chlorothionil appears to have a low toxicity potential for humans.

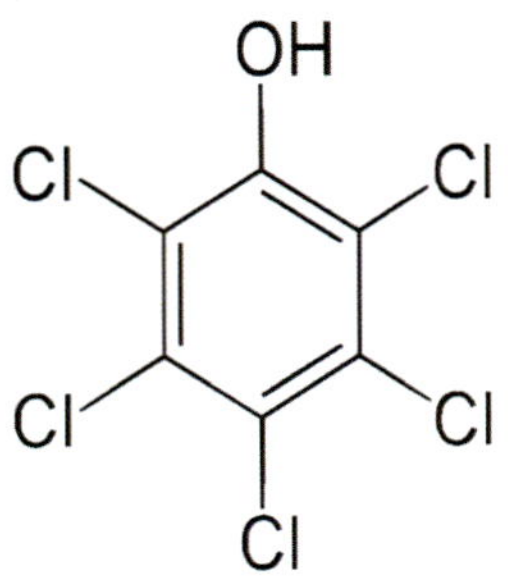

Figure 4.7. *Pentachlorophenol.*

Source: Wikipedia

4.5.3. Copper Compounds

Exposure to dust and powder formulations of copper-based fungicides has been reported to cause irritation to the skin, eyes, and respiratory tract. Systemic poisoning in humans from copper fungicides has been reported rarely. Ingestion of the compound has been reported to cause gastrointestinal irritation, nausea, and vomiting, diarrhea, headache, sweating, weakness, liver enlargement, hemolysis, and methemoglobinemia, albuminuria, hemoglobinuria, and occasionally renal failure. Treatment of copper intoxication may consist of an attempt to prevent absorption (e.g., lavage) followed by chelation therapy.

4.6. Rodenticides

Rodenticides, as the name suggests, are a class of compounds that specifically target rodents. In some cases, these compounds have taken advantage of physiological differences between rodents and other mammals (e.g., humans) that make rodents more susceptible to their toxic effects. The most effective route of exposure for these compounds is ingestion.

The action of this class of rodenticides is based on the suppression of vitamin K synthesis of blood coagulation factors II (prothrombin), VII, IX, and X. This anticoagulant property manifests itself in diffuse internal bleeding, which usually occurs several days after ingestion of the rodenticide bait. Warfarin (*see* Figure 4.8) is a commonly used coumarin rodenticide that exerts its toxic effects by inhibiting prothrombin formation and inhibiting vitamin K-dependent factors in the body. Other anticoagulant rodenticides are coumafuryl, brodifacoum, difenacoum, and proline. It is known that warfarin can be absorbed both through the skin and by ingestion. Signs and symptoms of warfarin poisoning include epistaxis, hemoptysis, bleeding gums, gastrointestinal, and genitourinary bleeding and ecchymosis.

In contrast to coumarins, indandiones cause effects on the nervous system, heart, and lungs in laboratory animals, which precede death due to the anticoagulant effect. These types of adverse effects have not been reported in human exposure. Examples of indandione rodenticides include diphacinone, diphacin, and chlorphacinone.

The most prominent clinical laboratory sign associated with the administration of these classes of compounds is an increased prothrombin time and a decrease in plasma prothrombin concentration. The treatment of the toxicity of coumarins and indanediones consists of the administration of vitamin K1.

4.6.1. Thallium Sulfate

Thallium sulfate is easily absorbed by ingestion, through the skin and by inhalation. Target organs of thallium sulfate include the gastrointestinal tract (hemorrhagic gastroenteritis), heart, and blood vessels, kidneys, liver, skin, and hair. Symptoms such as headache, lethargy, muscle weakness, numbness, tremor, ataxia, myoclonus, convulsions, delirium, and coma occur in thallium sulfate-induced encephalopathy. Death from thallium sulfate intoxication is due to respiratory paralysis or cardiovascular failure.

The concentration of thallium in serum, urine, and hair can be used to assess exposure to this compound. There is no specific treatment for thallium sulfate poisoning, and treatment is supportive. A syrup of ipecac and activated charcoal can be used to reduce gastrointestinal absorption.

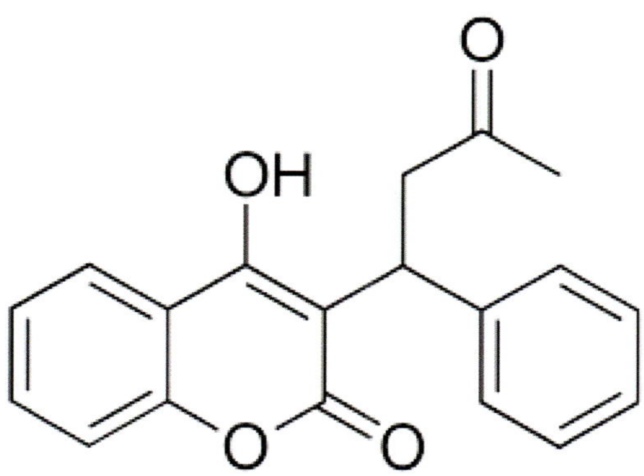

Figure 4.8. *Warfarin.*

Source: Wikipedia

4.6.2. Sodium Fluoroacetate

Sodium fluoroacetate is also known as 1080 (registered trademark). This compound is easily absorbed by ingestion, inhalation, and through the skin. The toxicity of sodium fluoroacetate is due to the reaction of three molecules of fluoroacetate that form fluorocitrate in the liver. Fluoroci-trat impairs cellular respiration by interfering with the tricarboxylic acid cycle (inhibition of the enzyme cis-aconitase). It is assumed that the accumulation of citrate in the tissues is also responsible for part of the acute toxicity of this compound. The target organs of sodium fluoroacetate are the heart (cardiac arrhythmias leading to ventricular fibrillation) and the brain (convulsions and twitching) following intoxication (typically following suicidal or accidental ingestion). There is no specific antidote for sodium fluoroacetate poisoning. Treatment consists of decontamination and supportive therapy, including gastric lavage and catharsis.

4.7. Fumigants

Fumigants (*see e.g.,* Figure 4.9) are a group of compounds that are volatile by nature. Some of the fumigants exist in a gas phase at room temperature, while others are liquid or solid.

Fumigants are generally readily absorbed through the skin, and respiratory tract and by ingestion. Treatment of overexposure to fumigants usually involves flushing the contaminated areas (skin, eyes). A doctor should be consulted after rinsing the eyes, as some of these compounds are highly corrosive to the cornea. Sufficient dermal absorption may occur, leading to systemic effects. Patients exposed to inhalation should be monitored for pulmonary edema and treated accordingly if edema develops. Contaminated clothing should be removed and disposed of. It should found that certain fumigants are able to penetrate rubber and neoprene (often used for personal protective equipment) (Bernhardt et al., 2017; Mesnage et al., 2021; Brühl et al., 2022).

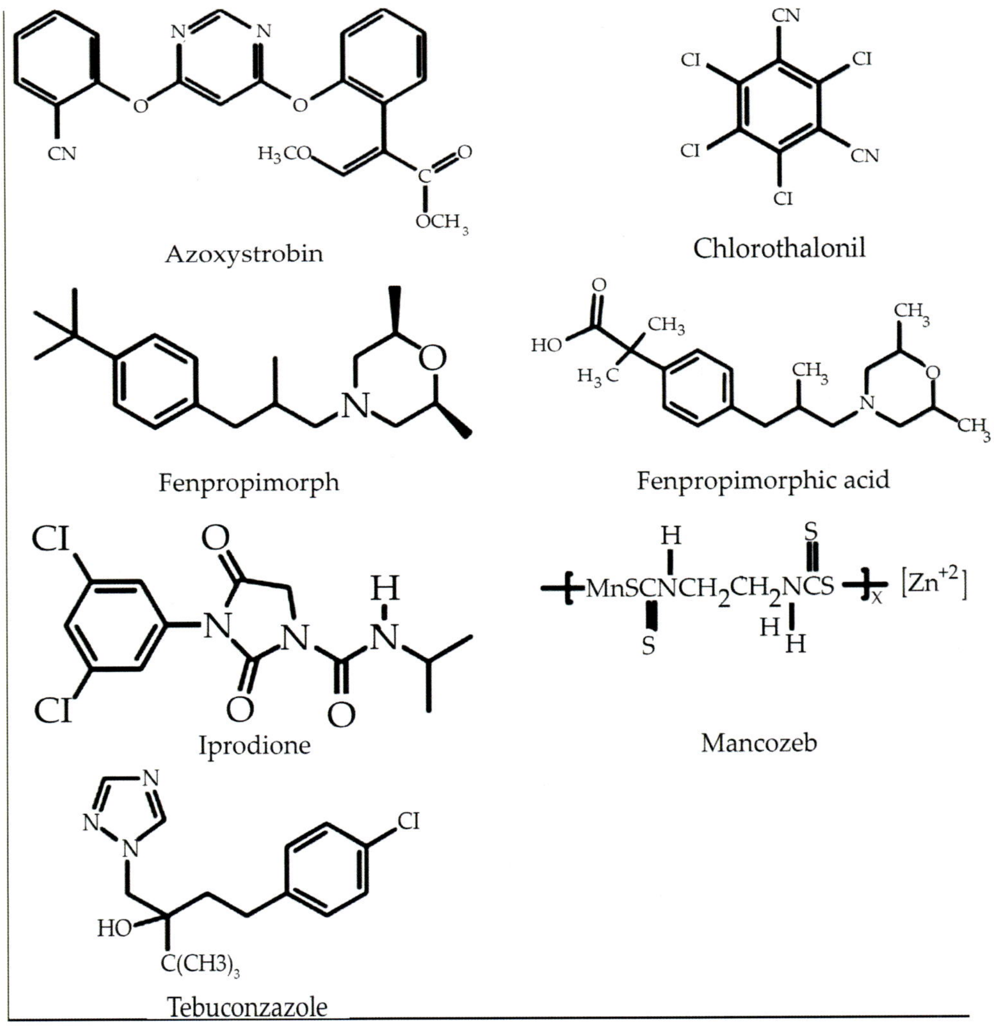

Figure 4.9. *Chemical structures of selected fumigants.*

Source: Wikipedia

4.7.1. Methyl Bromide

Methyl bromide (Brom-O-Sol, Terr-O-Gas) has been used as a fumigant since 1932 and is a colorless and virtually odorless compound (at low concentrations), with its low warning potential contributing to its toxicity. At higher concentrations, the odor of methyl bromide is similar to that of chloroform. Fatalities have been reported during application and from premature re-entry into treated areas. Methyl bromide has been used to treat dry packaged foods in mills and warehouses and as a soil fumigant to control nematodes and fungi.

Methyl bromide is very irritating to the lower respiratory tract. The parent compound is thought to be responsible for the toxicity of methyl bromide, with the mechanism of toxicity possibly related to its ability to bind with sulfhydryl enzymes. Exposure to high concentrations of methyl bromide can lead to pulmonary edema or hemorrhage, and intoxication is usually delayed (several hours after exposure) in affected individuals. Symptoms of acute poisoning include those associated with central nervous system depression, such as headache, dizziness, nausea, visual disturbances, vomiting, and ataxia. Exposure to very high concentrations can lead to unconsciousness. Death from exposure to lethal levels of methyl bromide usually occurs within 4–6 hours to 1–2 days after exposure; the cause of death is respiratory or cardiovascular failure due to pulmonary edema. Exposure of the skin to liquid methyl bromide can cause skin damage in the form of burning, itching, and blistering. Methyl bromide poisoning is treated symptomatically.

4.7.2. Ethylene Oxide

Ethylene oxide, also known as epoxyethane (ETO), is a sterilizing and fumigating agent that exists as a colorless gas and has a high odor threshold. Ethylene oxide is also a strong mucous membrane and skin irritant. Exposure of the skin in sufficient quantities can lead to edema, burns, blisters, and frostbite. Acute poisoning can lead to CNS depression characterized by headache, nausea, vomiting, drowsiness, weakness, and coughing. Exposure to extreme concentrations of ethylene oxide can lead to the development of pulmonary edema and cardiac arrhythmias.

4.7.3. Sulfuryl Fluoride

Sulfuryl fluoride (Vikane) (SO_2F_2), a colorless and odorless gas, is used for fumigation of buildings. There have been reports of deaths of people entering buildings that had recently been fumigated with sulfuryl fluoride before re-entry was permitted. Acute toxic effects of sulfuryl poisoning include mucous membrane irritation, nausea, vomiting, shortness of breath, coughing, severe weakness, restlessness, and seizures (Bernhardt et al., 2017; Mesnage et al., 2021; Brühl et al., 2022).

A Closer Look

Toxicity of Insecticides

Insecticides are essential tools for managing agricultural pests that have raised significant concerns regarding their toxicity and environmental impact. The chemical compounds in insecticides are designed to target and eliminate pests, but their non-selective nature often results in unintended harm to non-target species, including beneficial insects, wildlife, and even humans. Organophosphates, neonicotinoids, and pyrethroids are among the commonly used insecticides, each with distinct modes of action but shared toxicity concerns. Organophosphates, for instance, inhibit acetylcholinesterase, leading to the accumulation of acetylcholine and subsequent nervous system dysfunction in insects and mammals. Neonicotinoids, while targeting insect nicotinic acetylcholine receptors, have been implicated in the decline of pollinator populations, notably bees, which play a crucial role in ecosystem health and agriculture. Pyrethroids, synthetic analogs of pyrethrins, disrupt sodium channels in nerve cells but also pose risks to aquatic organisms due to runoff. Beyond immediate toxicity, chronic exposure to insecticides has been linked to long-term health effects, such as endocrine disruption and carcinogenicity, raising public health concerns. Moreover, the persistence and bioaccumulation of these chemicals in the environment exacerbate their impact, contaminating soil, water, and food supplies. The rise of insecticide resistance in pest populations further complicates their management, prompting higher doses and more frequent applications, which in turn heighten environmental and health risks. Integrated Pest Management (IPM) strategies, which emphasize the use of biological controls, cultural practices, and selective chemical use, offer a sustainable alternative to conventional insecticide reliance. Reducing toxicity and environmental impact requires a multifaceted approach, including the development of safer, target-specific insecticides, stricter regulatory measures, and increased awareness of the consequences of indiscriminate insecticide use. Addressing these challenges is crucial for safeguarding both agricultural productivity and ecological health.

Summary

- This chapter offers a detailed examination of the toxicology associated with various widely used groups of pesticides. These substances, crucial for pest control in agricultural, residential, and public health contexts, present a complex interplay of benefits and risks.
- Pesticides are employed for several purposes: they eliminate pests that threaten crops, control insects in homes and on pets, and combat vector-borne diseases like malaria. Their ubiquity in various spheres of life underscores their significance but also raises concerns about their potential health impacts on humans and the environment.
- The chapter underscores that individuals may encounter pesticides through various routes: inhalation, ingestion, and skin contact. Such exposures can occur in diverse settings, from agricultural fields and factories to homes, often categorizing exposure as occupational, dietary, accidental, or even intentional in cases of suicide attempts. This multifaceted exposure scenario complicates the assessment and management of risks associated with pesticides.
- In terms of mechanism, pesticides are designed to target specific physiological processes in pests, but these substances can also affect human and animal health. The biochemical pathways intended to harm pests can similarly disrupt cellular and physiological functions in non-target species, including humans, leading to acute and chronic health issues.
- Historically, persistent organochlorine insecticides were prevalent; however, due to their long-lasting environmental impacts and potential to bioaccumulate, there has been a shift towards organophosphate compounds. More recently, the focus has moved again toward substances such as pyrethrins, which are favored for their lower toxicity and reduced environmental persistence. This evolution in pesticide use reflects a growing awareness of and response to the environmental and health repercussions of pesticide residues.
- The chapter also discusses regulatory and safety frameworks that govern pesticide use. Industrial hygiene standards, such as the Occupational Safety and Health Administration's Permissible Exposure Limits (OSHA PELs), the American Conference of Governmental Industrial Hygienists' Threshold Limit Values (ACGIH TLVs), and Biological Exposure Indices (BEIs) are pivotal in establishing safe levels of exposure to various pesticides. These standards are essential for protecting workers and the public from the adverse effects of pesticides and are continually updated to reflect new scientific knowledge and technological advances.
- In addition to regulatory aspects, the chapter delves into the toxicological profiles of different pesticide classes. It highlights the acute and chronic effects of exposure, which can range from immediate symptoms like headaches and dizziness to long-term consequences such as neurotoxicity, reproductive harm, and cancer. The toxicological data not only inform safety guidelines but also guide the development of newer, safer pesticides.
- Moreover, the discussion extends to the challenges of balancing the need for effective pest control with the imperative to minimize health risks. This balance is crucial in global efforts to ensure food security, control disease vectors, and maintain biodiversity without compromising public health.

References

1. Bernhardt, E. S., Rosi, E. J., & Gessner, M. O. (2017). Synthetic chemicals as agents of global change. *Frontiers in Ecology and the Environment, 15*(2), 84–90. https://doi.org/10.1002/fee.1458.
2. Börner, H. (2009). *Pflanzenkrankheiten und Pflanzenschutz* (8th ed.). Springer.
3. Brühl, C. A., & Zaller, J. G. (2019). Biodiversity decline as a consequence of an inappropriate environmental risk assessment of pesticides. *Frontiers in Environmental Science, 7*, 177. https://doi.org/10.3389/fenvs.2019.00177.
4. Brühl, C. A., Bakanov, N., Köthe, S., Eichler, L., Sorg, M., Hörren, T., Mühlethaler, R., Meinel, G., & Lehmann, G. U. C. (2021). Direct pesticide exposure of insects in nature conservation areas in Germany. *Scientific Reports, 11*, 24144. https://doi.org/10.1038/s41598-021-03364-8.
5. Brühl, C. A., Zaller, J. G., Liess, M., & Wogram, J. (2022). The rejection of synthetic pesticides in organic farming has multiple benefits. *Trends in Ecology & Evolution, 37*, 113–114. https://doi.org/10.1016/j.tree.2021.09.015.
6. Cech, R. M., Jovanovic, S., Kegley, S., Hertoge, K., Leisch, F., & Zaller, J. G. (2022). Reducing overall herbicide use may reduce risks to humans but increase toxic loads to honeybees, earthworms and birds. *Environmental Sciences Europe, 34*, 44. https://doi.org/10.1186/s12302-022-00656-3.
7. Cech, R., Zaller, J. G., Lyssimachou, A., Clausing, P., Hertoge, K., & Linhart, C. (2023). Pesticide drift mitigation measures appear to reduce contamination of non-agricultural areas, but hazards to humans and the environment remain. *Science of The Total Environment, 854*, 158814. https://doi.org/10.1016/j.scitotenv.2022.158814.
8. Centner, T. J. (2021). Creating a compensation program for injuries from dicamba spray drift and volatilization. *Applied Economic Perspectives and Policy, 44*(4), 1068–1082. https://doi.org/10.1002/aepp.13101.
9. Clausing, P., Robinson, C., & Burtscher-Schaden, H. (2018). Pesticides and public health: An analysis of the regulatory approach to assessing the carcinogenicity of glyphosate in the European Union. *Journal of Epidemiology and Community Health, 72*(8), 668–672. https://doi.org/10.1136/jech-2017-210160.
10. EFSA Scientific Committee, More, S., Bampidis, V., Benford, D., Bragard, C., Halldorsson, T., & Naegeli, H. (2021). Statement on the derivation of Health-Based Guidance Values (HBGVs) for regulated products that are also nutrients. *EFSA Journal, 19*(11), e06479. https://doi.org/10.2903/j.efsa.2021.e06479.
11. EFSA, Arena, M., Auteri, D., Barmaz, S., Bellisai, G., Brancato, A., & Chiusolo, A. (2018). Peer review of the pesticide risk assessment of the active substance copper compounds copper(I), copper (II) variants namely copper hydroxide, copper oxychloride, tribasic copper sulfate, copper(I) oxide, Bordeaux mixture. *EFSA Journal, 16*(12), e05152. https://doi.org/10.2903/j.efsa.2018.e05152.
12. EFSA, Hernandez-Jerez, A., Adriaanse, P., Aldrich, A., Berny, P., & Millet, M. (2021). Statement of the PPR Panel on a framework for conducting the environmental exposure and risk assessment for transition metals when used as active substances in plant protection products (PPP). *EFSA Journal, 19*(12), e06498. https://doi.org/10.2903/j.efsa.2021.e06498.

13. Felgentreu, D., Herwig, N., & Hommel, B. (2017). Kupfergehalte in deutschen Obstbauregionen und deren Auswirkungen auf Regenwürmer. *Öko-Obstbau, 4*, 19–21.
14. Friis, K., Damgaard, C., & Holmstrup, M. (2004). Sublethal soil copper concentrations increase mortality in the earthworm *Aporrectodea caliginosa* during drought. *Ecotoxicology and Environmental Safety, 57*(1), 65–73. https://doi.org/10.1016/S0147-6513(03)00063-6.
15. Gill, J. P. K., Sethi, N., Mohan, A., Datta, S., & Girdhar, M. (2018). Glyphosate toxicity for animals. *Environmental Chemistry Letters, 16*(2), 401–426. https://doi.org/10.1007/s10311-018-0740-8.
16. Goulson, D. (2013). An overview of the environmental risks posed by neonicotinoid insecticides. *Journal of Applied Ecology, 50*(4), 977–987. https://doi.org/10.1111/1365-2664.12111.
17. Goulson, D. (2019). The insect apocalypse, and why it matters. *Current Biology, 29*(17), R967–R971. https://doi.org/10.1016/j.cub.2019.07.013.
18. Holzer, U., Kührer, E., & Blümel, S. (1994). Freilandversuche zur Wirkung verschiedener biologischer Pflanzenschutzmittel auf *Uncinula necator* (Oidium) und die Raubmilbenfauna im Weinbau. *Obst Wein Garten, 63*, 11–13.
19. Humann-Guilleminot, S., Binkowski, Ł. J., Jenni, L., Hilke, G., Glauser, G., & Helfenstein, F. (2019). A nation-wide survey of neonicotinoid insecticides in agricultural land with implications for Agri-environment schemes. *Journal of Applied Ecology, 56*(7), 1502–1514. https://doi.org/10.1111/1365-2664.13381.
20. Humann-Guilleminot, S., Laurent, S., Bize, P., Roulin, A., Glauser, G., & Helfenstein, F. (2021). Contamination by neonicotinoid insecticides in barn owls (*Tyto alba*) and Alpine swifts (*Tachymarptis melba*). *Science of The Total Environment, 785*, 147403. https://doi.org/10.1016/j.scitotenv.2021.147403.
21. IPBES. (2019). *Global Assessment Report on Biodiversity and Ecosystem Services of the Intergovernmental Science-Policy Platform on Biodiversity and Ecosystem Services*. IPBES Secretariat.
22. Karimi, B., Masson, V., Guilland, C., Leroy, E., Pellegrinelli, S., Giboulot, E., & Ranjard, L. (2021). Ecotoxicity of copper input and accumulation for soil biodiversity in vineyards. *Environmental Chemistry Letters, 19*(5), 2013–2030. https://doi.org/10.1007/s10311-021-01286-8.
23. Kruse-Plaß, M., Hofmann, F., Wosniok, W., Schlechtriemen, U., & Kohlschütter, N. (2021). Pesticides and pesticide-related products in ambient air in Germany. *Environmental Sciences Europe, 33*(1), 114. https://doi.org/10.1186/s12302-021-00500-5.
24. Kühne, S., Burth, U., & Marx, P. (2006). Biologischer Pflanzenschutz im Freiland. In *Pflanzengesundheit im Ökologischen Landbau*. Ulmer.
25. Lewis, K. A., Tzilivakis, J., Warner, D. J., & Green, A. (2016). An international database for pesticide risk assessments and management. *Human and Ecological Risk Assessment: An International Journal, 22*(4), 1050–1064.
26. Lopes, M. P., Fernandes, K. M., Tomé, H. V. V., Gonçalves, W. G., Miranda, F. R., Serrão, J. E., & Martins, G. F. (2018). Spinosad-mediated effects on the walking ability, midgut, and Malpighian tubules of Africanized honey bee workers. *Pest Management Science, 74*(6), 1311–1318.
27. Mackie, K. A., Müller, T., Zikeli, S., & Kandeler, E. (2013). Long-term copper application in an organic vineyard modifies spatial distribution of soil micro-organisms. *Soil Biology and Biochemistry, 65*, 245–253.

28. Marchand, P. A. (2016). Basic substances under EC 1107/2009 phytochemical regulation: Experience with non-biocide and food products as biorationals. *Journal of Plant Protection Research, 56*(4), 312–318.
29. Marchand, P. A. (2022). Evolution of plant protection active substances in Europe: The disappearance of chemicals in favor of biocontrol agents. *Environmental Science and Pollution Research, 30, 1–17.*
30. McCallan, S. E. A. (1949). The nature of the fungicidal action of copper and sulfur. *Botanical Review, 15*(10), 629–643.
31. Mesnage, R. (2021). Coformulants in commercial herbicides. In R. Mesnage, J. Zaller, & B. F. Thomas (Eds.), *Herbicides: Chemistry, Efficacy, Toxicology, and Environmental Impacts* (pp. 87–112). Elsevier.
32. Mesnage, R., & Zaller, J. G. (Eds.). (2021). *Herbicides: Chemistry, Efficacy, Toxicology, and Environmental Impacts.* Elsevier.
33. Mesnage, R., Szekács, A., & Zaller, J. G. (2021). Herbicides: Brief history, agricultural use, and potential alternatives for weed control. In R. Mesnage, J. Zaller, & B. F. Thomas (Eds.), *Herbicides: Chemistry, Efficacy, Toxicology, and Environmental Impacts* (pp. 1–20). Elsevier.
34. Mostafalou, S., & Abdollahi, M. (2017). Pesticides: An update of human exposure and toxicity. *Archives of Toxicology, 91*(2), 549–599.
35. Persson, L., Carney Almroth, B. M., Collins, C. D., Cornell, S., de Wit, C. A., Diamond, M. L., & Ryberg, M. W. (2022). Outside the safe operating space of the planetary boundary for novel entities. *Environmental Science & Technology, 56*(3), 1510–1521.
36. Portier, C. J., Armstrong, B. K., Baguley, B. C., Baur, X., Belyaev, I., Bellé, R., & Bruzzi, P. (2016). Differences in the carcinogenic evaluation of glyphosate between the International Agency for Research on Cancer (IARC) and the European Food Safety Authority (EFSA). *Journal of Epidemiology & Community Health, 70*(7), 741–745.
37. Riedo, J., Wettstein, F. E., Rösch, A., Herzog, C., Banerjee, S., Büchi, L., & Bucheli, T. D. (2021). Widespread occurrence of pesticides in organically managed agricultural soils—The ghost of a conventional agricultural past? *Environmental Science & Technology, 55*(5), 2919–2928.
38. Robin, D. C., & Marchand, P. A. (2021). The slow decrease of active substance candidates for substitution in the framework of the European pesticide regulation (EC) No 1107/2009. *European Journal of Risk Regulation, 2021*, 1–22.
39. Robin, D. C., & Marchand, P. A. (2022). Expansion of the low-risk substances in the framework of the European pesticide regulation (EC) No 1107/2009. *European Journal of Risk Regulation, 13*(3), 514–531.
40. Romanazzi, G., Orçonneau, Y., Moumni, M., Davillerd, Y., & Marchand, P. A. (2022). Basic substances, a sustainable tool to complement and eventually replace synthetic pesticides in the management of pre and postharvest diseases: Reviewed instructions for users. *Molecules, 27*(11), 3484.
41. Sanders, J., & Heß, J. (Eds.). (2019). *Leistungen des ökologischen Landbaus für Umwelt und Gesellschaft* (2nd ed.). Johann Heinrich von Thünen-Institut.
42. Schulz, R., Bub, S., Petschick, L. L., Stehle, S., & Wolfram, J. (2021). Applied pesticide toxicity shifts toward plants and invertebrates, even in GM crops. *Science, 372*(6537), 81–84.

43. SCNAT. (2021). Pestizide: Auswirkungen auf Umwelt, Biodiversität und Ökosystemleistungen. *Swiss Academies Factsheets, 16*(1), 12.

44. Senthil-Nathan, S. (2015). A review of biopesticides and their mode of action against insect pests. In P. Thangavel & G. Sridevi (Eds.), *Environmental Sustainability: Role of Green Technologies* (pp. 49–63). Springer.

45. Simon-Delso, N., Amaral-Rogers, V., Belzunces, L. P., Bonmatin, J. M., Chagnon, M., Downs, C., & Girolami, V. (2015). Systemic insecticides (neonicotinoids and fipronil): Trends, uses, mode of action and metabolites. *Environmental Science and Pollution Research, 22*(1), 5–34.

46. Steffen, W., Richardson, K., Rockström, J., Cornell, S. E., Fetzer, I., Bennett, E. M., & de Wit, C. A. (2015). Planetary boundaries: Guiding human development on a changing planet. *Science, 347*(6223), 736–746.

47. Stein-Bachinger, K., Preißel, S., Kühne, S., & Reckling, M. (2022). More diverse but less intensive farming enhances biodiversity. *Trends in Ecology & Evolution, 37*(5), 395–396.

48. Straw, E. A., & Brown, M. J. F. (2021). Co-formulant in a commercial fungicide product causes lethal and sub-lethal effects in bumble bees. *Scientific Reports, 11*, 21653.

49. Tang, F. H. M., Lenzen, M., McBratney, A., & Maggi, F. (2021). Risk of pesticide pollution at the global scale. *Nature Geoscience, 14*(4), 206–210.

50. Tarazona, J. V., González-Caballero, M. de C., Alba-Gonzalez, M. de, Pedraza-Diaz, S., Cañas, A., Dominguez-Morueco, N., & Katsonouri, A. (2022). Improving the risk assessment of pesticides through the integration of human biomonitoring and food monitoring data: A case study for chlorpyrifos. *Toxics, 10*(6), 313.

51. Topping, C. J., Aldrich, A., & Berny, P. (2020). Overhaul environmental risk assessment for pesticides. *Science, 367*(6476), 360–363.

52. van der Sluijs, J. P. (2020). Insect decline, an emerging global environmental risk. *Current Opinion in Environmental Sustainability, 46*, 39–42.

53. van Hoesel, W., Tiefenbacher, A., Koönig, N., Dorn, V. M., Hagenguth, J. F., Prah, U. A., & Bonkowski, M. (2017). Single and combined effects of pesticide seed dressings and herbicides on earthworms, soil microorganisms, and litter decomposition. *Frontiers in Plant Science, 8*, 215.

54. Zadoks, J. C. (2013). *Crop Protection in Medieval Agriculture: Studies in Pre-Modern Organic Agriculture*. Sidestone Press.

55. Zaller, J. G. (2020). *Daily Poison. Pesticides—An Underestimated Danger*. Springer Nature.

56. Zaller, J. G., König, N., Tiefenbacher, A., Muraoka, Y., Querner, P., Ratzenböck, A., & Koller, R. (2016). Pesticide seed dressings can affect the activity of various soil organisms and reduce decomposition of plant material. *BMC Ecology, 16*, 37.

57. Zaller, J. G., Kruse-Plaß, M., Schlechtriemen, U., Gruber, E., Peer, M., Nadeem, I., & Landler, L. (2022). Pesticides in ambient air, influenced by surrounding land use and weather, pose a potential threat to biodiversity and human. *Science of the Total Environment, 838*, 156012.

58. Zaller, J. G., Weber, M., Maderthaner, M., Gruber, E., Takács, E., Mörtl, M., & Leisch, F. (2021). Effects of glyphosate-based herbicides and their active ingredients on earthworms, water infiltration and glyphosate leaching are influenced by soil properties. *Environmental Sciences Europe, 33*, 51.

Chapter 5

EXPLORING ENVIRONMENTAL TOXICOLOGY: UNDERSTANDING THE IMPACT OF POLLUTANTS ON ECOSYSTEM AND HUMAN HEALTH

Contents

Introduction

The extensive utilization of various chemicals is fundamentally connected with agricultural and industrial practices. Historically, chemical wastes produced by industrial processes were often disposed of by being released directly into the environment. Gaseous emissions quickly dispersed into the atmosphere, whereas liquid wastes were diluted in bodies of water, swiftly transporting them away from their points of origin (Dai et al., 2020). Similarly, herbicides and other agricultural chemicals have played significant roles in enhancing forest and farm productivity. Initially, the environmental risks posed by these chemicals were considered negligible when weighed against the benefits they provided. However, the publication of Rachel Carson's "Silent Spring" in 1962 marked a pivotal moment. Carson, a scientist with the U.S. Fish and Wildlife Service, began her influential book by imagining a world without birds, using this scenario to highlight the dire consequences of pesticide use. Through her narrative, she detailed numerous instances of mass die-offs of fish and birds, attributing these to pesticide applications in diverse environments ranging from residential areas to national parks. She argued that the observable effects on wildlife could foreshadow similar detrimental impacts on human health (Rehman et al., 2019).

This increased public awareness about the potential hazards of chemical pollutants led to the initiation of several key environmental movements and legislative actions, including the first Earth Day, the creation of the United States Environmental Protection Agency (EPA), and the enactment of various laws aimed at controlling and limiting chemical discharges into the environment. Proper regulation of these discharges, without overly stringent constraints on agricultural and industrial activities, requires an in-depth understanding of the toxicological properties and environmental consequences of these chemicals. This need gave rise to the field of environmental toxicology (Bailer & Piegorsch, 2000).

Environmental toxicology is the study concerned with the destiny and effects of chemicals in natural settings. While it includes naturally occurring toxins—like microbial, animal venoms, and plant toxins—the field is predominantly associated with the analysis of chemicals derived from human activities, known as anthropogenic chemicals (Rittschof et al., 2005). Environmental toxicology is divided into two main areas: environmental health toxicology, which examines the adverse effects of natural and anthropogenic chemicals on human health, and ecotoxicology, which focuses on the impact of environmental pollutants on ecosystems and their constituents such as wildlife and aquatic organisms. The assessment of the harmful effects on human health often employs established animal models like rats and mice, alongside epidemiological studies of human populations exposed to these chemicals, such as factory workers and farmers (Matthews et al., 1996). Ecotoxicology, in contrast, studies the adverse effects of toxic substances on a broad array of ecosystem inhabitants, from microorganisms to apex predators.

Moreover, a comprehensive understanding of chemical impacts in the environment extends beyond toxicology to include studies of a chemical's fate in the environment and interactions with nonliving (abiotic) elements of ecosystems. Thus, the broad analyses of the detrimental effects of chemicals rely on interdisciplinary contributions from various scientific fields. The ultimate objectives of these studies are to identify the adverse effects of chemicals that are already present in the environment (retrospective hazard assessment) and to predict potential negative impacts before new chemicals are released (predictive hazard assessment) (Eason et al., 1999).

Orientation and Directional Terms

Term	Definition	Illustration
Non-Biological Breakdown Process	The process by which materials are broken down or degraded by physical or chemical means, rather than through the action of living organisms.	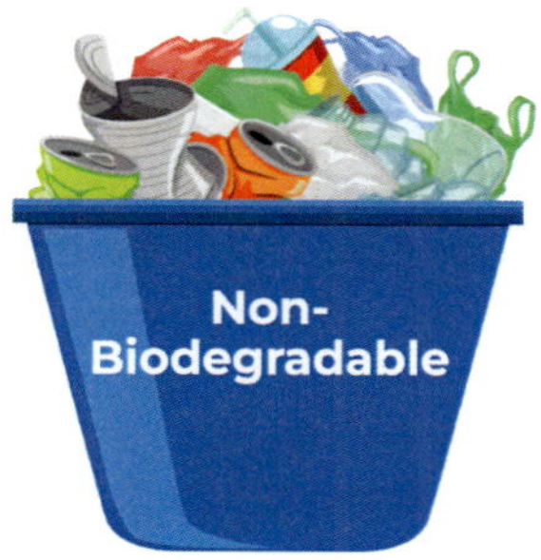
Biological Decomposition	The process by which organic substances are broken down into simpler organic or inorganic matter through the action of microorganisms, fungi, or other biological activity.	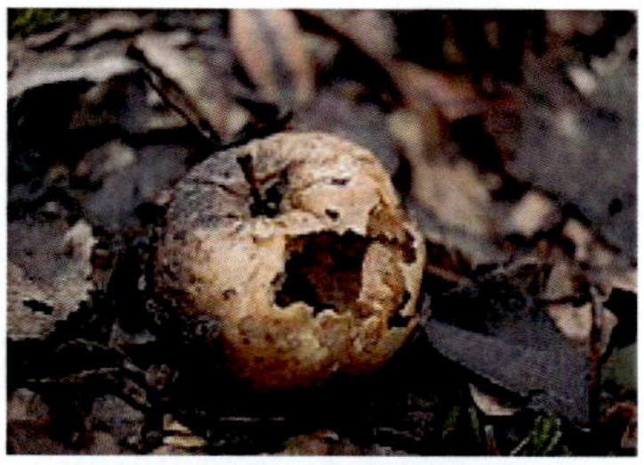
Biological Remediation Techniques	Methods that use biological organisms, such as plants, bacteria, or fungi, to remove or neutralize contaminants from soil, water, or other environments.	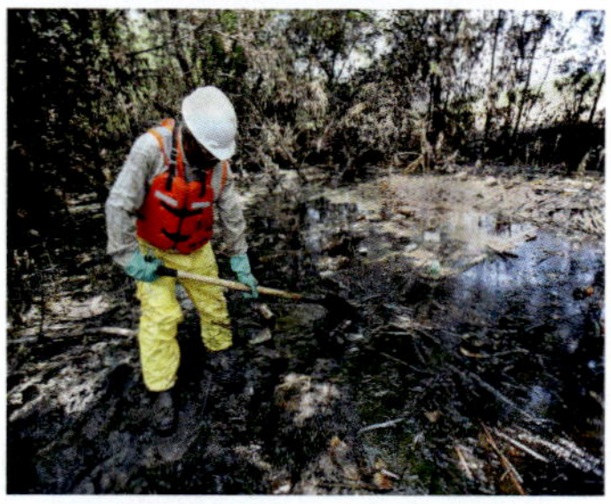
Bioaccumulation	The gradual accumulation of substances, such as pesticides or other chemicals, in an organism. This occurs when the organism absorbs a substance at a rate faster than it can be metabolized or excreted.	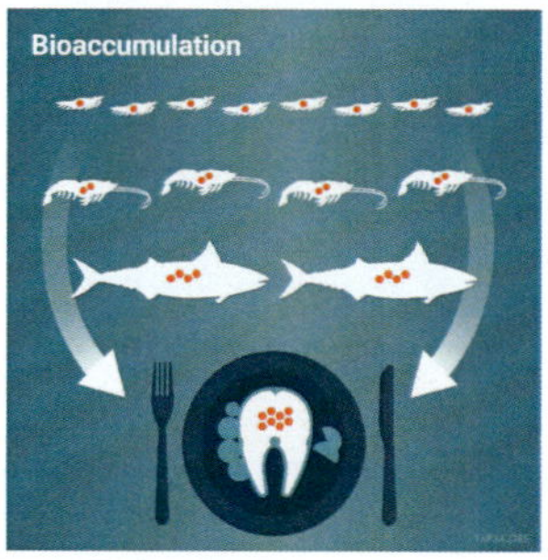
Environmental Toxicology	The study of the harmful effects of various chemical, biological, and physical agents on living organisms, including humans, within the context of the environment.	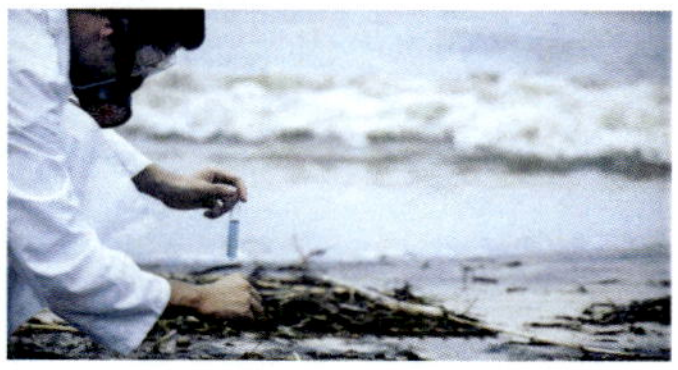

5.1. Environmental Persistence: The Enduring Presence and Impact of Chemicals in Ecosystems Over Time

In the natural environment, a variety of biotic (biological) and abiotic (non-biological) mechanisms work collaboratively to mitigate the impact of harmful substances by processes such as decomposition. Many chemicals that are released into the atmosphere have relatively short lifespans due to these mechanisms, leading to a minimal risk posed by their presence (Kotwal & Cannon, 2014). However, some chemicals have historically been a major environmental concern, such as TCDD (dioxin), PCBs (polychlorinated biphenyls), and DDT (dichlorodiphenyltrichloroethane), which are notoriously resistant to natural metabolic and decomposing processes (Figure 5.1).

Figure 5.1. *Persistence, environmental hazards, and mitigation of pharmaceutically active residual contaminants.*

Source: By Unknown author - EPS file pollu.eps from UNECE web site converted with ImageMagick convert and with potrace, edited in inkscape, Public Domain; https://commons.wikimedia.org/w/index.php?curid=4984008.

Consequently, these substances can remain in the environment for prolonged periods, as indicated in detailed studies like those summarized in Table 5.1.

The persistence of such chemicals in the environment means they can continue to accumulate over time, reaching levels that may induce toxicity in ecosystems. Even long after their initial discharge or disposal has ceased, these persistent environmental contaminants can continue to pose significant threats. A notable historical example of such contamination occurred during the 1950s and 1970s when Lake Ontario was heavily polluted by the herbicide mirex, leading to severe ecological damage (Webster et al., 1998).

This example underscores the lasting impact of persistent toxicants and highlights the critical need for ongoing vigilance and effective management strategies to protect environmental and public health from such enduring chemical hazards.

Table 5.1. *Certain Environmental Half-Lives of Chemical Pollutants*

Pollutant	Media	Half-Life
TCDD	Soil	9 Years
DDT	Soil	10 Years
Benzoperylene (PAH)	Soil	14 Months
Atrazine	Water	25 Months
Carbofuran	Water	45 Days
Phenanthrene (PAH)	Soil	138 Days

Source: *(Council et al., 2010)*

5.1.1. Non-Biological Breakdown Processes

The degradation of chemicals in the environment is influenced by a range of environmental factors that threaten their structural integrity. Among these, light (via photolysis) and water (via hydrolysis) play pivotal roles in several key abiotic degradation processes (Jakubowicz et al., 2006):

1. **Photolysis:** This process involves the breakdown of chemical bonds under the influence of light, particularly ultraviolet (UV) light, which plays a critical role in the environmental degradation of certain compounds. Photolysis is most effective in areas exposed to high light intensities, such as the atmosphere or surface waters. The susceptibility of contaminants to photolysis depends significantly on their ability to absorb photons, particularly those compounds with unsaturated aromatic structures like polycyclic aromatic hydrocarbons. These molecules are notably prone to photolysis due to their high photon absorption capabilities. Additionally, light energy can facilitate the oxidation of pollutants, leading to their transformation through oxidative or hydrolytic reactions. An illustrative example of this is the photooxidation of the organophosphorus (OP) insecticide parathion. (Albertsson et al., 1994).
2. **Hydrolysis:** In this process, water interacts with chemicals, often facilitated by heat and light, to break chemical bonds. Hydrolysis typically involves the insertion of an oxygen atom into a chemical structure, resulting in the loss of a fragment of the molecule. This reaction is particularly prevalent in compounds with ester bonds, such as those found in organophosphate pesticides (e.g., parathion). These bonds are highly susceptible to hydrolysis, significantly reducing the environmental persistence, or half-lives, of these chemicals. Factors such as temperature and pH levels in the water significantly influence the rate of hydrolysis; generally, increases in temperature and optimal pH levels accelerate the hydrolysis process (Gliksman et al., 2017).

These mechanisms of abiotic degradation are essential for understanding how chemicals disintegrate in the environment, which is critical for assessing their long-term impact on ecosystems and formulating strategies for pollution control and remediation.

5.1.2. Biological Breakdown and Decomposition

Whereas several environmental pollutants are amenable to abiotic degradative procedures, these procedures are frequently sluggish. The activities of microorganisms in the environment may dramatically accelerate the breakdown of chemical pollutants. Chemicals are degraded by microorganisms (mainly fungi and bacteria) to obtain energy from them. Such enzyme-mediated biotic degradative procedures often happen at rates considerably above abiotic disintegration (Gliksman et al., 2017). Chemicals may be completely mineralized by biotic degradative procedures resulting in carbon dioxide, water, and primary inorganic elements. Biotic disintegration comprises procedures like the scission of ringed structures (ring cleavage), the elimination of chlorine atoms (dehalogenation), and the elimination of carbon chains (dealkylation), as well as those connected with abiotic disintegration (e.g., oxidation and hydrolysis). Bioremediation is the technique of using microorganisms to aid in the release of toxins from the atmosphere (Hakkarainen, 2002) (Figure 5.2).

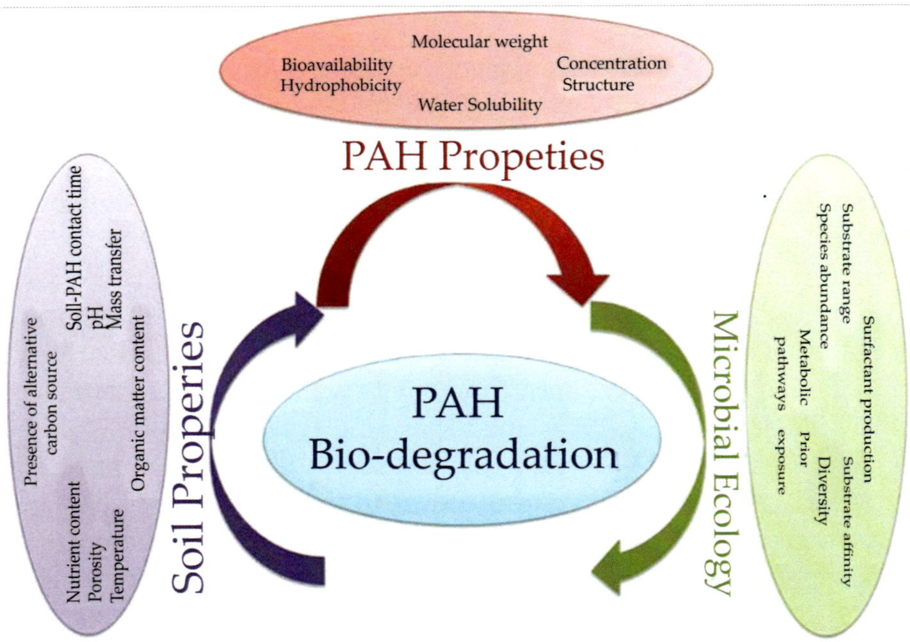

Figure 5.2. *Abiotic and biotic factors influencing the degradation of PAHs in soil.*

Source: Salari, M., Rahmanian, V., Hashemi, S. A., Chiang, W. H., Lai, C. W., Mousavi, S. M., & Gholami, A., (2022). Bioremediation treatment of polyaromatic hydrocarbons for environmental sustainability. Water, 14(23), 3980. https://doi.org/10.3390/w14233980.

5.1.3. Non-Degradative Elimination Processes

Several mechanisms are at work in the atmosphere that help to eliminate a pollutant from an area by shifting its distribution. Pollutants with a higher enough vapor pressure may evaporate from polluted aquatic or terrestrial divisions and be transported to other sites through the environment. Global distillation procedures have been thought to be substantially responsible for the largest spread of relatively volatile organochlorine pesticides like hexachlorobenzene and lindane (Lai et al., 2008). Pollutant distribution has been further aided by the entrainment of pollutant particles or dust upon which the pollutants have been sorbed via wind and higher environmental currents. The release of pollutants from the water column and their distribution into bottom sediments might arise from contamination sorption to suspended particles in an aquatic environment alongside concomitant sedimentation. Because a lipophilic chemical's propensity to segregate from sediments to organisms is substantially smaller than its propensity to split from water to organism, sediment sorption greatly lowers bioavailability. Soil percolation and r runoff may eliminate and disperse more extremely water-soluble pollutants. The herbicide atrazine, for instance, is among the most widely utilized herbicides in the U.S. (Kim et al., 2012). It is utilized in agriculture and landscaping to reduce weed and broadleaf grasses. Because of its widespread usage, atrazine is found in abundance in surface waters. Atrazine had been detected in 92% of the reservoirs tested in a study of midwestern states. Furthermore, due to its relatively higher water solubility and little proclivity to bind to soil particles, atrazine has a significant likelihood of migrating into groundwater. Furthermore, field investigations have demonstrated that atrazine spraying on the surface usually leads to aquifer pollution underneath the application site (Garcia et al., 1992).

5.2. Biological Remediation Techniques

Bioremediation is a technique for cleaning up contaminated environments by converting toxic heavy metals into less dangerous conditions utilizing enzymes or bacteria. The approach is both ecologically benign and cost-effective in terms of environmental regeneration. Heavy metal bioremediation involves limits. Microbes' generation of hazardous metabolites and heavy metals' non-biodegradability are two examples (Vidali, 2001).

Direct application of microorganisms having specific catabolic capabilities and their products, like enzymes and biosurfactants, is a new way to improve and augment its remediation effectiveness. Various options are also proposed to broaden the scope of microbiological methods' use in the heavy metal cleanup. The usage of a microbial fuel cell (MFC) to digest resistant heavy metals, for example, is investigated. Heavy metal-polluted environments may be cleaned up via biofilm-mediated bioremediation (Iwamoto & Nasu, 2001).

Microbial technologies are alive and well, and they're only getting started. The interaction of microorganisms with metals in natural and man-made settings has a long history. Metals elimination, for example, pollution removal and remediation, is the primary focus of microbial-metal interactions (Boopathy, 2000). The resurgence of solid-state electrodes as electron acceptors or donors for microorganism growth has ushered in new possibilities, leading to microbial-electrochemical technology (METs). It is claimed that microorganisms can be used to synthesize metallic nanoparticles (NPs) in a green way. As a remedial strategy, genetically engineered microbes have also been deployed. Chemical modification and g Genetic engineering may change the elements of a cell's surface, increasing adsorption capability and specificity for target metal species (Atlas, 1995) (Figure 5.3).

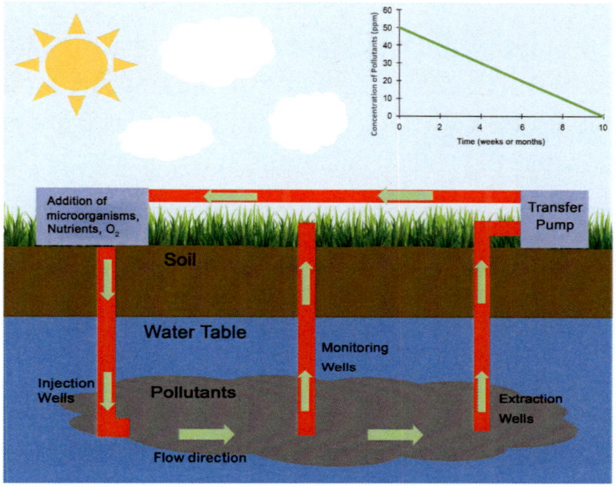

Figure 5.3. *Bioremediation.*

Source: By Hoodlind – Own work, CC BY-SA 4.0; https://commons.wikimedia.org/w/index.php?curid=64647624.

5.3. Bioaccumulation

A chemical's persistence in the environment doesn't make it a hazard to the environment. If a chemical can't penetrate the bodies of living beings, it poses no risk of toxicity. Once ingested, the chemical should build up in the body to the point where it causes toxicity. The mechanism through which organisms acquire chemicals both immediately from the abiotic environment (e.g., air, soil, and water) and via food resources is known as bioaccumulation (trophic transfer). Chemicals in the environment are mostly absorbed by organisms through passive diffusion. The membranes of the gills, lungs, and gastrointestinal system are the main routes of absorption. Whereas the integument (skin) and related structures (feathers, scales, hair, etc.) include a protective layer against several environmental assaults, certain substances may be absorbed through the skin. Since substances should pass through the lipid bilayer of membranes to penetrate the skin, their bioaccumulation potential is proportional to their lipid solubility (lipophilicity) (Franke et al., 1994).

Lipophilic substances cross the hurdle between the abiotic environment and the biota most often in the aquatic atmosphere. This is because (1) rivers, lakes, and seas serve as sinks for such chemicals, and (2) aquatic creatures transport massive amounts of water over their respiratory membranes (e.g., gills), enabling effective chemical extraction from the water (Bryan & Darracott, 1979).

Lipophilic substances may bioaccumulate in aquatic species, resulting in concentrations of the body that have been many orders of magnitude higher than the chemical's concentration in the environment (Table 5.2). Because body lipids act as the principal location of preservation of chemicals, the extent to which aquatic species acquire xenobiotics from the atmosphere is primarily determined by their lipid composition (Luoma & Rainbow, 2005).

Chemicals may also be passed down the food chain from the victim to the hunter (trophic transfer). For each successive link in the food chain, such transmission may result in rising amounts of highly lipophilic substances (biomagnification).

A chemical that bioaccumulates by a factor of two, irrespective of whether the pollutant has been detected in food or water, can amplify at every trophic level, resulting in higher levels in birds of prey compared to the abiotic environment (Van der Oost et al., 2003).

Table 5.2. *Fish Bioaccumulation of Certain Environmental Pollutants*

Chemical	Bioaccumulation Facto[r]a
TCDD	39,000
DDT	1,27,000
Pentachlorobenzene	5,000
Endrin	6,800
Trichlorobenzene	183
Lepthophos	750

Source: https://pubs.acs.org/doi/10.1021/es00064a008.

Notably, bioaccumulation is often far stronger in water than in food, and this is unusual that an organism will acquire the same amount of a chemical both from resources. Several bird-eating raptor communities declined due to the transmission of DDT via the food chain, which led to the decision to limit the usage of this pesticide in the U.S. (Morel et al., 1998).

Because the toxicant can be firstly stored in lipid deposits but then deployed to target areas of toxicity whenever these lipid reserves have been used, bioaccumulation may result in a delayed start of toxicity. Lipid storage, for instance, has been often deployed in readiness for regeneration. The loss of the lipid may lead to the discharge of lipophilic toxicants, allowing them to be toxic. Mature organisms may die when they reach reproductive maturity as a consequence of these impacts (Chojnacka, 2010).

5.3.1. Factors That Influence Bioaccumulation

Certain variables impact the likelihood of an environmental toxin bioaccumulating. The very first factor to examine is environmental stability. The amount of a chemical that bioaccumulates is determined by its concentration in the environment (Aladesanmi et al., 2019). Bioaccumulation would not be possible with pollutants that have been easily removed from the atmosphere. Instances, when the contamination is constantly delivered into the ecosystem, will be an exception (e.g., water that is treated after an effluent release has occurred) (Bryan & Darracott, 1979).

As previously stated, lipophilicity is an important factor in determining a chemical's bioaccumulation potential. Lipophilic compounds, on the other hand, have a higher proclivity for sorbing sediments, making them less bioaccumulate. The sorption of benzo[a]pyrene to humic acids, for instance, decreased its proclivity to bioaccumulate in sunfish about 3 times. Fish in oligotrophic lakes with low suspended solid levels are found to collect more DDT as compared to fish in eutrophic lakes with higher suspended solid concentrations (Menéndez-Pedriza & Jaumot, 2020).

The destiny of the pollutant once taken by the organism would impact its bioaccumulation. Chemicals that have been easily biotransformed become less lipid-soluble as well as more water-soluble. As a result, the biotransformed molecule is less likely to get into trouble in lipid partitions and is more prone to be excreted from the body (Rowan & Rasmussen, 1994). Chemicals that have been sensitive to biotransformation bioaccumulate far less than will be expected depending on lipophilicity, as shown in Table 5.3. By conjugating xenobiotics to glutathione and glucuronic acid, active transport mechanisms may target the xenobiotic for biliary clearance, considerably enhancing the rate of removal. Bioaccumulation differs between species due to variances in chemical removal rates (Frazier, 1979).

Table 5.3. *Measured and Predicted Bioaccumulation Factors in Fish of Chemicals That Differ in Susceptibility to Biotransformation*

Chemical Name	Measured Bioaccumulation Factor (BAF)	Predicted Bioaccumulation Factor (BAF)	Susceptibility to Biotransformation
Hexachlorobenzene	12,000	11,500	Low
DDT (dichlorodiphenyltrichloroethane)	15,000	14,000	Low
Atrazine	500	450	High
Bisphenol A	900	870	High
PCB 153 (polychlorinated biphenyl 153)	30,000	28,000	Low
Pyrene	1,800	1,700	Moderate

Source: (Blasco et al., 2016)

5.4. Toxicity

5.4.1. Acute Toxicity

The phrase "acute toxicity" refers to the kind of toxicity that may develop after only a brief encounter with a poisonous substance. Accidents (such as the derailing of a train that results in the release of a chemical into a river) and irresponsible usage of chemicals are typically to blame for instances of acute toxicity in the atmosphere (e.g., aerial drift of a herbicide to nontarget regions). Whenever adhered to, the discharge limitations that are put on urban and industrial wastes are largely effective in protecting species in waste-receiving regions against acute toxicity. It is usual practice to quantify the acute toxicity of a substance using either the LC_{50} or the LD_{50} (Lorke, 1983).

Such metrics don't give any insight into the amounts of pollutants that are considered to be ecologically tolerable (It is difficult to tolerate a concentration that kills 50% of the organisms that are exposed to it). The LD_{50} and LC_{50} values, on the other hand, do offer statistically reliable and reproducible measurements of the comparative acute toxicity of substances. LD_{50} and LC_{50} and LD_{50} levels, correspondingly, for both terrestrial and aquatic animal species (Kaise et al., 1985).

Experiments are conducted with certain species which act as representations of certain levels of trophic organization inside an ecosystem to evaluate the acute toxicity of environmental contaminants (such as birds, mammals, invertebrates, fish, algae, and vascular plants). When determining the standards for the quality of water, the United States Environmental Protection Agency (EPA), for instance, mandates that acute toxicity tests be conducted with representatives of minimum 8 distinct species of marine and freshwater organisms (sixteen tests), (Johnson, 2005) which may contain plants, invertebrates, and fish. Although it is common practice to try to classify different groups of creatures according to their sensitivity to toxicants, the reality is that no organism is uniformly less or more vulnerable to the acute toxicity of chemicals. In addition, the usage of standard species in the evaluation of toxicity tests on the assumption that such species have been "representative" of the sensitivity exhibited by other individuals belonging to that degree of ecological structure. These kinds of assumptions are frequently flawed (Gaines, 1969).

5.4.2. Chronic Toxicity

Chronic toxicity has been described as toxicity caused by repeated exposure to a toxicant over a lengthy period. Chronic toxicity is frequently accompanied having sublethal outcomes. Reproductive, endocrine, immunological, and developmental issues are among them. Chronic exposure, on the other hand, may lead to direct mortality that is not seen after acute exposure (Bernot et al., 2005). Chronic exposure to extremely lipophilic compounds, for instance, may lead to the chemical's bioaccumulation to levels that have been fatal to the organisms. Alternatively, as stated previously, during reproduction, the release of lipophilic toxins from lipid compartments can be fatal. It is vital to remember that while all substances can cause acute toxicity at a sufficiently large dosage, they aren't all chronically harmful (Wollenberger et al., 2000).

Chronic toxicity has been evaluated using endpoints like the greatest degree of a chemical that doesn't cause toxicity while continuous, extended exposure (no observed impact level, NOEL), the smallest degree of a chemical that causes toxicity while continuous, extended exposure (smallest observed impact level, LOEL), or the chronic value (CV), which has been the geometric mean of the LOEL and the NOEL. The acute chronic ratio (ACR), which has been computed by dividing the acute LC_{50} value by the CV, has been frequently used to assess a chemical's chronic toxicity. Chemicals having an ACR of fewer than ten are often linked with minimal or no long-term toxicity (Table 5.4) (Hu et al., 1998).

Table 5.4. *Chronic and Acute Toxicity of Pesticides Measuring Fish Exposures in the Laboratory*

Chlordecone	10	Extremely toxic	0.3	33	Yes
Endosulfan	166	Extremely toxic	4.3	39	Yes
Carbaryl	15,000	Moderately toxic	378	40	Yes
Malathion	3,000	Very toxic	340	8.8	No

Source: https://www.wiley.com/.

When determining a chemical's chronic toxicity, the following factors ought to be taken into account: (1) ACR-based simple numerical estimations of chronic toxicity are merely rough indications of the chemical's probable chronic toxicity. The majority of laboratory exposures used to determine CVs concentrate on a few basic endpoints including growth, survival, and reproductive potential (Smith, 1968; Kociba et al., 1978). Examining more subtle chronic toxicity endpoints can yield dramatically various 'CV.' (2) Laboratory exposures have been carried out on a limited number of test species which can be manipulated in the lab. With these species, the determination of chronic and ACR values must not be taken as absolute. Chronic toxicity can be elicited by toxicants in certain species but not in others. (3) Interactions between biotic and abiotic elements of the ecosystem can assist in chemical chronic toxicity, even if these interactions are unlikely to happen in laboratory tests of direct chemical toxicity. The below incidence of chronic toxicity of substances in the atmosphere exemplifies such factors (Scheuhammer, 1987).

5.4.3. Species-Specific Chronic Toxicity

Imposex in Neogastropods Induced by Tributyltin. In the 1970s, scientists discovered that dogwhelks on the English coast had a hermaphroditic-like condition in which females had a penis in addition to typical female genitalia. Whereas other molluscan species use hermaphroditism as a survival mechanism, dogwhelks are dioecious. About one hundred and forty species of neogastropods have been found to have this pseudohermaphroditic trait known as imposex. Imposex is linked to lower neogastropod population fertility, population reductions, and local elimination of afflicted populations (Bussiere et al., 2009).

The fact that imposex was mostly found at marinas identified a link to a pollutant that came from those establishments. Experiments in the field revealed that neogastropods moved from pristine areas to more often establish imposex. Tributyltin, a biocide utilized in marine paints, was finally identified as the cause of imposex in laboratory experiments. At low parts-per-billion quantities, tributyltin is harmful to most marine species tested in the lab. Exposed neogastropods to lower parts-per-trillion quantities, on the other hand, may produce imposex. As a result, neogastropods are particularly vulnerable to tributyltin toxicity, having impacts that have not been visible in normal laboratory toxicity characterizations (Lewis, 1990).

Frogs with Atrazine-Induced Hermaphroditism. The herbicide atrazine has long been thought to be ecologically harmless, as it is found to be just mildly to moderately hazardous in routine wildlife and fish toxicity tests. Surface water atrazine concentrations seldom surpass 0.04 mg/L. Atrazine's chronic and acute toxicity to aquatic species has been often more than 1 mg/L. As a result, this chemical appears to have plenty of safety margins. In current experiments involving frogs, it was shown that exposure to 0.0001 mg/L atrazine at the larval stage enabled the frogs to grow an ovary and a testis. Such chemical-induced hermaphroditic condition's toxicological relevance is unknown. Environmentally relevant doses of the herbicide, on the other hand, seem to can harm such creatures' reproductive success (Eldridge et al., 1999).

5.4.4. Biotic and Abiotic Interactions

Interactions between ozone, chlorofluorocarbons, amphibians, and UV-B radiation. The loss of the earth's stratospheric ozone layer, which acts as a filter against damaging UV radiation, is linked to the emission of chlorofluorocarbons into the atmosphere. UV-B radiation has been shown to rise with time, posing an increased risk of several diseases in both animal and plant life (Unrine et al., 2012).

Several amphibian populations have declined in tandem with the rise in UV-B radiation degrees at the earth's surface. Loss of habitat, contaminants, and increasing disease incidence are all possible explanations for such decreases; although, new research shows that rises in UV-B radiation can be a substantial factor in the fall in certain populations (Atkinson & Urwin, 2012). Field observations in Oregon's Cascade Mountains indicated a significant rate of death amongst western toad and Cascade frog embryos. The laboratory incubation of eggs acquired from the environment, together with the pond water wherein the eggs had been gathered, resulted in minimal mortality, indicating that pollutants in the water had not been directly responsible for the mortality. Moreover, placing UV-B filters over the embryos and incubating them in ambient settings dramatically boosted their vitality (Singh et al., 2009)

Photolyase activity was tested in a variety of amphibian species. This enzyme is in charge of repairing UV-B radiation-induced DNA damage. Between the species studied, there was an eighty-fold variability in photolyase activity. When contrasted to species with stable population numbers, photolyase activity had been much lower in species referred to be in decline. Current research has also revealed that high amounts of UV-B radiation in the environment might increase the vulnerability of frog embryos to fungal infection-related death (Plénet et al., 1995).

Such findings show that chlorofluorocarbons can play a role in amphibian population reduction. This toxicological impact, on the other hand, is the product of abiotic interactions (e.g., chlorofluorocarbons diminishing atmospheric ozone levels, increasing UV-B radiation absorption and leading to embryo death). Biotic (fungus) and Abiotic (UV-B) interactions might have a role in the toxicity. Direct laboratory analyses of chlorofluorocarbon toxicity to frogs will not anticipate these consequences, highlighting the need to consider indirect toxicity related to environmental pollutants (Bone et al., 2012). Microbial interactions having Kraft Pulpmill Effluent cause fish to become more masculine. Females with male features like male-type mating behavior and the alteration of the anal fin to mimic the sperm-transmitting gonopodium of males were discovered in field surveys of mosquito fish populations in the state of Florida (Kelts & Talbot, 1990). Masculinized females have been detected downstream of kraft pulp mill effluents, implying that effluent elements are to blame for the masculinizing impact. These impacts were not observed in direct toxicity studies using the wastewater. The addition of microbes to the wastewater, on the other hand, resulted in masculinization. Further research indicated that microorganisms may convert phytosterols in kraft pulp mill effluent to androgenic C19 steroids, which are able to masculinize female fish (Jeon et al., 2016).

Therefore, before this covert toxicity linked with the kraft pulp mill wastewater has been revealed, abiotic (phytosterols): and biotic (microorganisms) interactions in the atmosphere need to occur (Guillou, 1996).

Pollutants in the Disease and Atmosphere in Marine Mammals. Over the last twenty years, bottlenose dolphins, populations of harbor seals, and other marine animals all over the world have seen enormous mortality. Such mortality is ascribed to illness in several cases. In the 1980s, the phocine distemper virus killed over eighteen thousand harbor seals in the Irish, North, and Baltic seas. The illness epidemic was most severe in places with high levels of pollution, and seals who died from the sickness had significant amounts of polychlorinated biphenyls in their tissues (PCBs) (Sannino et al., 1999; Sloan et al., 2011). PCBs and other organochlorine chemicals like hexachlorobenzene, DDT, and dieldrin are found to decrease immune function in laboratory animals, and the exposure to such chemicals may have enhanced their vulnerability to the virus. This idea had been investigated by feeding fish to seals for 93 weeks, either from a reasonably pristine location or from a contaminated coastal area, and then evaluating the seals' immune systems. The immunological responses of seals fed the polluted fish were compromised, adding support to the theory that organochlorine toxins in the marine environment are leaving certain animals immunodeficient. Death happens as a result of increased vulnerability to infections, not as a direct result of chemical toxicity (Manyala & Ojuok, 2007).

5.5. Environmental Toxicology on Human Health

Compounds are increasingly being used, and human exposure to such chemicals and the toxicity that results has long been a worry. Toxicology is always related to poisons from a historical standpoint. Toxicology is derived from two Greek words: Toxicon, a deadly material used to dip arrowheads, and toxicos, a bow. Any chemical that hurts a biological system is considered a poison. In this regard, one of the most influential pioneers in the history of toxicology, Paracelsus (1493–1541), recognized the relevance of the dosage response connection. In this famous phrase, he neatly articulated this concept (Genchi et al., 2020):

"Every chemical is a poison; there isn't one that isn't poison.

The appropriate dose distinguishes between a poison and a cure."

—(Paracelsus)

Animal venoms, plant extracts, and minerals, such as lead, arsenic, opium, and cyanogenic glycosides, were among the first poisons employed for hunting, warfare, and governmental execution. Poisons nowadays include both hazardous naturally occurring compounds such as those found in plants, animals, and microbes, as well as manmade chemicals (Morais et al., 2012). Toxins are the name for the former, whereas toxicants are the word for the latter. Toxicants comprise manmade pharmaceuticals/chemicals with commercial value, like insecticides or medications, as well as those produced by anthropogenic activity, like incomplete combustion by-products (Zahir et al., 2005).

Toxicology can include a wide range of topics, including the detection, occurrence, characteristics, consequences, and control of dangerous chemicals. Toxicology, like medicine, has been a multidisciplinary field with various sub-disciplines, one of which is environmental toxicology. However, particularly in the realms of environmental, occupational, and regulatory toxicology, there is a lot of overlap across the many aspects of toxicology (Jaggi & Freedman, 1992; Asha et al., 2022). The mobility and influence of toxicants and their metabolites in food chains, in the environment, and on the function and structure of biological systems are the primary concerns of environmental toxicology. Every living system, like humans and other plants, animals, other species, and their surroundings, is included in biological systems. Biodiversity loss is among the most serious consequences of an environmental hazard. Biodiversity is a term that refers to genes, species, and ecosystems (Rehman et al., 2019). It has been derived from the word "biological diversity." Species from the animal and plant kingdoms, bacteria, fungi, viruses, protozoa, and ecological complexes like the tundra, coral reefs, and the rainforest all contribute to the variety. The focus of this issue would be on the negative consequences of environmental toxicants on the health of humans, instead of on ecological changes in the climate. In this regard, environmental health, a relatively young and related profession, plays a vital role in generating information about the negative health impacts of environmental stressors (Bols et al., 2005).

5.6. Environmental Toxicology's Historical Effects on Human Health

Environmental health refers to the characteristics of people's health, such as life quality, which are influenced by environmental variables such as biological, physical, psychological, and social factors. It also includes the idea and practice of identifying, addressing, and preventing environmental issues that may harm the health of current and future generations. Environmental toxicology has been a relatively new field, and Rachel Carson (1962), the author of Silent Spring, is credited with its quick growth and improvement (Oberdörster et al., 2007). Carson's main goal at the time had been to stop pesticides and other chemicals from being used widely and without regard. This has the effect of raising public awareness about the hazards of chemical pollution to the environment. In a short, she conveyed her elevated effect message: Spring is the season of rebirth and bird song for as far as man is on this earth. Several birds have died as a result of our reckless effort to control our atmosphere through the usage of chemicals that pollute not just insects against which they have been directed, but also the birds in the air, the fish in the rivers, the earth that provides our meals, and, invariably (to the what degree is still unidentified), the man himself (Nordberg, 2009; Völker & Kistemann, 2011).

In the 1970s, scientists concerned with environmental toxins increasingly concentrated their study on the effects of biological warfare agents, industrial pollution, and mine discharge. In the following decade, the importance of environmental toxicology to contemporary society became apparent with the discharge of forty-five tons of toxic methyl isocyanate gas from a plant and the discharge of huge amounts of radioactive material into the environment following the blast of a nuclear reactor (Calabrese, 2011). The Bhopal tragedy murdered between fifteen thousand and twenty thousand people and left tens of thousands more with severe illnesses. The Chornobyl disaster resulted in the deaths of thousands of people and the poisoning of millions of acres of land across Europe. Environmental toxicology grew in popularity in the late twentieth and early twenty-first centuries. The disposal of medical and radioactive waste, as well as the effect of compounds that had been routinely discharged into environmental reservoirs, were among its main concerns (Sudakin, 2003).

As a result, the US Environmental Protection Agency established various regulatory rules to safeguard human health and the environment beginning in 1970. The rise of environmental consciousness in business has resulted in the birth of yet another major specialty known as occupational medicine. This discipline entails a thorough study of diseases that arise as a consequence of human exposure and are either professional or commercial in origin, and also methods for controlling and preventing the diseases. Furthermore, in recent ages, toxicologic plagues and disasters have become more prevalent occurrences, whether intentional or unintentional (Collins et al., 2008).

5.7. Environmental Chemicals and Human Health

Humans come into touch with a wide range of chemicals, either by accident due to their presence in the environment, through contact during occupational or leisure activities, or through the consumption of food ingredients. Whenever chemicals have been released into the atmosphere, all exposures are unavoidable, however, exposure to chemicals utilized in the industry is regulated via industrial hygiene and occupational safety, as well as the health standards and practices of such an industry (LaKind et al., 2004). Certain chemicals may be discharged into the atmosphere accidently, posing a hazard to public health. With the rising level of progress and the increased usage of industrial chemicals, it appears that no employment is completely free of exposure to a range of chemicals that might have negative impacts on biological tissues. Currently, over ten thousand chemical entities contribute to over 500 thousand items that have been employed in industries to manufacture a wide range of non-durable and durable goods. Most such compounds have certain toxicity data available, and the bulk of chemical makers consider it vital to get a minimum of a basic level of toxicity data on every substance they employ (Zeise et al., 2013; Bourdon-Lacombe et al., 2015). Drugs for medicinal reasons, as well as herbicides and insecticides, can be included in animal feed. If the animals are utilized for human consumption, there are restrictions on the number of chemicals that can be used and how long they must be removed. The usage of insecticides and pesticides in agriculture has allowed farmers to create more and the best products (Van der Schali et al., 1999), but there has been a risk that residues of such chemicals will be present whenever the food is eaten. Chemical preservatives added to processed foods have allowed some food preparations to persist and have a longer shelf life. Environmental toxicologists are interested in the constraints that should be respected for food additives, as well as the assessment of safety from the negative impacts of such compounds (Sexton et al., 2004; Clarkson et al., 2003).

5.8. Impact of Pollution

Human populations have been more urbanized as the world has become more industrialized. More than 50% of the population of the US lives on less than 5% of the total land area. Pollution of water via industrial products and inappropriate sewage disposal, and also contamination of the environment via industry and cars in densely populated regions, have produced a significant human health hazard (Nazir et al., 2019). While civilization has relied on the vast volume of the environment to dilute contaminant concentrations below efficient levels, it has now been clear that environmental dilution is restricted and is reliant upon meteorological conditions as well as the amount and scope of pollution produced. Gases, dust, and aerosols, as well as CO, acids, and alkalis, all contribute to pollution. Air pollution and water are not only unattractive, but they also expose vast populations to an infinite number of potentially dangerous compounds capable of causing recognized immediate injury and chronic debilitating sickness in people (Graff Zivin & Neidell, 2012).

Environmental toxicology is the field of

toxicology that deals with the unintentional exposure of biological tissue, particularly human tissue, to chemicals that have been essentially pollutants in the atmosphere, water, and food. This is the study of the causes, circumstances, consequences, and safety limitations of exposure to chemicals (Rusznak et al., 1994).

A Closer Look

Toxicity of Benzene

Benzene is a ubiquitous industrial chemical that poses significant toxicity risks due to its widespread use and presence in the environment. It is primarily found in petroleum products, making it a common pollutant in air, water, and soil. Benzene exposure occurs through inhalation, ingestion, and dermal contact, with the respiratory route being the most concerning due to its rapid absorption. Acute exposure to high levels of benzene can cause central nervous system effects, including dizziness, headaches, and unconsciousness. Chronic exposure, even at lower levels, is more insidious and alarming. Benzene is a well-established carcinogen, primarily linked to hematological malignancies such as leukemia. Its toxic mechanism involves the formation of reactive metabolites that damage bone marrow cells, leading to aplastic anemia and pancytopenia. Benzene also disrupts the normal functioning of the immune system, exacerbating the risk of infections and diseases. Furthermore, benzene's impact extends to the liver and kidneys, causing biochemical disruptions that affect their detoxifying capabilities. The genetic damage induced by benzene metabolites can result in mutations and chromosomal aberrations, contributing to its carcinogenic potential. Regulatory bodies have set exposure limits to minimize these risks, yet occupational and environmental exposures remain a concern, particularly in industries like petrochemicals, rubber, and plastics manufacturing. The persistence of benzene in the environment, combined with its high volatility, underscores the need for stringent monitoring and protective measures. Advances in analytical techniques have improved the detection of benzene and its metabolites, aiding in early diagnosis and intervention. Despite these measures, the pervasive nature of benzene and its potent toxicity necessitate ongoing research and policy efforts to mitigate its impact on public health.

Summary

- Environmental toxicology, often termed ecotoxicology, is a multidisciplinary field that integrates toxicology and environmental sciences to study the effects of natural or synthetic pollutants on the health of organisms and ecosystems. The discipline primarily addresses the toxic impacts of chemical, physical, and biological agents on living organisms, particularly animals, plants, and microbial species, and extends to include their potential impacts on human health and the environment.
- Environmental toxicology is the assessment of the levels at which environmental exposures to chemicals become harmful, understanding the mechanisms through which these chemicals exert their effects, and evaluating the long-term consequences of these exposures on ecosystems and human populations. The scope of this field covers a range of pollutants including heavy metals, organic compounds, pesticides, industrial chemicals, and emerging contaminants such as pharmaceuticals and nanomaterials.
- Environmental toxicologists study the pathways through which chemicals enter and affect biological systems. Common routes of exposure include inhalation, ingestion, and dermal absorption. Once inside an organism, toxic substances can undergo biotransformation, leading to the production of metabolites that may be more or less toxic than the original substance. These chemicals can affect individual organisms directly, or indirectly influence them through changes in their habitat and food sources.
- On the organism level, toxicants can cause acute or chronic health effects ranging from minor irritations to severe illnesses and death. For example, pesticides can disrupt the endocrine systems of wildlife, leading to reproductive failures and population declines. At the ecosystem level, the introduction of toxic substances can lead to biodiversity loss, shifts in species composition, and altered nutrient cycling. The infamous case of DDT, a pesticide that led to the decline in bird populations due to eggshell thinning, exemplifies the broader ecological impacts of toxic chemicals.
- The implications for human health are a significant concern of environmental toxicology. Humans can be exposed to environmental toxins through contaminated air, water, soil, or food. Long-term exposure to certain chemicals, such as asbestos or benzene, is known to cause serious health issues including cancers, respiratory illnesses, and neurological disorders. The discipline uses risk assessment methodologies to evaluate the potential health risks associated with environmental exposures and to guide public health policies.
- To mitigate the impacts of toxic substances, environmental toxicology informs regulatory standards and pollution control strategies. Regulations such as the U.S. Clean Air Act and the REACH (Registration, Evaluation, Authorization, and Restriction of Chemicals) legislation in the European Union are underpinned by toxicological data that dictate safe levels of chemical exposures. These regulations aim to protect both environmental and human health by controlling the release of pollutants into the environment and ensuring the safe use of chemicals.

- Therefore, environmental toxicology plays a crucial role in our understanding of the impacts of pollutants on the natural world and human health. By advancing our knowledge of toxic mechanisms and effects, it supports the development of strategies to prevent and mitigate pollution, ensuring a safer, healthier environment for future generations.

References

1. Azeredo, D. B. C., de Sousa Anselmo, D., Soares, P., Graceli, J. B., Magliano, D. C., & Miranda-Alves, L. (2023). Environmental endocrinology: Parabens hazardous effects on hypothalamic–pituitary–thyroid axis. *International Journal of Molecular Sciences, 24*, 15246.
2. Bai, Z., He, Y., Han, Z., & Wu, F. (2022). Leaching mechanism and health risk assessment of As and Sb in tailings of typical antimony mines: A case study in Yunnan and Guizhou Province, Southwest China. *Toxics, 10*, 777.
3. Beg, M. A., Beg, M. A., Zargar, U. R., Sheikh, I. A., Bajouh, O. S., Abuzenadah, A. M., & Rehan, M. (2023). Organotin antifouling compounds and sex-steroid nuclear receptor perturbation: Some structural insights. *Toxics, 11*, 25.
4. Bernard, A., & Dudler, V. (2022). Health risk assessment of dermal exposure to polycyclic aromatic hydrocarbons from the use of infant diapers. *International Journal of Environmental Research and Public Health, 19*, 14760.
5. Bianchi, J., Mantovani, M. S., & Marin-Morales, M. A. (2015). Analysis of the genotoxic potential of low concentrations of malathion on the *Allium cepa* cells and rat hepatoma tissue culture. *Journal of Environmental Science, 36*, 102–111.
6. Caicedo-Rivas, G., Salas-Moreno, M., & Marrugo-Negrete, J. (2023). Health risk assessment for human exposure to heavy metals via food consumption in inhabitants of middle basin of the Atrato River in the Colombian Pacific. *International Journal of Environmental Research and Public Health, 20*, 435.
7. Demir, E., & Kacew, S. (2023). Drosophila as a robust model system for assessing autophagy: A review. *Toxics, 11*, 682.
8. Demir, E., & Turna Demir, F. (2022). Drosophila: A promising model for evaluating the toxicity of environmental pollutants. *Karaelmas Science and Engineering Journal, 12*, 101–118.
9. Duess, J. W., Gosemann, J. H., Kaskova Gheorghescu, A., Puri, P., & Thompson, J. (2023). Y-27632 impairs angiogenesis on extra-embryonic vasculature in post-gastrulation chick embryos. *Toxics, 11*, 134.
10. Eom, H. (2023). Development of an improved sulfur-oxidizing bacteria-based ecotoxicity test for simple and rapid on-site application. *Toxics, 11*, 352.
11. Espino-Valdés, M. S., Rodríguez-Lozano, D. F., Gutiérrez, M., & Silva-Hidalgo, H. (2022). Relationship of fluoride concentration to well depth in an alluvial aquifer in a semiarid area. *Environments, 9*, 155.
12. Gloekler, L. E., de Gandiaga, E. J., Binczewski, N. R., Steimel, K. G., Massarsky, A., Kozal, J., Vincent, M., Zisook, R., LaGuardia, M. J., Dotson, S., et al. (2022). Evaluation of the safety and efficacy of hand sanitizer products marketed to children available during the COVID-19 pandemic. *International Journal of Environmental Research and Public Health, 19*, 14424.

13. Guan, Q., Li, Y., Wang, Z., Cao, J., Dong, Y., Ren, F., & Chen, Y. (2022). Monochromatic light pollution exacerbates high-fat diet-induced adipocytic hypertrophy in mice. *Cells, 11*, 3808.

14. Guerrero-Limón, G., Nivelle, R., Bich-Ngoc, N., Duy-Thanh, D., & Muller, M. (2023). A realistic mixture of persistent organic pollutants affects zebrafish development, behavior, and specifically eye formation by inhibiting the condensing I complex. *Toxics, 11*, 357.

15. Huang, X., Su, Z., Li, J., He, J., Zhao, N., Nie, L., Guan, B., Huang, Q., Zhao, H., Lu, G. D., et al. (2023). Downregulation of LncRNA GCLC-1 promotes microcystin-LR-induced malignant transformation of human liver cells by regulating GCLC expression. *Toxics, 11*, 162.

16. Jia, R., Han, J., Liu, X., Li, K., Lai, W., Bian, L., Yan, J., & Xi, Z. (2023). Exposure to polypropylene microplastics via oral ingestion induces colonic apoptosis and intestinal barrier damage through oxidative stress and inflammation in mice. *Toxics, 11*, 127.

17. Laganà, A., Visalli, G., Facciolà, A., Celesti, C., Iannazzo, D., & Di Pietro, A. (2023). Uptake of breathable nano- and micro-sized polystyrene particles: Comparison of virgin and oxidized nPS/mPS in human alveolar cells. *Toxics, 11*, 686.

18. Lee, H., Park, J., & Park, K. (2023). Mixture effects of bisphenol A and its structural analogs on estrogen receptor transcriptional activation. *Toxics, 11*, 986.

19. Malm, E., Vilhelmsson, A., Högfeldt, H., Deshayes, I., Källén, K., Hansson, S. R., Lindh, C. H., & Rylander, L. (2023). Maternal serum concentrations of per- and polyfluoroalkyl substances in early pregnancy and small for gestational age in Southern Sweden. *Toxics, 11*, 750.

20. Nazari, A., Hong, J., Taghizadeh-Hesary, F., & Taghizadeh-Hesary, F. (2022). Reducing virus transmission from heating, ventilation, and air conditioning systems of urban subways. *Toxics, 10*, 796.

21. Pan, Z., Huang, J., Hu, T., Zhang, Y., Zhang, L., Zhang, J., Cui, D., Li, L., Wang, J., & Wu, Q. (2023). Protective effects of selenium nanoparticles against bisphenol A-induced toxicity in porcine intestinal epithelial cells. *International Journal of Molecular Sciences, 24*, 7242.

22. Salk, J. J., & Kennedy, S. R. (2020). Next-generation genotoxicology: Using modern sequencing technologies to assess somatic mutagenesis and cancer risk. *Environmental and Molecular Mutagenesis, 61*, 135–151.

23. Sawadogo, B., Konaté, F. O., Konaté, Y., Traoré, O., Sossou, S. K., Sawadogo, E., Sourabié Ouattara, P. B., & Karambiri, H. (2023). Transfer of bisphenol A and trace metals from plastic packaging to mineral water in Ouagadougou, Burkina Faso. *International Journal of Environmental Research and Public Health, 20*, 6908.

24. Seyyedsalehi, M. S., Mohebbi, E., Tourang, F., Sasanfar, B., Boffetta, P., & Zendehdel, K. (2023). Association of dietary nitrate, nitrite, and N-nitroso compounds intake and gastrointestinal cancers: A systematic review and meta-analysis. *Toxics, 11*, 190.

25. Taylor, B. K., Smith, O. V., & Miller, G. E. (2023). Chronic home radon exposure is associated with higher inflammatory biomarker concentrations in children and adolescents. *International Journal of Environmental Research and Public Health, 20*, 246.

26. Wu, X., Li, P., Tao, J., Chen, X., & Zhang, A. (2023). Subchronic low-dose methylmercury exposure accelerated cerebral telomere shortening in relevant with declined urinary aMT6s level in rats. *Toxics, 11*, 191.

27. Xu, X., Wu, H., Terry, P. D., Zhao, L., & Chen, J. (2022). Impact of paraben exposure on adiposity-related measures: An updated literature review of population-based studies. *International Journal of Environmental Research and Public Health, 19*, 16268.

28. Xue, J., Xiao, Q., Zhang, M., Li, D., & Wang, X. (2023). Toxic effects and mechanisms of polybrominated diphenyl ethers. *International Journal of Molecular Sciences, 24*, 13487.

29. Yao, T., Sun, P., & Zhao, W. (2023). Triazine herbicides risk management strategies on environmental and human health aspects using in-silico methods. *International Journal of Molecular Sciences, 24*, 5691.

Chapter

TOXICITY AND MECHANISMS OF OCCUPATIONAL POLLUTANTS

6

Contents

Introduction

Occupational toxicology is a specialized branch of toxicology that focuses on the study and understanding of the health risks associated with chemical, biological, and physical agents encountered in the workplace. This field plays a critical role in ensuring workplace safety by identifying potential hazards, assessing risks, and helping to implement effective control measures to protect workers from harmful exposures.

The primary objective of occupational toxicology is to understand how occupational exposures affect worker health and to determine safe exposure levels. Toxicologists in this field study the effects of various substances that workers might be exposed to in industries such as manufacturing, agriculture, healthcare, and construction. Common hazards include solvents, metals, dust, gases, and radiation, each posing unique risks requiring specific safety measures.

Occupational exposures can occur through inhalation, skin contact, or ingestion. The route of exposure significantly influences the toxicity of a substance. For instance, inhalation of asbestos fibers can lead to severe respiratory diseases, including lung cancer and mesothelioma, while dermal exposure to chemicals like benzene can cause skin irritation or systemic toxicity.

Effects of occupational exposures can range from mild, acute reactions such as skin irritation and respiratory distress to severe, chronic outcomes including neurotoxicity, reproductive toxicity, and carcinogenicity. Occupational toxicologists work to identify both the immediate and delayed health effects of substance exposures. For example, prolonged exposure to lead can cause severe damage to the nervous system and kidneys over time.

Occupational toxicologists perform risk assessments to evaluate the likelihood and severity of adverse health outcomes resulting from workplace exposures. These assessments are critical for setting regulatory standards and workplace safety guidelines. They involve hazard identification, dose-response assessment, exposure assessment, and risk characterization. Based on these assessments, appropriate risk management strategies, such as engineering controls, personal protective equipment (PPE), and administrative controls, are implemented to minimize risks.

A significant part of occupational toxicology is ensuring compliance with workplace safety regulations. Regulatory bodies such as the Occupational Safety and Health Administration (OSHA) in the United States and the Health and Safety Executive (HSE) in the United Kingdom set exposure limits and guidelines to protect workers. Occupational toxicologists often collaborate with these agencies to develop and update safety standards based on the latest scientific research.

Continuous monitoring and surveillance are essential components of occupational toxicology. These practices help in detecting harmful exposures early and assessing the effectiveness of implemented safety measures. Biomonitoring, which involves measuring chemicals or their metabolites in biological specimens like blood or urine, is a common method used to assess exposure levels and health risks in workers.

Educating employers and employees about the risks associated with workplace exposures and training them in proper safety practices are also key aspects of occupational toxicology. This includes training on the use of PPE, safe handling and storage of hazardous materials, and emergency response procedures.

As industrial processes evolve and new materials and chemicals are developed, occupational toxicology faces ongoing challenges. The emergence of nanotechnology, biotechnology, and new manufacturing technologies requires continuous research to understand potential new health risks. Moreover, the global nature of many industries necessitates international collaboration to standardize safety practices and exposure limits. Through rigorous scientific research, risk assessment, regulatory efforts, and educational initiatives, occupational toxicologists contribute significantly to the prevention of workplace-related diseases and injuries, ensuring a healthier workforce.

Orientation and Directional Terms

Term	Definition	Illustration
Occupational Exposure	The potential contact or absorption of a hazardous substance by a worker during the course of their job. This can include exposure to chemicals, biological agents, or physical hazards.	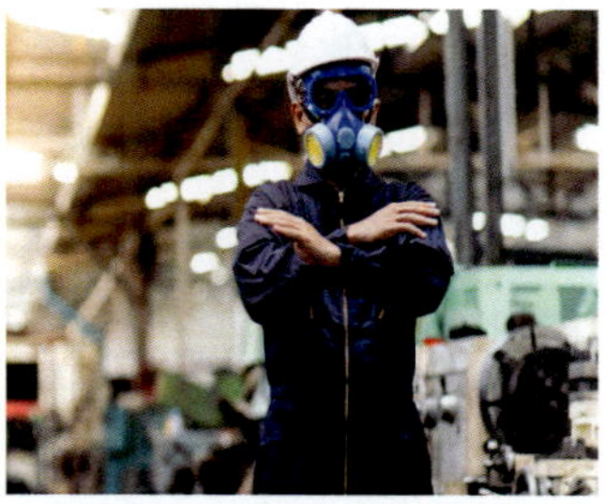
Chronic Toxicity	The adverse health effects that occur after prolonged exposure to a substance, typically at lower levels, over an extended period of time, often resulting in long-term or permanent damage.	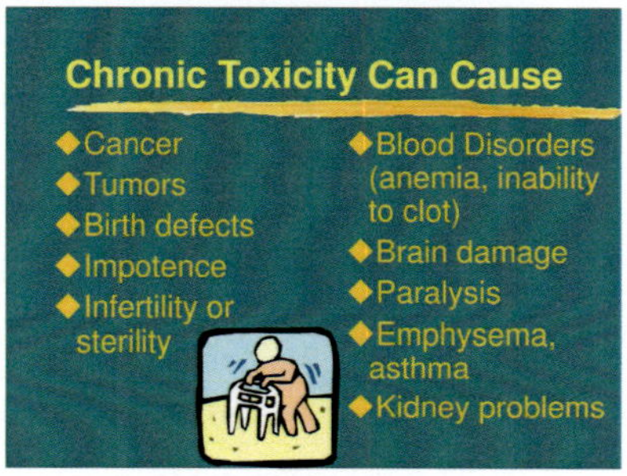
Occupational Toxicologists	Specialists who study the effects of workplace chemicals and other agents on workers' health, aiming to understand and prevent occupational diseases and injuries through risk assessment, safety evaluations, and regulatory compliance.	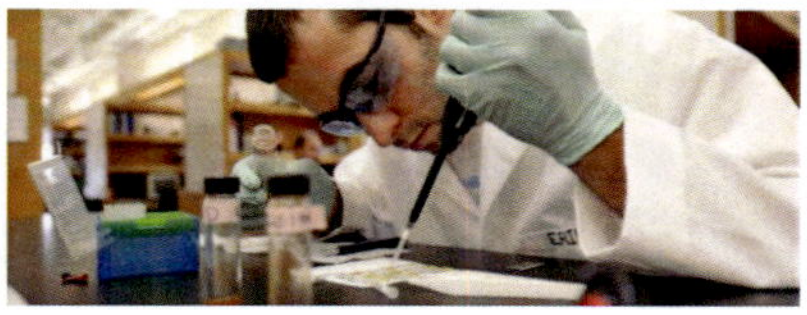
Personal Protective Equipment (PPE)	Equipment worn by workers to minimize exposure to specific occupational hazards. Examples include gloves, goggles, respirators, and protective clothing designed to protect from chemicals, biological agents, and physical hazards.	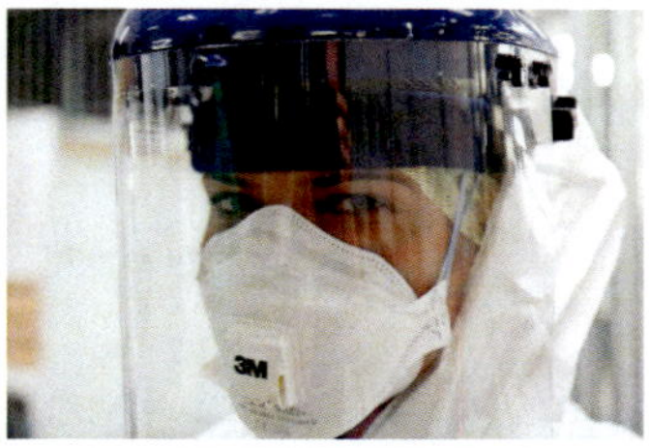
Occupational Safety and Health Administration (OSHA)	A U.S. government agency under the Department of Labor responsible for setting and enforcing workplace safety and health regulations to ensure safe and healthy working conditions for employees by enforcing standards and providing workplace safety training.	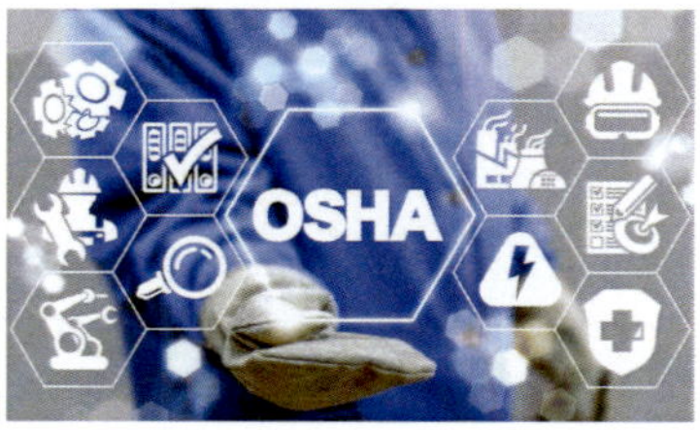

6.1. Occupational Exposure and Toxicity

In the domain of occupational health, "exposure" encapsulates any interaction between a substance and the body, suggesting the potential reception of a dose. This interaction does not guarantee a medically significant dose, as this is influenced by various factors such as the intensity, route, and duration of exposure. According to research by James et al. (2000), to mitigate the risk associated with these exposures, workplaces employ a variety of engineering and process controls designed to reduce contact with potentially hazardous agents. These controls are crucial for maintaining safety in environments where chemical, physical, or biological hazards are present (Figure 6.1).

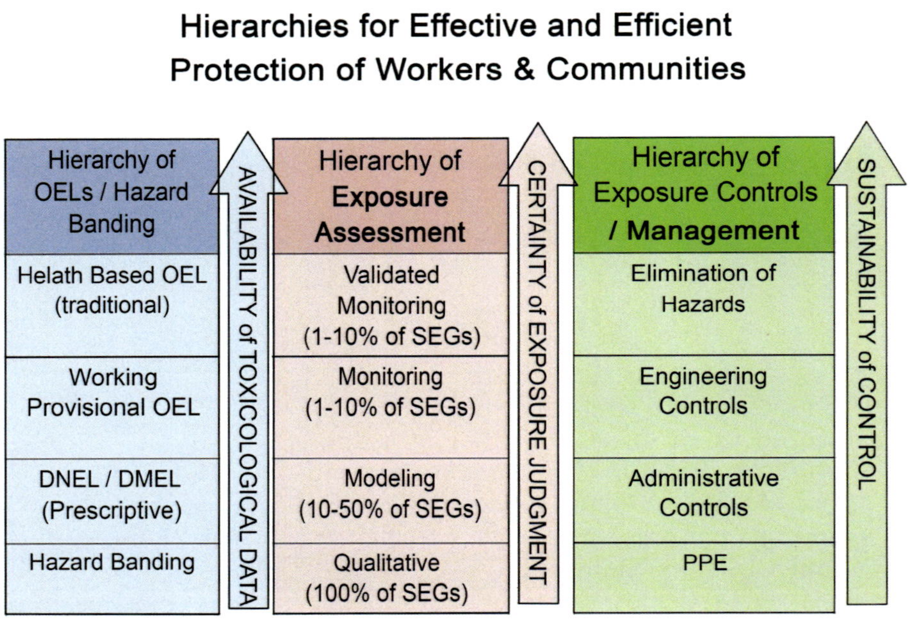

Figure 6.1. *Occupational exposure and toxicity.*

Source: By Exposurescientist – Own work, CC BY-SA 3.0; https://commons.wikimedia.org/w/index.php?curid=30360592.

The concept of "dose" is central to occupational toxicology and refers to the amount of a substance that enters the body and is transported to locations where it may produce specific biological effects. The actual measurement of an absorbed dose is complex and often impractical in occupational settings; therefore, surrogate indicators such as exposure duration and intensity are frequently used (Mutti, 1999). These indicators help in estimating the potential toxic load that might reach critical body systems and organs.

Personal Protective Equipment (PPE) plays a pivotal role in altering the dose-response dynamics. Even when exposure levels are similar, PPE can significantly reduce the dose that an individual absorbs, leading to markedly different health outcomes between protected and unprotected workers. This differential protection underscores the importance of proper PPE usage and adherence to safety protocols to mitigate the risks associated with hazardous substances. The biological response elicited by a toxin is typically specific to the toxin itself and varies according to the dose and the individual's sensitivity to the toxin. Sensitivity can be influenced by genetic factors, pre-existing health conditions, age, and even lifestyle choices, which can all modify how a toxin is processed by the body. The response to a toxin's dose can vary from negligible effects to severe outcomes, including death, illustrating the critical nature of understanding and managing toxic exposures (Landrigan, 1990).

Moreover, the relationship between the dose of a substance and its biological impact is often characterized by a dose-response curve, which can help identify the threshold level below which no adverse effects are observed. This threshold is crucial for determining safe exposure limits in the workplace and is supported by toxicological studies such as those by Arble & Wachs (2004), who illustrate these relationships and thresholds in their research.

In occupational toxicology, the goal is not only to understand these interactions and effects but also to implement strategies that can preemptively reduce or eliminate exposures. Regulatory frameworks are put in place to enforce these safety measures, requiring continuous monitoring and compliance to ensure worker protection. This regulatory compliance is supported by ongoing research and technological advancements that aim to improve the accuracy of exposure assessments and the effectiveness of intervention strategies (Figure 6.2).

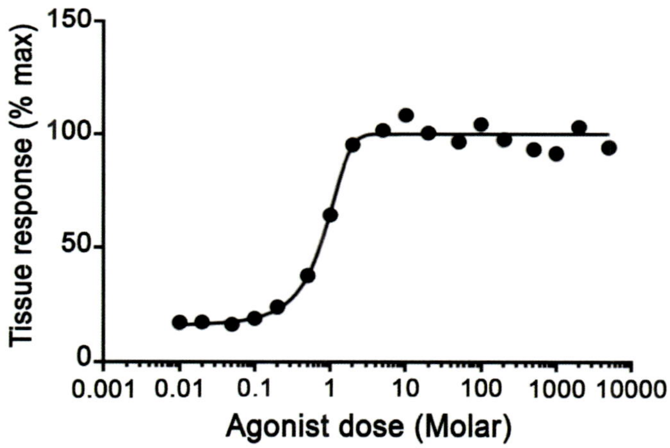

Figure 6.2. *Representation of dose-response relationship.*

Source: By Jamgoodman – Own work, CC BY-SA 4.0; https://commons.wikimedia.org/w/index.php?curid=79749638.

6.2. Acute versus Chronic Toxicity

Toxins can have either acute or long-lasting negative effects. Chronic effects could need a particular cumulative dose or happen after a latency period, whereas acute effects typically occur quickly after exposure. After sustained exposure to toxins below the threshold for acute toxicity, chronic consequences may develop (Bhardwaj & Gupta, 2012).

Because the diagnosis is not always straightforward, an emergency physician must retain high suspicion for occupational disorders. Only chronic toxicity exacerbation may be visible to the emergency physician, possibly years after exposure has ended. Exacerbations of occupational asthma and the development of myelodysplastic syndrome in patients with remote, excessive benzene exposure are two instances (Smith, 1968). Acute toxicity resulting from workplace exposure is often quickly identifiable and avoided by both employers and employees. Hence, acute toxicity typically manifests after an exceptional exposure, such as chemical spill, a failure to employ appropriate personal protective equipment, a system failure, and an accident (Zhao et al., 2009) (Figure 6.3).

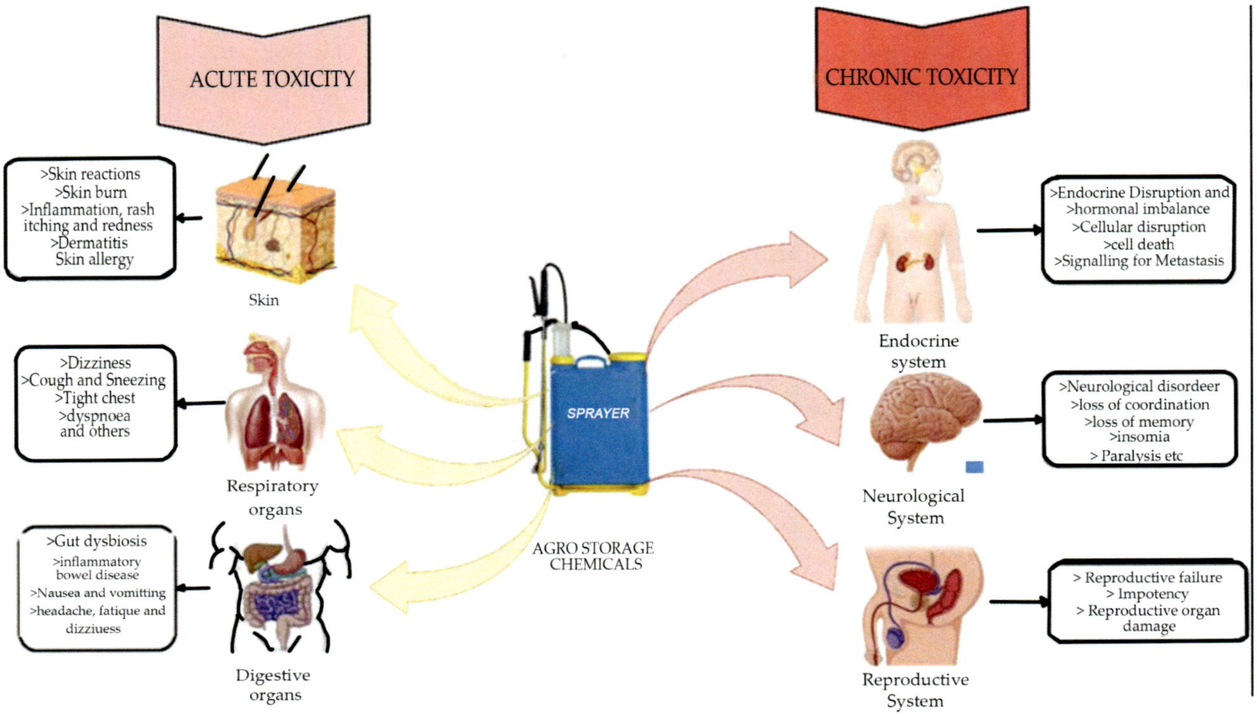

Figure 6.3. *Acute and chronic health effects of toxic chemicals.*

Source: Dali Wang; Creative Commons License.

On the other hand, it may be challenging to identify chronic toxicity and correctly link it to a working exposure. As recognized occupational toxicants that cause disease were gradually discovered, numerous organizations and regulatory bodies established limitations as either recommendations or legislation to protect workers' health. These restrictions are referred to as limitations for occupational exposure as a whole. The Occupational Safety and Health Administration (OSHA) has established permissible exposure limits (PELs) as legally enforceable thresholds. The American Conference of Governmental Industrial Hygienists (ACGIH) establishes threshold limit values (TLVs), while the National Institute for Occupational Safety and Health (NIOSH) recommends exposure limits (RELs) (ACGIH). RELs and TLVs are created solely with attention to worker safety and health; technical and economic concerns aren't considered, even though they are not legally enforceable (Arble & Wachs, 2004). Because of this, TLVs and RELs may offer a higher margin of safety than OSHA's PELs because they are often more conservative (Hood & Larranaga, 2007).

The term "time-weighted averages" refers to all of the occupational exposure limits that were previously discussed (TWAs). These controls are designed to consider short-term fluctuations in exposure concentration brought on by adjustments to job duties, processes, and ventilation settings.

The TWA takes into account both the duration of exposure as well as its concentration (McCluskey et al., 2003). By balancing various short-term concentrations against their respective exposure times, a TWA can calculate the average concentration throughout an entire work shift.

The most typical exposure limit may be an eight-hour TWA. These numbers are used to account for daily exposure level variations (Arble & Wachs, 2004). While NIOSH bases its regulations on 40-hour workweek with a maximum of 10 hours of exposure per day, the ACGIH & OSHA 8-hour TWAs are designed to protect employees for an 8-hour workday & 40-hour workweek (McCluskey et al., 2003; Nielsen & Ovrebo, 2008). These upper limits also indicate safety for a 40-year worker who works up to 50 weeks annually.

Short-term exposure limits (STELs), as opposed to 8-h TWAs, relate to exposures that last no longer than 15 minutes. Even though average exposure, calculated using time-weighted average, falls within allowable limits, these levels are not to be exceeded. A ceiling limit is a maximum concentration that may not be reached at any point throughout the working day, not even for a moment (Arble & Wachs, 2004; Nielsen & Ovrebo, 2008). There are other exposure limits, although they are less prevalent and not specified for most of the substances. These labels include median LD/lethal concentration (LC), the lowest observable adverse effect level (LOAEL), immediately dangerous to life and health (IDLH) level, and no observable effect level (NOEL) (Zhao et al., 2009).

A few key terms in occupational toxicology need to be defined. When approaching a patient with occupational exposure, it is important to clearly understand dose, exposure, dose-response relationship, and acute versus chronic toxicity.

6.3. Medical Approach

6.3.1. Acute Stabilization and Decontamination

When presented to an emergency room, an emergency physician must first determine if an occupationally exposed patient was exposed acutely or it is been more than weeks, months, or even years. Individuals who have chronic exposures typically don't need emergency care and can be released without risk of follow-up care with an occupational health doctor or regular care doctor. Further analysis of acute toxicity is frequently necessary to rule out rare but potentially fatal diseases (Gallo & Doull, 1996).

Terminating the exposure and lowering the total dose received is one of the most crucial treatments for acute toxicity. The emergency physician is supposed to actively look for sources of ongoing exposure, like contaminated work gear or chemical residue on conjunctivae, hair or skin. However, this is frequently done on the scene. When a patient may be contaminated, isolation, and decontamination safeguard the patient and other people nearby, including medical personnel. In this regard, managing incident scenes involving hazardous materials and acute occupational toxicity are frequently similar.

Decontamination is typically only necessary after exposure to solid or liquid chemicals. Very water-soluble irritating gasses, such as anhydrous ammonia, are an exception, especially in diaphoretic patients (Burgess et al., 1999; Walter, 2006). While starting decontamination, it is best to keep or move afflicted individuals outside. If it becomes necessary to bring these people indoors and if a decontamination room with the requisite equipment is unavailable, the single sizable room can be used. This room needs to well-ventilated and close to the emergency room, with less to no recycled air leaving the building to other hospital areas (Burgess et al., 1999).

Decontamination is a two-step process when deemed required. Patient's clothes, shoes, and jewelry should all be taken off and bagged before anything else. The polluted area should be where these belongings are left. If a patient can, they should be allowed to decontaminate themselves. Brush away any clinging solid particles, and blot any adherent liquids. The patient is given a thorough bath with lots of water in the second decontamination stage (Burgess et al., 1999; Walter, 2006). A moderate liquid detergent should be applied if exposed substances are unknown or non-water soluble. Decontaminating open wounds is a priority; surgical drapes can cover exposed skin. The axillae, vaginal region, foot, and skin folds need special attention. Mild water pressure should be used to apply lukewarm water methodically from head to toe After that, flush the exposed areas for at least 10–15 minutes, preferably longer, while gently scrubbing to prevent breakdown of skin. Open wounds should receive an extra 5–10 minutes of irrigation. The removal of contact lenses is advised. Ideally, it is imperative to liberally irrigate eye exposures using Morgan lenses (Schwartz et al., 2014).

Several types of personal equipment for protection may be required in decontamination scenarios are available for doctors and hospital employees. The amount of protection is differentiated using an A–D classification scheme. A self-contained breathing device is worn underneath vapor-protective, airtight, enclosed, chemical-resistant suit as part of Level A equipment, providing the maximum level of respiratory and cutaneous protection. Only this equipment offers complete protection from gasses and vapors. The maximum level of respiratory protection is provided by Level B equipment (either self-contained breathing apparatus or positive-pressure supplied-air respirators) (Vale, 1992). Nonetheless, despite the fact that it has a hood and is resistant to chemicals, the suit does not provide vapor protection for the skin. In oxygen-deficient situations, both levels A and B are acceptable. Level C offers less protection for the respiratory system while providing the same cutaneous protection as level B. Air-purifying respirators are utilized at this level. Therefore, oxygen-deficient situations cannot be used with this equipment. Standard attire makes up Level D. There is no respiratory protection, and only little skin protection is provided at this level (Walter, 2006). The selection of protective equipment must made by the doctor on a case basis with the help of a medical toxicologist if one is available.

Securing the polluted location must become the emergency physician's first responsibility while decontaminating. All unnecessary equipment should, if possible, be removed from nearby spaces. Clearly marked zones must be constructed by using tape on the floor to distinguish between polluted hot zones and cold/warm zones. The hospital supervisors, emergency department director, hospital security, and exposure-appropriate staff like chemical spill officers or hospital radiation control should all be informed immediately. A medical toxicologist or neighborhood poison control center ought to be contacted. Contamination must be continuously evaluated by staff. Also, the level of contamination must be determined, and if necessary, the emergency department must be evacuated (Burgess et al., 1999). Although uncommon, emergency department evacuations are thought to happen in up to 13% of hospitals over five years, with an annual frequency of 2.5% (Burgess et al., 1997; Burgess, 1999). If patients or staff members outside the isolation room are exhibiting symptoms or if there have been primary toxic spills inside the emergency department, evacuation should be considered. If it is decided to evacuate, a different triage and treatment location must be set up. For help and divert status, it is advised to notify the emergency medical services system and fire department, respectively (Burgess et al., 1999).

In addition to treatment requirements, isolation, and decontamination must be carried out. Lifesaving interventions must be carried out as soon as feasible, but this requirement needs to be balanced against hospital staff safety measures. The protection of providers comes first and foremost. The attending physician must try to identify the compounds in question and determine their toxicity (Pons & Dart, 1999). Unfortunately, it is sometimes inaccurate or not immediately available to identify the substance in question, and emergency department staff should be trained to identify toxic syndrome (toxidrome) (Burgess et al., 1999). Patients should also be checked for trauma; if necessary, the relevant alerts should be summoned. Supportive care should be provided, including extra oxygen. If necessary, specific antidote therapy may be used (Greenberg, 2002).

6.3.2. Occupational History

A focused history, as well as physical examination, might start when initial stabilization and documentation are finished or if it is determined that they are not essential. Identifying the conditions that led to the patient's admission to the emergency room is crucial, especially if an evident acute exposure or more subdued chronic exposure happened (Lax et al., 1998).

The exposure must be defined as precisely as feasible in the case of acute exposures. It is important to describe the task the person was working on at the time of exposure, note the incident's timing, and quantify the exposure's route, duration, and intensity as exactly as possible. The time between the initial exposure and the beginning or progression of symptoms must be precisely defined. The use of activated charcoal is something that should be considered if there was an oral exposure and the consumption occurred recently (within the last hour). However, it will be useless for many agents and is contraindicated for caustic ingestion (Chyka & Serger, 1997). The most frequent type of occupational exposure, chemical inhalations, necessitates emergency room attendance and a complete evaluation of the patient's ventilatory and oxygenation capability (Rosenberg & Israel, 1997). The emergency physician must carefully assess the patient's respiratory condition in cases of hydrocarbon ingestion because these exposures carry a significant risk of aspiration and subsequent chemical pneumonitis. Exposures to the skin and eyes necessitate decontamination and irrigation as away. The doctor must assess whether the worker employed personal protective equipment appropriately and with all sorts of occupational exposures, both acute and chronic.

A doctor needs a precise disease progression timeline when a potential chronic occupational exposure is revealed. It is important to assess whether the patient's condition worsened gradually over time or developed suddenly. Evaluation of the frequency and intensity of symptoms during work-free periods is a necessary component of a thorough occupational history. Because longer working hours raise the risk of bioaccumulation of drugs with extended half-lives, this assessment will be helpful if the patient works more than typical eight-hour shifts or forty-hour weeks. The conclusion of the workday or workweek would be predicted for such individuals to experience worsening symptoms, but as a disease progresses, this pattern can disappear, necessitating careful history taking. At the time of evaluation, the connection between work and symptom onset and relief in some occupational disorders, such as occupational asthma, may have become muddled or even unrecognizable (Tarlo, 2003).

To determine the source of an unknown exposure, asking coworkers if they have experienced similar symptoms can be helpful. Determine the severity of any symptoms coworkers may have reported. It is well known that some inhalational exposures, including H_2S, can swiftly knock out employees. This result, often known as the knockdown effect, can indicate an asphyxiant intoxication. Patients should be questioned about peculiar smells associated with their symptoms and their persistence or absence. The concept of olfactory extinction occurs when some substances cause olfactory nerve paralysis or olfactory tiredness in sufficient amounts (McCunney & Rountree, 2004). If the toxicant was encountered in ever higher doses, a patient might have described an initial odor that later vanished. Patients should be questioned about previous or ongoing employment, especially if it involves handling chemicals. The duties the employee completes at work, and the possibility of occupational exposure should be the main focus points. It is important to take note of the employee's hand-washing practices at work and any eating or smoking that occurs outside of permitted places. Last but not least, a doctor should question patients about the environment of their home, diet, drinking water source (if the availability of well water is a concern in the surrounding communities), hobbies, and activities, contact with others exposed to chemicals, use of tobacco, alcohol, and drugs to assess for a potential non-occupational exposure (Nikkanen & Burns, 2004).

6.3.3. Toxicologically Focused Physical Examination

Well, every emergency physician should be at ease conducting a typical physical examination, patients with occupational exposures require extra care. A few parts of physical examination are quite important for particular exposure pathways. Patients with dermal exposures should certainly have their skin thoroughly examined. Particularly cyanosis, sloughing, erythema, pallor, dryness, ulceration, and hypersalivation should be observed in the mucosal regions. Visual acuity testing, a possible slit-lamp examination, and if necessary, fluorescein staining are all required for ocular exposures. Note any nystagmus or disconjugate gazing (Hendrickson et al., 2021). Pulmonary findings should get special consideration throughout the cardiopulmonary examination. In patients exposed to wheezing, rales, pulmonary irritants, or rhonchi may be present. During an abdominal exam, you should look for distention, discomfort, and bowel activity signs. It is possible that an anticholinergic toxidrome is the cause of your substantial bladder distention. Reflexes should be evoked, and extremities must be examined for clubbing or cyanosis. A thorough examination of the integument should also be done, looking for signs of alopecia, anomalies in the nail beds or their absence, and skin irregularities or rashes.

6.3.4. Laboratory and Radiographic Evaluations

Laboratory and radiographic examinations are patient- and exposure-dependent, like physical exams. Blood chemistry analysis can determine whether an anion gap exists in a patient who has experienced an unknown exposure. Blood gas analysis, including co-oximetry, might be helpful if there is evidence of an anion gap or if the patient looks to have a cardiac compromise. In certain cases, chest radiography might also be necessary. If the doctor thinks an ingested chemical might be radio-opaque, plain abdominal radiographs might be advised (Tobin, 2005).

Unknown exposures should be monitored with electrocardiography, which should pay close attention to rhythm, rate, and interval anomalies. Quantitative assessment of a toxicant's concentration in urine or blood for occupational exposures is rarely feasible in a timely manner or helpful in an emergency. Samples might be retained for later forensic, medical, medicolegal, analysis in serious or rare instances. Complete blood count and liver function testing that may be done in an outpatient clinic may occasionally benefit patients with unknown potential chronic occupational exposures.

6.3.5. Information Resources

If a medical toxicologist is unavailable, the doctor should contact the poison control center first. An attempt should be made to get in touch with the health or safety officer at the workplace after a major known exposure to learn more about the chemicals involved and the nature and probable exposure routes. (Goldsman & Peters, 1981).

You can also get material safety data sheets (MSDS) from these officers. OSHA orders employers to maintain MSDS for every chemical used at work that poses a risk of injury. While treating a patient who has been exposed at work, the emergency physician may find the MSDS to be a useful resource. MSDS offers helpful information during a chemical spill or accident, including physical data, reactivity, storage, and disposal information, spill procedures, and information about first aid, health effects and toxicity. For employees or first responders to easily obtain MSDS in an emergency, it should be kept at the workplace. The doctor should try to contact site's safety or health officer if MSDS is not readily available (Thorne, 2008).

MSDS usually explain themselves. The parts on health impacts, toxicity, and 1st aid are helpful for the emergency physician. Even though it is not a comprehensive resource, the MSDS can be a good place to start for a medical professional unfamiliar with a certain chemical. Another quick resource is the National Fire Protection Association's 704 system, frequently displayed as placard on or close to allegedly hazardous substance. This placard is made up of four diamond-shaped boxes that have color-coded designations and numbers ranging from 0 (little or no harm) to 4 (moderate injury) (greatest harm) (Laamanen et al., 2008).

Table 6.1. *Tabular Representation of Environmental Causes of Medical Problems*

	Agent	Potential Exposures
Immediate or short-term effects. Dermatoses (allergic or irritant).	Metals (chromium, nickel), fibrous glass, epoxy resins, cutting oils, solvents, caustic alkali, soaps.	Electroplating, metal cleaning, plastics, machining, leather tanning, housekeeping.
Headache	Carbon monoxide, solvents	Firefighting, automobile exhaust, foundry, wood finishing, dry cleaning.
Asthma or dry cough	Formaldehyde, toluene diisocyanate, animal dander.	Textiles, plastics, polyurethane kits, lacquer use, animal handling.
Acute psychoses	Lead (especially organic), mercury, carbon disulfide de.	Gasoline handling, seed handling, fungicide, wood preservative, viscose rayon industry.
Pulmonary edema, pneumonitis	Nitrogen oxides, phosgene, halogen gasses, cadmium.	Welding, farming ("silo filler's disease"), chemical operations, smelting.
Angina	Carbon monoxide.	Traffic exhaust, foundry, wood finishing, car repair.

Abdominal pain	Lead	Smelting, painting, welding, ceramics, plumbing, battery making, enameling.
Cardiac arrhythmias	Solvents, fluorocarbons	Solvent use, refrigerator maintenance, metal cleaning.
Latent or long-term effects chronic dyspnea, pulmonary fibrosis.	Silica, beryllium, coal, asbestos, aluminum.	Pipefitting, quarrying, metal alloy work, aircraft or electrical parts, sandblasting, mining, insulation.
Chronic bronchitis, emphysema.	Cadmium, coal dust, organic solvents, cigarettes, cotton dust.	Battery production, soldering, the textile industry, mining, solvent use.
Hepatitis (may become a long-term effect)	Halogenated hydrocarbons (e.g., carbon tetrachloride), virus.	Solvent use, lacquer use, hospital workers.
Bladder cancer	β-Naphthylamine, benzidine dyes.	Dye industry, leather, rubber working, chemists.
Peripheral neuropathy	Lead, methyl butyl ketone, acrylamide, arsenic, n-hexane.	Battery production, painting, shoemaking, solvent use, plumbing, smelting, insecticides.
Lung cancer	Asbestos, uranium, coke oven emissions, arsenic, nickel.	Insulation, smelting, shipyard workers, pipefitting, nickel refining, uranium mining, coke ovens.
Behavioral changes	Lead, carbon disulfide, solvents, mercury, manganese.	Dental amalgam workers, battery production, smelting, viscose rayon industry, manufacture/repair of scientific instruments, degreasing.
Aplastic anemia, leukemia	Benzene, ionizing radiation.	Cleaning, degreasing, radiation workers, furniture refinishing, chemists.
Extrapyramidal syndrome	Manganese, carbon disulfide.	Steel production, battery production, foundry, viscose rayon industry.

Source: Kim & Kim; Creative Commons License.

Red boxes indicate a substance's flammability. Yellow boxes indicate chemical reactivity, whereas blue boxes indicate the health risk to individuals exposed. White boxes provide additional details about the substance in question. Typically, they describe a substance's reactivity with water or other properties, such as whether it is alkaline, acidic, corrosive, radioactive, or oxidizing. If no particular information is available for that chemical, this box is left empty (Walter, 2006).

The Internet is a great tool for finding relevant medical and toxicological information in the modern emergency room (Table 6.2). TOXNET is a gateway to numerous databases, including the Hazardous Substance Data Bank (http://toxnet.nlm.nih.gov/cgi-bin/sis/htmlgen?HSDB), which is very helpful.

Table 6.2. *Graphical Representation of Resources for Further Toxicological Information*

http://www.cdc.gov/niosh/npg/	NIOSH (National Institute for Occupational Safety and Health) Pocket Guide to Chemical Hazards
http://toxnet.nlm.nih.gov/	TOXNET
http://www.atsdr.cdc.gov/	Agency for Toxic Substances and Disease Registry
http://www.ilpi.com/msds/http://siri.uvm.edu/	Material safety data sheets (search engines)
1-800-222-1222	AAPCC (National Poison Control Center Line)
http://www.osha.gov/	Occupational Safety and Health Administration
http://www.cdc.gov/NIOSH/	NIOSH
http://www.acgih.org/home.htm	American Conference of Governmental Industrial Hygienists
http://www.epa.gov/	Environmental Protection Agency

Source: Kim & Kim; Creative Commons License.

6.4. Disposition and Treatment

Although specific antidotes are typically not easily accessible, strong supportive care is the cornerstone of effective toxicological care. Seldom will the treatment of a patient who has been poisoned at work deviate from regular emergency room procedures, including adhering to rules of advanced cardiac life support. A specific treatment may be necessary when poisoning by a particular substance is suspected or proven. Still, in most circumstances, a physician toxicologist's advice or data from a poison center should be used to guide treatment (Maier et al., 2020).

The most common treatments for respiratory distress brought on by occupational exposure are corticosteroids, supplementary oxygen, and -agonists. A detailed medical history and the right diagnostics may be able to spot cases that may need particular antidotes such as sodium nitrite, hydroxocobalamin, or methylene blue (for methemoglobinemia) (for poisoning with cyanide or cyanogen). Benzodiazepines titrated to response are commonly used to treat toxicant-induced seizures, although occasionally, particular antidotes such as pyridoxine are needed.

The clinical state should be used to gauge patient disposition initially. A suitable observation time is often between 4 and 6 hours. It is important to set up proper follow-up care with an occupational physician, specifically when exposure could result in impairment. Certain toxins can potentially cause severe, delayed poisoning, sometimes with just minor early symptoms. Patients whose substantial delayed toxicity is a worry, as well as those whose severe symptoms persist after initial decontamination and treatment, should be admitted to the hospital (Kim & Kim, 2011).

A Closer Look

Toxicity of Carbon Monoxide

Carbon monoxide (CO) is a colorless, odorless gas that poses a significant threat to human health due to its high toxicity. This gas is produced by the incomplete combustion of carbon-containing fuels such as gasoline, natural gas, oil, coal, and wood. When inhaled, CO binds with hemoglobin in the blood, forming carboxyhemoglobin, which severely reduces the blood's capacity to carry oxygen to cells and tissues. This hypoxic effect can lead to a range of symptoms including headache, dizziness, weakness, nausea, confusion, and, in severe cases, loss of consciousness and death. The brain and heart are particularly vulnerable to CO poisoning because of their high oxygen demands. Chronic exposure to low levels of CO can result in long-term neurological effects such as cognitive impairment and emotional instability. Moreover, certain populations, including unborn babies, infants, the elderly, and individuals with chronic heart disease, anemia, or respiratory conditions, are at increased risk of adverse health effects from CO exposure. Preventive measures are crucial to mitigate CO poisoning risks. These include the proper maintenance and venting of combustion appliances, the use of CO detectors in homes and workplaces, and ensuring adequate ventilation in enclosed spaces. Understanding the sources and effects of CO is vital for implementing effective safety measures and reducing the incidence of CO poisoning.

Summary

- This chapter provides an extensive and thorough examination of the fundamental concepts within this specialized area of study. It begins by outlining the various sources of toxins found within workplace environments, exploring the different pathways through which individuals may be exposed to these harmful substances, and delving into toxicokinetics—the study of how these substances behave once they enter the body. A pivotal aspect of the chapter is its detailed explanation of the dose-response relationship, a critical principle that illustrates how the intensity and nature of toxic effects vary directly with the level and duration of exposure to the toxin.
- Moreover, the chapter distinguishes between acute and chronic toxicological impacts, clarifying that acute exposure results in immediate symptoms, whereas chronic exposure is characterized by prolonged health consequences that may develop slowly over time. This distinction is vital for understanding the full spectrum of potential health impacts stemming from exposure to workplace toxins.
- The significance of occupational toxicology within the realm of medical science is also highlighted, with a particular focus on its role in the identification and prevention of toxic exposures in occupational settings. Strategies for managing and mitigating exposure risks are discussed, alongside methods for the effective treatment and disposition of toxins from the body. The chapter emphasizes the necessity of developing and implementing effective detoxification protocols and treatment plans tailored to specific toxins and exposure scenarios.

References

1. Arakawa, T., Aota, T., Iitani, K., Toma, K., Iwasaki, Y., & Mitsubayashi, K. (2020). Skin ethanol gas measurement system with a biochemical gas sensor and gas concentrator toward monitoring of blood volatile compounds. *Talanta, 219*, 121187.
2. Baishya, N., Momouei, M., Budidha, K., Qassem, M., Vadgama, P., & Kyriacou, P. A. (2020). Near infrared spectrometric investigation of lactate in a varying pH buffer. *Journal of Near Infrared Spectroscopy, 28*(5), 328–333.
3. Bihar, E., Deng, Y., Miyake, T., Saadaoui, M., Malliaras, G. G., & Rolandi, M. (2016). A disposable paper breathalyzer with an alcohol sensing organic electrochemical transistor. *Scientific Reports, 6*, 1–6.
4. Boushel, R., Langberg, H., Olesen, J., Gonzales-Alonzo, J., Bülow, J., & Kjaer, M. (2001). Monitoring tissue oxygen availability with near infrared spectroscopy (NIRS) in health and disease. *Scandinavian Journal of Medicine & Science in Sports, 11*(4), 213–222.
5. Cederbaum, A. I. (2012). Alcohol metabolism. *Clinics in Liver Disease, 16*(4), 667–685.
6. Chapp, A. D., Mermelstein, P. G., & Thomas, M. J. (2021). The ethanol metabolite acetic acid activates mouse nucleus accumbens shell medium spiny neurons. *Journal of Neurophysiology, 125*(2), 620–627.
7. Davies, A., & Rutland, S. G. (1988). Identification of an OH, CH combination band in the near infrared spectrum of ethanol. *Spectrochemical Acta Part A: Molecular Spectroscopy, 44*(11), 1143–1145.

8. Davis-Martin, R. E., Alessi, S. M., & Boudreaux, E. D. (2021). Alcohol use disorder in the age of technology: A review of wearable biosensors in alcohol use disorder treatment. *Frontiers in Psychiatry, 12*, 642813.

9. Dong, Q., Yu, C., Li, L., Nie, L., & Li, D. (2019). Near-infrared spectroscopic study of molecular interaction in ethanol-water mixtures. *Spectrochimica Acta Part A: Molecular and Biomolecular Spectroscopy, 222*, 117183.

10. Egmond, K. V., Wright, C., Livingston, M., & Kuntsche, E. (2020). Wearable transdermal alcohol monitors: A systematic review of detection validity, and relationship between transdermal and breath alcohol concentration and influencing factors. *Alcoholism: Clinical and Experimental Research, 44*(9), 1918–1932.

11. Ferguson, S. A., Traube, E., Zaouk, A., & Strassburger, R. (2009). Driver alcohol detection system for safety (DADSS)—A non-regulatory approach in the research and development of vehicle safety technology to reduce alcohol-impaired driving—A status update. In *Proceedings of the 21st International Technical Conference on the Enhanced Safety of Vehicles, Stuttgart, Germany, 15–18 June 2009.*

12. Giles, H. G., Meggiorini, S., & Vidins, E. I. (1986). Semiautomated analysis of ethanol and acetate in human plasma by head space gas chromatography. *Canadian Journal of Physiology and Pharmacology, 64*(6), 717–719.

13. Hlastala, M. P., & Anderson, J. C. (2007). The impact of breathing pattern and lung size on the alcohol breath test. *Annals of Biomedical Engineering, 35*(2), 264–272.

14. Jones, A. W. (1982). How breathing technique can influence the results of breath-alcohol analysis. *Medicine, Science and the Law, 22*(4), 275–280.

15. Ljungblad, J., Hök, B., Allalou, A., & Pettersson, H. (2017). Passive in-vehicle driver breath alcohol detection using advanced sensor signal acquisition and fusion. *Traffic Injury Prevention, 18*(sup1), S31–S36.

16. McGuire, L. C., Cruickshank, A. M., & Munro, P. T. (2006). Alcoholic ketoacidosis. *Emergency Medicine Journal, 23*(6), 417–420.

17. Memon, S. F., Wang, R., Strunz, B., Chowdhry, B. S., Pembroke, J. T., & Lewis, E. (2022). A review of optical fiber ethanol sensors: Current state and future prospects. *Sensors, 22*(3), 950.

18. Paprocki, S., Qassem, M., & Kyriacou, P. A. (2022). Review of ethanol intoxication sensing technologies and techniques. *Sensors, 22*(18), 6819.

19. Querido, W., Kandel, S., & Pleshko, N. (2021). Applications of vibrational spectroscopy for analysis of connective tissues. *Molecules, 26*(4), 922.

20. Ridder, T. (2008). Noninvasive determination of alcohol in tissue. *U.S. Patent US7403804B2*, 22 July 2008.

21. Ridder, T. D., Steeg, B. J. V., & Price, G. L. (2014). Robust calibration transfer in noninvasive ethanol measurements, Part I: Mathematical basis for spectral distortions in Fourier transform near-infrared spectroscopy (FT-NIR). *Applied Spectroscopy, 68*(8), 852–864.

22. Ridder, T. D., Steeg, B. J. V., Vanslyke, S. J., & Way, J. F. (2009). Noninvasive NIR monitoring of interstitial ethanol concentration. In *Optical Diagnostics and Sensing IX* (pp. 55–65). SPIE.

23. Ridder, T. D., Ver Steeg, B. J., & Laaksonen, B. D. (2009). Comparison of spectroscopically measured tissue alcohol concentration to blood and breath alcohol measurements. *Journal of Biomedical Optics, 14*(5), 054039.

24. Roger, J. M., Mallet, A., & Marini, F. (2022). Preprocessing NIR spectra for aquaphotomics. *Molecules, 27*(21), 6795.

25. Selvam, A. P., Muthukumar, S., Kamakoti, V., & Prasad, S. (2016). A wearable biochemical sensor for monitoring alcohol consumption lifestyle through Ethyl glucuronide (EtG) detection in human sweat. *Scientific Reports, 6*, 23111.

26. Siesler, H. W., Ozaki, Y., Kawata, S., & Heise, H. M. (2002). *Near-infrared spectroscopy: Principles, instruments, applications*. John Wiley & Sons.

27. Simpson, G. (1989). Do breathe tests really underestimate blood alcohol concentration. *Journal of Analytical Toxicology, 13*(2), 120–123.

28. Sorbello, J. G., Devilly, G. J., Allen, C., Hughes, L. R., & Brown, K. (2018). Fuel-cell breathalyzer use for field research on alcohol intoxication: An independent psychometric evaluation. *PeerJ, 6*, e4418.

29. Sordillo, D. C., Sordillo, L. A., Sordillo, P. P., Shi, L., & Alfano, R. R. (2017). Short wavelength infrared optical windows for evaluation of benign and malignant tissues. *Journal of Biomedical Optics, 22*(4), 45002.

30. Tiscione, N. B., Alford, I., Yeatman, D. T., & Shan, X. (2011). Ethanol analysis by headspace gas chromatography with simultaneous flame-ionization and mass spectrometry detection. *Journal of Analytical Toxicology, 35*(7), 501–511.

31. Tsukamoto, S., Muto, T., Nagoya, T., Shimamura, M., & Saito, M. (1989). Determinations of ethanol, acetaldehyde and acetate in blood and urine during alcohol oxidation in man. *Alcohol and Alcoholism, 24*(2), 101–108.

32. Wright, B. M., Jones, T. P., & Jones, A. W. (1975). Breath alcohol analysis and the blood: Breath ratio. *Medicine, Science and the Law, 15*(4), 205–210.

Chapter 7

PROPERTIES AND EFFECTS OF NATURAL TOXINS AND VENOMS

Contents

Introduction

Our world is replete with a vast array of organisms—ranging from animals and plants to microbes—that contain substances potentially hazardous to our health. Despite the risks posed by naturally occurring toxins, urban residents typically face relatively minor threats of developing serious or lethal responses to these toxins. Nonetheless, even within the confines of urban environments, we are not completely shielded from the threats posed by natural toxins. These can be found in various common sources, including food, decorative plants, and even within our own homes. As urban boundaries extend into more rural areas, the human populations migrating into these zones are increasingly exposed to a variety of poisonous species. In this chapter, we will explore some of the most prevalent natural toxins, their biological mechanisms of action, and discuss contemporary strategies for managing and treating exposures to these toxins.

Orientation and Directional Terms

Term	Definition	Illustration
Cytotoxins	Cytotoxins are toxic substances that have a specific toxic effect on certain cells, often leading to cell damage or cell death.	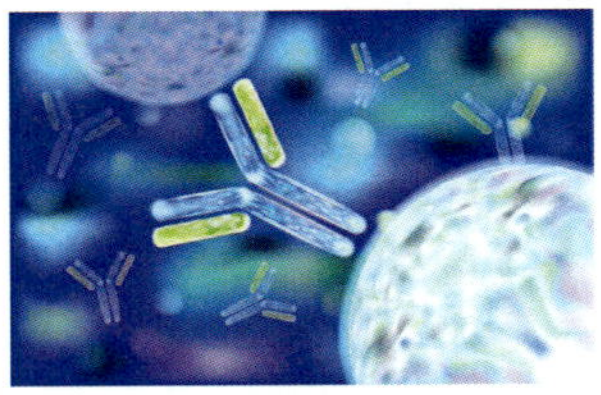
Cardiovascular Toxins	Cardiovascular toxins are toxic substances that adversely affect the heart and blood vessels, potentially causing conditions like arrhythmias and heart failure.	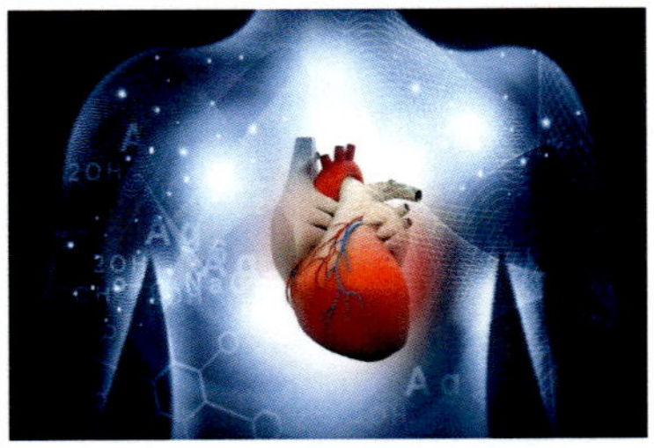
Bacterial Toxins	Bacterial toxins are harmful substances produced by bacteria that can cause disease and damage tissues in the host organism.	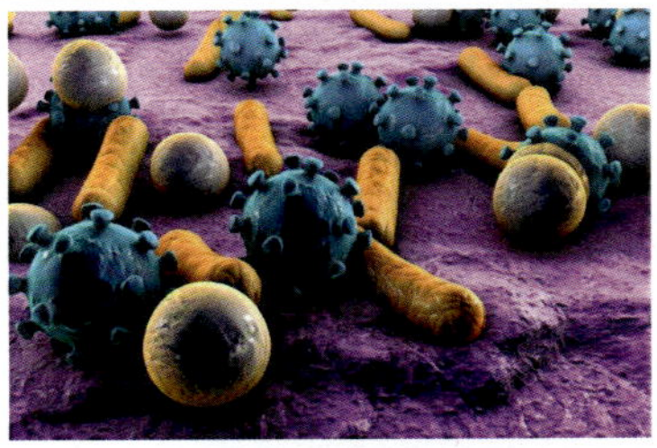
Dinoflagellate (Shellfish) Toxins	Dinoflagellate toxins are toxic compounds produced by certain species of dinoflagellates, often leading to shellfish poisoning when humans consume contaminated shellfish.	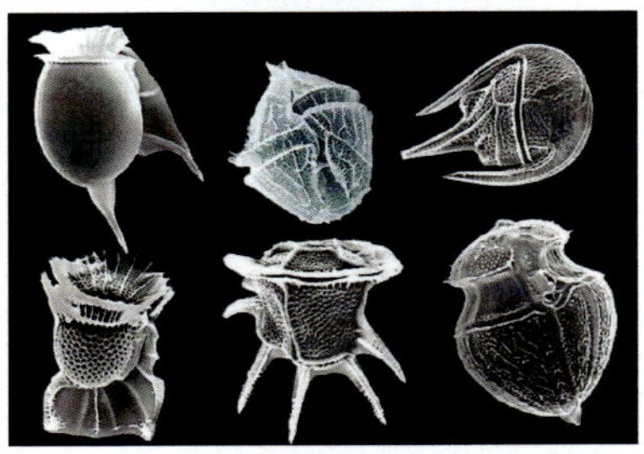
Animal Venoms	Animal venoms are complex mixtures of toxins produced by various animals, such as snakes, spiders, and scorpions, which they use for defense or to immobilize prey.	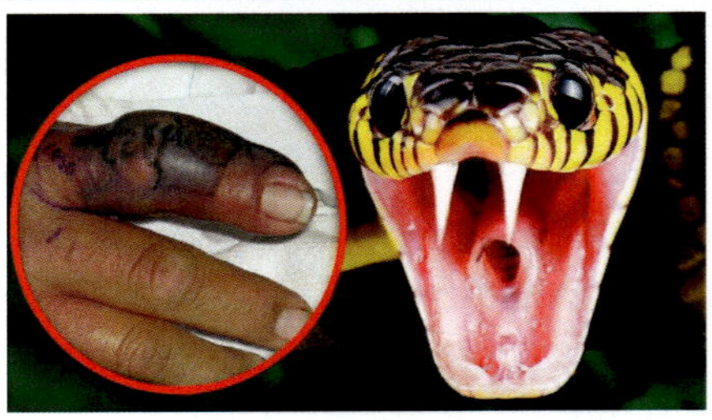

7.1. Poisons, Toxins, and Venoms

First, it is necessary for us to comprehend the meanings of the terms poison, toxin, and venom. Any chemical or combination of substances that has the potential to cause one's death is considered to be a poison. Poisonous organisms either emit or contain one or more compounds (toxins) that can cause significant disruptions to the normal physiological activities of the organism. An individual chemical that has molecular features that can be defined and that disrupts normal function is referred to as a toxin. Toxins are typically exogenous compounds that are produced by one organism to have a negative impact on another creature. Endogenous toxins, such as complement and defensins, are produced by humans as well, to protect themselves from being attacked by invading organisms like bacteria and viruses. Venoms are secretions that contain a variety of physiologically active molecules, such as enzymes, poisons, neurotransmitters, and other compounds. Venoms are secretions that are produced by different animals. In general, they are utilized not only for the purpose of capturing prey but also as a chemical defensive mechanism against other predators. Toxins are frequently secreted from relatively basic integumentary glands and may even be maintained within visceral organs when they are employed only for the purpose of providing a chemical defense against predators. In these instances, the toxins possess a specific function. Pufferfish toxin is an example of this type of toxin, and it will be explored further down in this article (Lalloo & Theakston, 2003; Alirol et al., 2010; Bolt, 2021).

7.2. Molecular and Functional Diversity of Natural Toxins and Venoms

Every major class of molecules that are synthesized by living organisms, including proteins, lipids, carbohydrates, nucleosides, and alkaloids, have been utilized by certain species to produce a toxic drug. Listed in Table 7.1 are some of the natural toxins that will be discussed in this chapter that are considered to be of greater significance.

Generally speaking, proteins are the most powerful toxins. This is probably since proteins have larger molecular surfaces, which allows for greater bonding contact with the receptors on which they act. There is an additional possible explanation for why many toxins are peptides or proteins, in addition to the high potency of these substances. The biosynthesis of protein toxins does not require any unusual substrates or catalysts; all that is required is a messenger RNA template that specifies the amino acid sequence of the toxin. The remaining components of the necessary biosynthetic machinery, such as ribosomes, messenger RNA, transfer RNA, nucleotides, and RNA polymerase, are already present. To this day, it is not entirely clear how the protein toxins came into existence during the course of evolution. On the other hand, certain polypeptide toxins found in snakes have amino acid sequences that are extremely similar to those of endogenous polypeptides that function as proteolytic enzyme inhibitors. It is hypothesized that these toxins originated from duplicated (extra) genes that were responsible for the production of these enzyme inhibitors.

The production of toxins that are chemically similar by organisms that are not related to one another in terms of taxonomy is a relatively common occurrence. Therefore, certain echinoderms, such as starfish and sea cucumbers, are capable of producing sterol glycosides. These glycosides are chemically and pharmacologically very similar to the saponins that are identified in certain plants. The alkaloid toxin known as anabaseine, which is found in certain marine worms, is almost identical to the alkaloid known as anabasine, which is found in tobacco. In light of the fact that enzymes, which act as catalysts for metabolic pathways that are common in living organisms, are responsible for the synthesis of a great number of toxins, it is possible that this evolutionary convergence at the molecular level is something that should be anticipated. Since the beginning of time, it has been known that plants produce an incredible variety of "secondary" metabolic products that contain nitrogen. These products are typically referred to as alkaloids. To protect themselves from herbivores, many of these metabolites are produced. These compounds are also produced by protozoans and animals, and some of these compounds will be discussed further down in this article.

Table 7.1. *Mouse Lethality of Skeletal Natural Toxins*

Toxin Name	Source	Lethal Dose (LD_{50})	Mode of Action	Symptoms in Mice
Tetrodotoxin	Puffer fish	10 μg/kg	Sodium channel blocker	Paralysis, respiratory failure
Saxitoxin	Certain algae	11 μg/kg	Sodium channel blocker	Paralysis, respiratory distress
Batrachotoxin	Poison dart frogs	2 μg/kg	Sodium channel modulator	Cardiac arrest, muscle spasms
Conotoxin	Cone snail	30 μg/kg	Calcium channel blocker	Muscle paralysis, respiratory arrest
Ricin	Castor beans	22 μg/kg	Protein synthesis inhibitor	Severe abdominal pain, death
α-Amanitin	Death cap mushrooms	0.1 mg/kg	RNA polymerase inhibitor	Severe liver damage, renal failure

Source: Modified from Middlebrook (1989).

Different organs, such as plant vacuoles and animal venom glands, are responsible for the storage of toxic substances by organisms that are toxic for a variety of reasons. In the first place, the toxic organism might be exposed to its own poison if it were not for this. It is possible to protect the other tissues of the organism from being exposed to the substance or collection of substances (venom) by enclosing the toxin within a membrane sac that acts as an impermeable barrier to the toxin. When it comes to the second point, it is typically beneficial to store the chemical in a concentrated form. This allows for the chemical to be injected into the victim effectively, with the assistance of a fang or barb. Last but not least, the venom apparatus needs to be linked up with an effector system that can detect the presence of the person who is supposed to be the target of the venom. However, in certain venomous invertebrates, such as jellyfish, the entire sensory and motor apparatus for activating venom release is built into each venom-emitting cell. This is in contrast to the majority of venomous animals, which release their venom in response to instructions from the central nervous system.

7.3. Natural Roles of Toxins and Venoms

In the majority of instances, the practical value of any venom is rather obvious, whether it be to acquire prey or to protect against predators. To consume relatively large prey animals at a more leisurely pace, a venomous predator can immobilize them and consume them instead. The consumption of a plant or animal that is sufficiently toxic but not venomous is avoided in the same manner. Even if the toxicity of a single individual is not sufficient to protect its own life, an herbivore or predator will be compelled to consume a smaller number of individuals than it would otherwise to avoid becoming fatally intoxicated by the substance. It is through this method that the survival of the species that is not desirable will be improved.

There is a possibility that the biological function of a toxin in prokaryotic organisms that are toxic was not at all obvious. Dinoflagellate organisms and red tide organisms are two examples that immediately come to mind. Dinoflagellate populations can sometimes reach such high densities in aquatic communities that the concentrations of toxins in the seawater are sufficient to cause massive fish kills. However, these postulated endogenous functions have not yet been discovered, although it has been hypothesized that these toxins typically act as regulators of cell growth or metabolism and only infrequently act as toxins.

7.4. Major Sites and Mechanisms of Toxic Action Neurotoxic Actions

Because the nervous system serves primarily as a master communication network that swiftly coordinates the operation of virtually all of the body's cells, tissues, and organs, it is an ideal target for toxins, which are designed to rapidly alter the functioning of the organism that they are intended to affect. The production of two distinct kinds of electrical signals is essential for the expeditious communication that occurs within the nervous system. Dendrites, which are small processes that emanate from the cell body of the neuron, initially generate a relatively slow depolarizing junctional potential in response to neurotransmitters that are released from neighboring neurons. This elicits an action potential, which then rapidly travels to the end of the axon, where neurotransmitter is released once more to either activate or inhibit some effector cell.

A wide range of toxins canexert their influence on electrically active tissues, such as neuronal cells and muscle cells, which generate their electrical signals through the utilization of neurotransmitter- and voltage-gated ion channels. No blood–brain barrier protects the peripheral nervous and muscular systems from being exposed to toxins, which makes them particularly vulnerable cellular targets for rapidly acting toxins.

Around the year 1920, a physiologist by the name of Langley demonstrated for the first time that the tobacco alkaloid nicotine acted at a few discrete sites along the length of a muscle cell. He did this by applying nicotine locally at only a few locations along the length of the muscle. When these nicotinic receptors were purified from electric fishes in 1971, it was a particularly rich source of information regarding their molecular properties. Before that time, there was very little information available. Each muscle-like nicotinic receptor is a pentameric complex that is composed of five polypeptide subunits. These subunits are only held together by noncovalent bonds. There is a similarity between two of the five subunits. They are actually the acetylcholine (ACh) binding sites that are contained within these so-called alpha subunits. Agonists are substances that activate the receptor, such as acetylcholine and nicotine. On the other hand, competitive antagonists are substances that bind to the same site in a reversible manner without activating the receptor. Some examples of competitive antagonists include tubocurarine, which is a poison found in South American Indian arrows, and certain components of snake venom. Toxins have the potential to exert their influence on this large membrane protein complex in a number of different locations, in addition to the ACh recognition site. To give just one example, numerous alkaloid toxins that are relatively small canphysically block the ion channel. It is likely that other toxins bind at the interface that exists between the polypeptide subunits and the lipid bilayer that is adjacent to them.

An action potential must be able to be generated in response to the depolarization that is induced by acetylcholine (ACh). The membrane of the muscle cell, which is continuous with the postsynaptic membrane of the muscle cell, is electrically excitable. The phenomenon known as an action potential is characterized by the sequential opening and closing of two distinct ion channels in response to the depolarization of the membrane. In the beginning, the sodium-selective channel opens, which allows sodium ions to enter the cell. This causes the cell's electrical potential to be reversed, which results in the interior of the cell temporarily becoming electropositive. This results in the depolarization of the membrane that is adjacent to it, which in turn triggers the opening of additional sodium channels. In this way, a wave of electrical charge travels along the length of the muscle fiber in a very rapid manner. This wave of depolarization is immediately followed by a wave of repolarization as a result of the opening of potassium ion-selective channels. This opens the door for potassium to flow out of the cell, allowing it to flow down its concentration gradient. As a result of the fact that it would be counterproductive for the sodium channels to remain open while the potassium channels were opening, an additional process known as sodium channel inactivation takes place while the potassium channels are opening. In some muscle cells, a calcium-selective channel either replaces the sodium channel (in smooth muscle) or supplements its ability to depolarize the cell (in cardiac muscle). This occurs more frequently in smooth muscle than in cardiac muscle.

Calcium channels that are voltage-gated take the place of sodium channels in smooth muscles and in a large number of neurons. This is because sodium channels are responsible for causing at least a portion of the initial cationic influx that drives action potentials. The exocytotic release of neurotransmitters is also mediated by calcium ions that are flowing through these calcium channels at the terminals of nerves within the body. The calcium ion-passing channels will be discussed in more detail later on. There are many extremely powerful toxins that can either activate or inhibit these channels. The sarcoplasmic reticulum membranes of muscle cells contain intracellular calcium channels. These calcium channels must be able to rapidly release calcium ions for the muscle to contract. Ryanodine, a plant toxin, canblock these calcium channels.

Each and every ion channel appears to be a potential target for some natural toxin, which typically exerts its effects at a concentration that is significantly lower than that of drugs that act on the same site (ion channel). For example, tetracaine, which is considered to be one of the most powerful local anesthetics, can block sodium channels of nerves at concentrations that are greater than 10–6 M. On the other hand, the pufferfish toxin tetrodotoxin can achieve the same blockade at a concentration that is one thousand times lower!

7.4.1. Cardiovascular Toxins

The cardiovascular system is also quite susceptible to the effects of a large number of naturally occurring toxins that can act on ion channels in smooth or cardiac muscles, as well as on the terminals of autonomic nerves. There is a high probability that the rapid action of venoms on excitable cells is responsible for many of their lethal effects. After the victim has been envenomated, the active constituents immediately begin to spread throughout the area in accordance with their molecular size and other chemical properties. If they rapidly spread into the tissues surrounding the bite, their entry into the systemic circulation will be greatly enhanced.

This can be enhanced by a venom enzyme called hyaluronidase, which breaks down the hyaluronic acid that is present in connective tissue. Certain venoms also contain proteins that induce hemorrhage, act as anticoagulants, and have hemolytic properties. These proteins, when combined, can result in a significant loss of blood volume, tissue edema, and cytolysis. Therefore, venoms and the toxic components that they contain have the potential to influence the cardiovascular system in a variety of different ways (Lalloo & Theakston, 2003; Alirol et al., 2010; Bolt, 2021).

7.4.2. Toxins Affecting the Liver and Kidneys

Furthermore, the liver and the kidney are two additional organs that are particularly susceptible to the effects of toxins. In the beginning, substances that have been absorbed from the gastrointestinal tract are transported to the liver by the hepatic portal venous system. This organ contains many catabolic enzymes and is thus capable of metabolizing practically any type of exogenous compounds, usually to a less active or toxic form. On the other hand, metabolites might be even more hazardous than the molecules that they are derived from. Because they are able to gain easy entry into the hepatic cells through a special solute transport system that is normally used for the reabsorption of bile salts, certain cyclic peptide toxins that are found in poisonous mushrooms (amatoxins) and freshwater algae (microcystins) are considered to be relatively selective hepatotoxins. Certain toxins, particularly those that enter the renal tubule through glomerular filtration but are not readily reabsorbed, are particularly dangerous to the kidney because of its relatively high susceptibility to them. They become more concentrated in the nephron and the urine as a result of this, which increases their capacity to cause damage to renal structures.

7.4.3. Cytotoxins

This is most likely the most widespread category of toxic substances. Generally speaking, cytotoxins have an effect on processes that are necessary for life, such as the synthesis of proteins, the replication of DNA, the synthesis of RNA, oxidative phosphorylation (metabolism), or the electrolyte balance of the cell. Cytolysins are a type of cytotoxin that induces an osmotic imbalance, which in turn leads to the swelling of cells and, ultimately, the lysis of those cells. Cytolysins that are particularly powerful are able to create large holes in the cell membrane, which allows for the release of a wide variety of proteins and substances with a low molecular weight.

The lipid bilayer organization of cell membranes is disrupted by other substances, which behave similarly to detergents. In spite of the fact that the majority of cytotoxins are capable of attacking a wide range of cells, many of them are cardiotoxic when they are present in sublytic concentrations. This is because they candirectly contract muscle cells by depolarizing the resting membranes of excitable cells.

7.4.4. Toxins Affecting Secondary Messengers

7.4.4.1. Signal Transduction

The majority of slow receptor-mediated responses are indirectly coupled to an effector, such as an ion channel, utilizing a "second messenger" signal, which is typically a cyclic nucleotide or some phosphoinositide. This signal is responsible for locating another effector molecule and modifying its activity. Cyclic AMP stimulates various phosphoryl kinase enzymes, which catalyze the phosphorylation of ion channels and other signaling systems, thereby modulating their function.

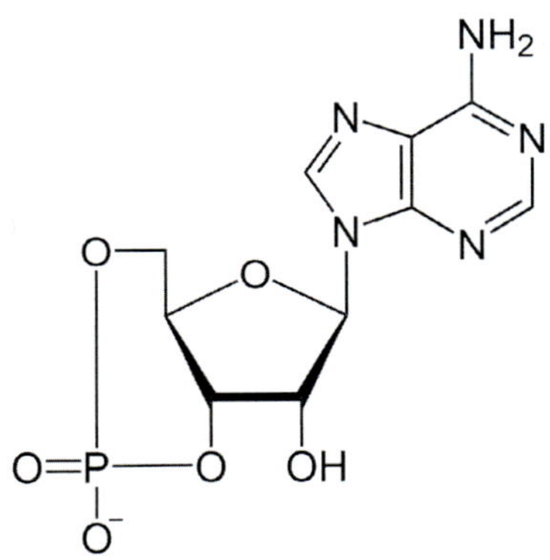

Figure 7.1. *Cyclic AMP.*

Source: By NEUROtiker – Own work, Public Domain; https://commons.wikimedia.org/w/index.php?curid=2220446.

Numerous toxins have been discovered to specifically alter the system that is responsible for producing cAMP. Some molecules exert their influence in a roundabout way by influencing guanosine nucleotide-binding proteins, also known as G proteins, which modulate adenylate cyclase. For example, cholera toxin stimulates the formation of Gs, which is the stimulatory G protein subunit, and consequently increases the amount of cAMP that is produced. On the other hand, pertussis toxin inhibits the binding of the inhibitory G protein subunit Gi to the cyclase, which also results in the stimulation of cAMP production. On the other hand, the sponge toxin okadaic acid acts in a completely different manner. It does this by inhibiting specific phophatases, which are enzymes that normally reverse the phosphorylation that is catalyzed by cAMP. This results in an increase in the concentration of cAMP (Figure 7.1) (Lalloo & Theakston, 2003; Alirol et al., 2010; Bolt, 2021).

7.4.5. Inflammatory and Carcinogenic Toxins

In most cases, the purpose of these kinds of toxins is to discourage consumption or even contact with the toxic organism. A wide variety of sedentary organisms, such as plants and certain marine animals, are capable of producing inflammatory substances. These may be analogous to endogenous chemical mediators, such as histamine, prostaglandins, or phospholipids, or they may be able to liberate endogenous mediators from basophils and other cells that are responsible for mediating inflammatory processes.

As an example, the ochratoxins are examples of natural substances that are among the most powerful carcinogens. In a great number of instances, their mechanisms of action are not yet determined. The provocative hypothesis that Ames has presented is that the risks associated with exposure to certain industrial carcinogens may not be any more severe than the risks associated with the daily consumption of small amounts of natural carcinogens that occur in certain food plants.

7.5. Toxins in Unicellular Organisms

7.5.1. Bacterial Toxins

Due to the fact that there are so many bacterial toxins, we are only able to focus on a few of the most prevalent and fascinating ones here. The most powerful naturally occurring toxins are neurotoxins that are bacterial proteins.

Anaerobic *Clostridium botulinum* bacterial spores can survive and multiply in food that has been improperly canned, which can lead to botulinum poisoning. Botulinum poisoning is primarily a foodborne disease. Several different strains of this anaerobe are capable of producing toxins that are related to one another. Each and every one of the botulinum toxins exerts its effects by inhibiting the release of neurotransmitters at the neuromuscular junction of the skeletal muscle. If the symptoms are not alleviated, this peripheral action, which is dominated by botulinum toxins, will eventually result in flaccid paralysis and subsequent death. Therapy is a challenging process. After it has bound, the toxin is then internalized at the motor nerve terminal, where it begins to exert its effects on the body. It is possible for botulinum antiserum to neutralize toxins that have not yet been absorbed by the body. The administration of an acetylcholinesterase inhibitor, such as neostigmine, to the patient at the time of treatment has the potential to improve neuromuscular transmission. It is possible that the patient will require artificial respiration until they can regain their new transmitter release sites.

Clostridium tetani, an additional anaerobe, is the causative agent of tetanus poisoning. Once more, a number of strains produce closely related toxins. In spite of the fact that they all inhibit neurotransmitter release in a manner that is superficially comparable to that of botulinum toxin, the tetanus toxins that are found in mammals primarily inhibit the release of glycine, which is an inhibitory neurotransmitter, within the central nervous system. This inhibition of an inhibitory influence on central motor neurons, which is referred to as " disinhibition," enables full expression of the excitatory synaptic input to these neurons, which in turn causes peripheral excitation of all skeletal muscles. It is possible for victims to become immobilized in a contorted contraction that poses a threat to their lives. This is because extensor muscles are typically the most powerful. The only symptom of this condition is referred to as "lockjaw." A "booster" vaccination should also be taken approximately once every ten years, particularly for various outdoor persons who are more likely to be exposed to this bacterium (gardeners, farmers, trash handlers, etc.). Since the majority of us have received a tetanus toxoid vaccination when we were children, the likelihood of developing tetanus poisoning is significantly reduced.

Cytotoxic proteins are frequently responsible for the fever, vasodilation, and tissue damage that are normally associated with an infection. These proteins are produced by infectious bacteria. One of the representatives of this group that is the most well-known and understood is the staphylococcal alpha-toxin. Multiple molecules of this toxin clump together on the membrane of the target cell, resulting in the formation of a large pore that enables the release of a variety of cellular constituents, including large proteins. Cytolytic toxins are not typically fatal, but they do contribute to the symptoms that are associated with bacterial infections being present.

The GS protein coupling to adenylate cyclase is activated by the cholera toxin. Because of this, the intestinal ion and water secretion is stimulated, which ultimately leads to dehydration and death if the condition is not properly treated.

Different bacterial cytotoxins have a completely different mechanism of action, which is to inhibit the production of proteins in the cell that they are targeting. Toxins caused by Pseudomonas and diphtheria are two effective examples. It has been determined that a single molecule of one of these toxins is sufficient to inhibit sufficient protein synthesis to the point where the cell is unable to replenish the proteins that are also being continuously broken down. Fortunately, the process by which the cytotoxin is internalized and gains entry into the cytoplasmic compartment is not as efficient as one might think. In fact, it takes thousands of toxin molecules that are bound to the cell membrane for a single molecule to reach its ribosomal destination in a manner that is lethal.

Because the spores of many bacteria are widely dispersed by the movement of air and water around the earth, these bacteria are capable of being found almost everywhere. On the other hand, the distribution of certain species is significantly more restricted to a specific area. One example is the marine bacterium known as *Vibrio vulnificus*, which has the potential to cause infections that are potentially fatal in individuals who consume raw marine shellfish or swim in the ocean with skin abrasions that are susceptible to infection. Approximately 20% of the patients who participated in a recent study passed away as a result of necrotic tissue or liver disease. Vibriolysin, a cytolytic protein with a molecular weight of 56 kilodaltons, is thought to be the mediator of the tissue damage.

Despite the fact that it was initially believed that pufferfish and certain newts (amphibians) were the only organisms capable of producing the alkaloidal neurotoxin tetrodotoxin, it has been discovered in a wide variety of marine animals over the course of the last ten years. These marine animals include worms, crabs, and an Australian octopus. Because it was recently discovered that some different species of marine bacteria are capable of producing tetrodotoxin, it is highly probable that the animals obtain the toxin from microbial symbionts within their bodies (Lalloo & Theakston, 2003; Alirol et al., 2010; Bolt, 2021).

7.5.2. A Toxin Implicated in Amebic Dysentery

For example, an infection caused by the freshwater amoeba known as *Entamoebae histolytica* can result in meningitis, which is a potentially fatal condition, as well as inflammation of the colon and abscesses in the intestinal tract. The direct contact caises osmosis, swelling, and lysis of the target cell through the amobapre (a pore-forming peptide).

7.5.3. Dinoflagellate (Shellfish) Toxins

In the presence of conditions that are particularly favorable for the growth of populations, toxic algal blooms are caused by several different toxic marine dinoflagellate species. In addition to causing a significant number of fish and other marine animals to perish, these "red tides," which are so called because the water that contains high concentrations of these dinoflagellates can sometimes have a reddish color, can also cause massive mortality. Blooms of algae are more likely to occur along coastlines that are negatively impacted by pollution caused by human and agricultural waste. The ability to concentrate a significant number of these toxins without becoming intoxicated is possessed by filter-feeding mollusks. Consuming poisonous clams, mussels, and other organisms can result in a variety of symptoms, the nature of which is determined by the toxins that are present in the organisms. Among the intoxications that can occur are paralytic shellfish poisoning (PSP), neurotoxic shellfish poisoning (NSP), and diarrheic shellfish poisoning (DSP), all of which will be discussed further down in this article.

There is a dinoflagellate known as Gonyaulax catenella that is responsible for one of the most common red tides in the northern hemisphere.

This dinoflagellate secretes a family of over 30 related toxins known as saxitoxins, which block sodium channels. Saxitoxins are considered to be paralytic shellfish poisons (PSPs) because their detrimental effects on the nervous system can be reversed if the individual is able to avoid having their death occur. The consumption of shellfish that contain high concentrations of these toxins is the only occasion on which they become hazardous to human health. Since shellfish filter feeds on poisonous dinoflagellates, their tissues retain the toxins that are present in the saxitoxins. Shellfish are relatively resistant to the saxitoxins. This guanidinium toxin binding site on the sodium channel was formerly referred to as "site 1" on the sodium channel (Table 7.2). It has been demonstrated that these toxins, such as the pufferfish toxin tetrodotoxin, interact with a pore-forming segment on the sodium channel protein alpha-subunit. When compared to the sodium channels found in nerves and skeletal muscles, the sodium channel found in the heart of mammals is pharmacologically distinct in that it is approximately 500 times less sensitive to the toxins that are present. This is probably a fortunate circumstance for us.

Table 7.2. *Toxins Affecting Voltage-Gated Sodium Channels*

Toxin Name	Source	Description of Effect
Tetrodotoxin (TTX)	Pufferfish, blue-ringed octopus	Blocks sodium channels, preventing nerve impulses; can be lethal.
Saxitoxin	Certain marine dinoflagellates	Similar to TTX, blocks sodium channels leading to paralysis.
Batrachotoxin	Poison dart frogs	Forces sodium channels open, causing persistent nerve firing.
Aconitine	Monkshood plant	Binds to and persistently activates sodium channels.
Grayanotoxin	Rhododendrons, azaleas	Modifies sodium channel activation, leading to altered firing.
Veratridine	Lilies, false hellebore	Keeps sodium channels open, increasing nerve cell excitability.

Source: *(Zalups & Koropatnick, 2000)*

Off the coast of Nova Scotia in 1987, a typical instance of neurotoxic shellfish poisoning (NSP) was described as having taken place. The victims suffered from amnesia, which is characterized by a loss of the ability to recall information. A toxin known as domoic acid, which is an active analog of the excitatory neurotransmitter glutamic acid, was discovered to be the chemical in question. This toxin causes neuron degeneration by persistently activating glutamate ion channels, most likely by causing an excessive influx of calcium ions. This ultimately leads to neuron cell death. Ciguatoxin and okadaic acid are the two factors that lead to DSP.

The dinoflagellate *Gymnodinium breve* is responsible for the production of brevetoxins, which are able to open sodium channels rather than block them (Table 7.2). This organism is responsible for the massive fish kills that occur every few years and can be found in warmer waters, such as those that are found along the coastline of Florida. Brevetoxins, which are similar to ciguatoxin, are complex polycyclic ether molecules that cause the sodium channel to open even when the body is in a resting state. Because of this, nerve and muscle cells are able to generate action potentials on their own without being stimulated, which is, of course, a potentially fatal condition. It is unlikely that humans will become poisoned by eating fish that have been exposed to these toxins because fish are killed by relatively small amounts of these toxins. Nevertheless, during a bloom, some of the Gymnodinium becomes airborne in the spray from the ocean, and individuals may experience respiratory distress as a result of inhaling these toxic droplets.

7.6. Toxins of Higher Plants

7.6.1. Mushrooms and Other Fungi

There are fewer than 1% of the species of mushrooms that are toxic to humans, but those that are can be extremely hazardous. As a result of the growing interest in mushroom hunting, it is anticipated that the number of people who become intoxicated will also rise. It is the mushrooms belonging to the genus Amanita that pose the greatest threat. These contain approximately equal amounts of two cyclic peptide toxins known as amatoxins and phallotoxins. Both of these toxins are relatively small, consisting of seven amino acids. Because these cyclic peptides are relatively stable at high temperatures, they can survive exposure to cooking. Ingestion of even a single *Amanita phalloides* mushroom has the potential to result in death. The amatoxins are about 20 times more toxic than the phallotoxins, so they are the toxins that must be reckoned with the most. Due to the fact that they can be absorbed through the bile acid transport mechanism, they are especially harmful to the liver. After they have entered the hepatic parenchymal cell, they inhibit the essential transcriptional enzyme RNA polymerase that is located within the nucleus. This prevents the cell from being able to replace cellular proteins, which are constantly being broken down. For 10% to 30% of those who are intoxicated, this leads to necrosis of the liver and ultimately death. It is a significant challenge to diagnose and treat amanita poisoning because the symptoms that are characteristic of amatoxin do not appear until approximately 15 hours after ingestion, regardless of the amount of amatoxin that is consumed. The minimum amount of time required for the toxin to be absorbed and inhibit enzymes, as well as for the hepatic protein depletion to start having an effect on hepatic function, is precisely this amount of time. The phallotoxins cause one to experience gastric distress and diarrhea approximately six to ten hours after the ingestion of the substance. The actin filaments that are located on the inner surface of the cell membrane are bound to them, and this prevents the actin filaments from dissociating into monomeric actin, which is necessary for the normal functioning of the cell.

The presence of amatoxins in the blood and urine can be determined through a variety of methods, which can be used to determine the origin of the poisoning experience. Ingestion of activated charcoal through the mouth is effective in absorbing a significant amount of toxins, provided that it is done within four hours of the ingestion of the charcoal. Naturally, it is possible that the victim had not yet experienced a significant number of symptoms at that crucial time.

Certain species of mushrooms are capable of producing alkaloidal toxins, which are significantly less dangerous to human life. One such example is muscarine, which was first isolated more than a century ago and is utilized in the categorization of cholinergic receptors. The actions that it takes are not only quick but also quite predictable. Certain antidotes, such as the muscarinic antagonist atropine, are available, which is a fortunate development. Psilocybin and bufotenin are two examples of biogenic amines that are produced by other types of mushrooms. Bufotenin was initially isolated from the venom glands of the toad Bufo. These are hallucinogenic compounds, which primarily stimulates certain serotonin receptors in the brain. Finally, several mushrooms are capable of producing ibotenic acid, which is a glutamate receptor agonist that is comparable to domoic acid and has the potential to be neurotoxic.

Besides mushrooms, there are a few other types of fungi that are poisonous. Ergot is a type of fungus that thrives in moist environments and grows on specific grains. This particular fungus is responsible for the production of a wide range of biogenic amines, which are agonists on alpha-type adrenergic receptors. One of these agonists is ergotamine, which is clinically employed for the treatment of migraine headaches. There is a high probability that the primary hallucinogenic component of ergot is methylsergide, which is a serotonin antagonist. It has been discovered that certain molds are capable of producing carcinogenic substances known as aflatoxins and ochratoxins. Ensuring that vegetable crops that are susceptible to these molds are stored properly eliminates conditions that are favorable for the growth of these molds.

7.6.2. Flowering Plants

7.6.2.1. Cardiac Glycosides and Saponins

Additionally, cardiac glycosides can be found in both plant and animal sources. In the Western world, the foxglove, which is a stunning flowering plant that is now widely cultivated in many countries, has traditionally been the source of these compounds for medicinal purposes. The glycosides that are most important to the foxglove are referred to as digitoxin and digoxin. The venom glands of toads were utilized as a significant source of medicinal compounds (bufotoxins) that were very similar to those found in the Orient. The treatment of congestive heart failure, a condition that is characterized by a loss of myocardial contractility, is the primary therapeutic application of digitalis glycosides. The heart is unable to pump blood adequately to prevent the blood from pooling in the lungs and extremities for a variety of reasons, including long-term hypertension, atherosclerosis, kidney failure, and other conditions (Figure 7.2).

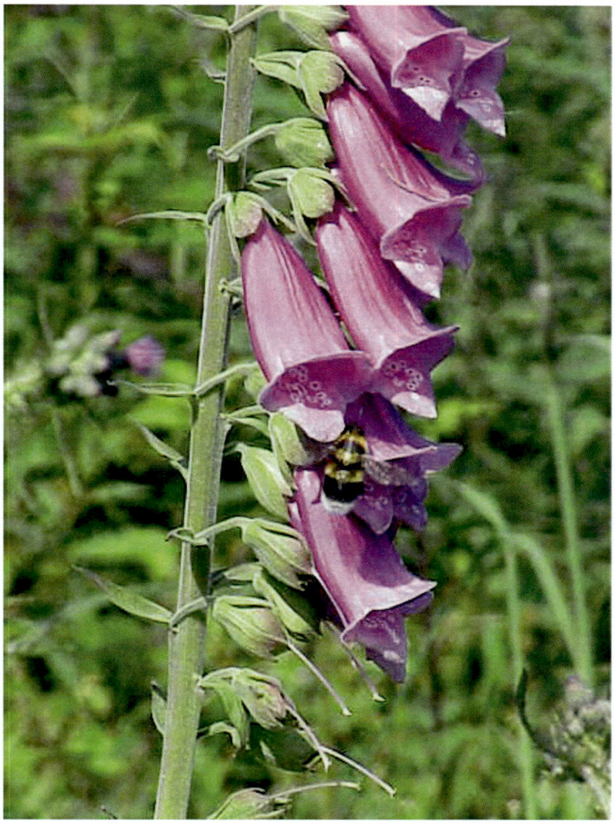

Figure 7.2. *Foxglove flowering plant.*

Source: By Kurt Stüber [1] – caliban.mpiz-koeln.mpg.de/mavica/index.html part of www.biolib.de, CC BY-SA 3.0; https://commons.wikimedia.org/w/index.php?curid=6516.

More than three hundred years ago, Withering discovered that the leaf of the foxglove was an extremely effective treatment for this condition, which was referred to as dropsy at the time. It is unfortunate that digitalis glycosides are also among the most toxic drugs, as they frequently cause cardiac arrhythmias at concentrations that are necessary to significantly increase the cardiac output. The Na, K-activated Mg-ATPase, which is also referred to as the sodium, potassium pump, is located in the cell membrane and is the site where their action takes place. Every cell has an intracellular environment that is high in potassium and low in sodium, and this active transport system is responsible for ensuring that this environment is maintained. In contrast, it seems that the blockade of a portion of the pumping sites in the heart by digitalis causes the intracellular sodium concentration to momentarily rise above normal during each myocardial action potential. This elevated sodium is then exchanged with calcium that is brought in from the outside of the cell by a membrane carrier that is referred to as the sodium–calcium exchanger. During the beating of the heart, this results in an increase in the amount of calcium that is found inside the cells, which in turn stimulates the actomyosin system to contract with greater force. Taking into consideration the fact that every cell possesses sodium and potassium pumps that are inhibited by digitalis, it is quite remarkable that these glycosides can be used as inotropic drugs at all.

The oleander bush (Nerium), which is an extremely common ornamental shrub in the southeastern United States, the lily-of-the-valley (Convallaria) ornamental flower, and the butterfly weed (Asclepias), which is a wildflower, are an additional examples of plants that produce dangerous quantities of digitalis compounds. An adult human being could be killed by the cardiac glycoside that is contained in a single leaf of the oleander plant. During the nonflowering season, the leaves of the foxglove plant are often confused with those of the common comfrey plant, whose leaves are commonly used in the preparation of herbal teas. This foxglove plant poses a potential risk because of this confusion. Many people have lost their lives as a result of the accidental consumption of foxglove leaves.

Certain members of the Solanaceae family, including potato spuds, green tomatoes (which contain the major saponin known as α-tomatine), and other members, contain toxic saponins. Moreover, sea cucumbers and starfish are also capable of producing them. Many saponins can disrupt the normal bilayer packing of phospholipids in cell membranes. This can cause the cells that are affected to become abnormally leaky to ions, which ultimately leads to lysis, which is the death of the cell. The primary saponin that can be found in foxglove is known as digitonin, and it features a high level of detergent activity.

Ginseng, also known as Panax, is a traditional herbal medicine that appears to be effective in treating a wide range of conditions, including but not limited to fatigue, sexual impotence, heart disease, and even cancer. Glycyrrhizins are a type of saponin that can be found in significant quantities in the roots of ginseng. These natural products are apparently safe when administered orally atrecommededdoses, usually as a tea or a tablet. On the other hand, people who consume excessive amounts of ginseng on a regular basis may experience negative side effects such as trouble sleeping, skin eruptions, diarrhea, and high blood pressure.

The majority of saponins, in their glycoside form, are not easily absorbed from the gastrointestinal tract, which is a fortunate circumstance for us. Glycosidase enzymes found in the intestinal tract are responsible for cleaving away the sugar groups that are attached to the 3-B–OH group on the sterol skeleton. This effectively eliminates the toxicity of the sterols completely. In addition to being easily absorbed, the non-polar aglycones are likely to be components that have pharmacological active properties. A large and chemically diverse group of compounds is known as saponins. Despite the fact that chemists have made a significant amount of effort to decipher their intricate structures, very little is currently known about the pharmacological mechanisms of action of these substances. Probably through a number of different cell receptors, they are able to exert a variety of actions. In spite of their popularity, their clinical efficacy has to be confirmed.

7.6.2.2. Alkaloid Toxins

It has been possible to isolate and investigate thousands of compounds of this type, and in many cases, the investigation has been quite superficial. In general, the majority of these substances can also be referred to as heterocyclic compounds because they have a ring structure that typically contains at least one atom that is not carbon, typically either nitrogen or oxygen. Flowering plants have been a particularly rich source of alkaloids. With the exception of antimicrobial drugs, which are primarily derived from bacteria, the majority of drugs have originated either directly or indirectly from alkaloids that are found in flowering plants.

One of the alkaloids that is utilized the most frequently is nicotine, which is a substance that stimulates cholinergic receptors that are known as "nicotinic." Additionally, nicotine and related compounds are useful toxins for controlling certain insect pests. This is in addition to the fact that nicotine can be self-administered as tobacco. This substance can be quite toxic to farm workers who apply it as an insecticide or to laboratory scientists who are handling the free base. This is because the free base form of nicotine rapidly diffuses across the skin. An additional heterocyclic compound that is said to have been consumed by the Greek philosopher Socrates is coniine, which is a significant alkaloid found in poison hemlock potion. More than two thousand years after its discovery, the mechanism of action of this notorious poison is still a mystery! Tubocurarine, an alkaloid found in South American arrow poison, functions as a competitive antagonist of acetylcholine and nicotine at the neuromuscular junction of skeletal muscle when it is present.

In recent years, a significant number of alkaloids have also been isolated from sources that are not as conventional, such as marine organisms; some of these alkaloids are also toxic.

7.6.2.3. Flowering Plants Containing Peptide and Protein Toxins

There are several plants that contain protein toxins that are fatal when taken orally or when administered parenterally if they are administered. Necklaces are frequently made from rosary bean seeds, which are a very attractive red seed with a black spot. As the name suggests, these seeds are frequently used to make necklaces. Abrin, a protein with a molecular weight of 70 kilodaltons, is found in these seeds. Abrin is a ribosomal protein synthesis inhibitor. A bean known as castor, which is now naturalized in southern California, is similar and is also used for making decorative necklaces. Ricine is a homologous protein that has the same mechanism of action and has the potential to be lethal. It is present in this substance. The A chain is the active inhibitor of protein synthesis, and the B chain is required to bind to the cell membrane and stimulate the internalization of the toxin. These different types of toxins, such as the diphtheria toxin, are made up of two different polypeptide chains. The symptoms of poisoning caused by these two toxins appear relatively slowly during the first twenty-four hours after ingestion; however, if the victim has consumed a large number of seeds, they may experience a great deal of suffering over the subsequent couple of days before ultimately succumbing to a terrifying death. Because the toxins are embedded within the fibrous seed pit, it is possible that the individual will not receive a significant amount of the toxin if they do not chew the seed pit. As soon as possible within the first few hours after ingestion, it is recommended that ipecac syrup be used to induce vomiting, which should then be followed by gastric lavage. If this is not possible, the only treatment that can be administered is symptomatic treatment because the toxins are internalized within the cell.

As herbal medicines, mistletoe leaves and berries have been used to prepare teas and extracts that are taken orally for the treatment of a wide range of conditions. Some of these conditions include high blood pressure, tachycardia, insomnia, depression, sterility, ulcers, and cancer, to name just a few. At this time, there are no medical reports that support the therapeutic use of mistletoe extracts. This is although a few of these conditions, such as hypertension and tachycardia, might ostensibly be alleviated based on the current knowledge of the contents of mistletoe. Ingestion of mistletoe extracts is likely to be harmful to one's health due to the presence of a toxin known as viscumin, which has an action that is comparable to that of ricin and abrin, as well as smaller peptide toxins known as viscotoxins. These viscotoxins depolarize the membranes of muscle cells, which can lead to hypotension, bradycardia, and other complications.

7.6.2.4. Plants Causing Contact Dermatitis

There is a wide range of living things, both plants and animals that are known to cause inflammatory responses. At the beginning of the twentieth century, the Nobel-prize-winning French physiologist Edward Richet initiated a study of natural inflammatory substances. While he was conducting research on the toxicity of the Portuguese man-o'war jellyfish, he made the discovery of anaphylaxis, which is an acute immune inflammatory response that poses a significant risk to one's life. It is possible for certain venoms to cause large inflammatory responses of comparable magnitude even in the absence of an immune component. Other naturally occurring compounds, because they are allergenic, are responsible for a delayed hypersensitivity response that is known as contact dermatitis. A response to poison ivy, poison oak, or poison sumac is one of the most well-known examples of this type of response.

In certain countries, such as the United States and Canada, where these plants are abundant in both urban and rural settings, this poses a significant risk to the majority of the people who live there. By coming into contact with these plants, a mixture of compounds that are very similar to one another is released. These compounds are known as urushiols, and they are catechols that are 4-alkyl-substituted dihydroxyphenyl compounds. The initial exposure to these substances does not typically result in inflammation; however, subsequent exposure to them does result in a delayed immune response. An initial oxidation process leads to the formation of quinone, which then undergoes a reaction with proteins found in the skin and transforms into an immunogen. The Langerhans cells of the skin that have been stimulated migrate to the thymus, where they, in turn, stimulate the production of thymic lymphocytes that are capable of responding to urushiol. The lymphocytes that originate in the thymus then move to the skin, where they take part in the inflammatory response that occurs in response to subsequent exposures to the urushiol compounds. It is fascinating to learn that the lacquer that is used to give Japanese pottery a glossy surface is derived from a plant that is related to poison ivy and also contains urushiols. Urushiols are rendered inactive when the lacquered surface is allowed to dry in the heat for an extended period of time.

The workers are unable to completely avoid being exposed to the urushiols that are present in the fluid that they initially apply. After prolonged exposure, many people develop hyposensitization or resistance to the substance.

7.7. Animal Venoms and Toxins

7.7.1. Reptiles and Amphibians

The scientific investigation of snake venom and the treatment of envenomation are both quite difficult to accomplish since snake venom is a complex mixture of active components. The vast body of literature that covers folklore, natural history, scientific investigation, and medical treatment of poisonous snake bites has piqued the interest of the majority of "toxicologists." Neon venom is the subject of a significant number of presentations that are given at meetings of the International Society of Toxinology (which are announced in the journal of the Society, Toxicon).

Toxic snakes can be classified into four different families. Both pit vipers, which belong to the family Crotalidae, and vipers, which belong to the family Viperidae, will have their venoms compared first. After that, we will investigate the venoms of the cobra (Elapidae) and the sea snake (Hydrophiidae), which are also closely related in terms of their biochemical and pharmacological properties (Figure 7.3).

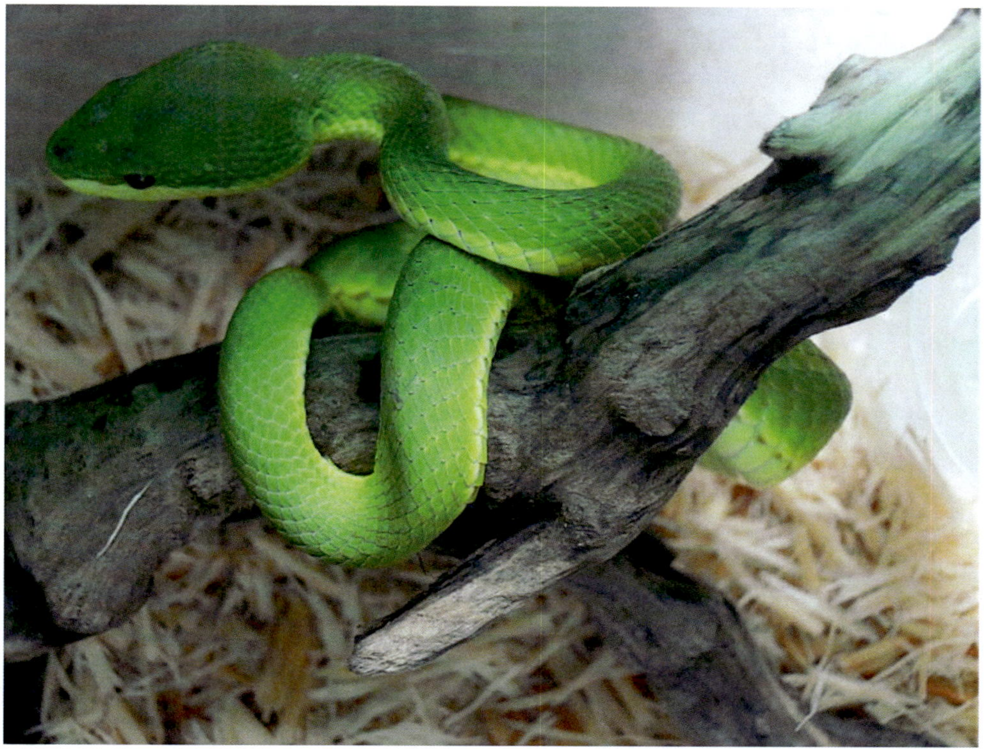

Figure 7.3. *Indian pit viper.*

Source: By Biomedicinal – Own work, CC BY-SA 3.0; https://commons.wikimedia.org/w/index.php?curid=29436267.

The pit vipers (Figure 7.3) have a heat-sensitive sensory organ that is located within a pit next to each eye. This organ is used to detect the presence of warm-blooded prey. Other members of this group include rattlesnakes, water mocassins, and copper-headed vipers. North and South America are home to a significant number of pit vipers, whereas vipers are only found in continental Africa and Europe. In general, pit viper and viper venoms have greater local effects on the tissues where the bite occurs and on the cardiovascular system. However, there are some exceptions to this rule. Protein hemorrhagic toxins are responsible for the development of localized tissue swelling, also known as edema. These toxins attack the capillary endothelium, causing it to breach and allow plasma proteins and blood cells to pass through. Protein myotoxins are believed to be responsible for the pathological release of intracellular calcium stores in skeletal muscle, which can lead to the development of muscle necrosis. Enzymes such as hyaluronidase and collagenase are responsible for the breakdown of connective tissue elements, which in turn facilitates the spread of venom from the site where the bite was initially made. In the absence of a medical emergency involving the cardiovascular system, motor paralysis is extremely rare; however, there is one notable exception to this rule. One of the most potent neurotoxins is called crotoxin, and it can be found in the venom of the Brazilian rattlesnake, which is also referred to as *Crotalus durissus terrificus*. Crotoxin causes a loss of neuromuscular transmission and flaccid paralysis by paralyzing the nerve terminals in the periphery of the body.

The majority of immunotherapeutic treatments for pit viper bites make use of a polyvalent horse antivenin that was initially prepared with an antigenic mixture of several different crotalid venoms. This is because crotalid venom, for the most part, contains similar toxins and enzymes, and it is frequently impossible to identify the species. The results of this strategy have been quite favorable.

In many cases, respiratory arrest is the first symptom of envenomation caused by a cobra or sea snake, which occurs before any signs of local tissue or systemic cardiovascular damage are visible. Elapid and hydrophiid venoms contain α-neurotoxin, which is the most prominent neurotoxin found in these venoms. This is a basic polypeptide that contains an amino acid residue count ranging from 65 to 80 and is crosslinked with four or five disulfide bonds. By acting as a competitive antagonist of the neurotransmitter acetylcholine (ACh) at the neuromuscular junction of skeletal muscle, the toxin serves to inhibit its activity. In contrast to the nondepolarizing muscle relaxants that are utilized in surgical procedures, which exert their effects at the same site, α-neurotoxin exhibits a high degree of adherence due to its larger molecular size, which allows for numerous interactions with the nicotinic receptor. The Taiwanese krait, also known as *Bungarus multicinctus*, contains a toxin known as alpha-bungarotoxin. This toxin binds to the nicotinic receptor in the skeletal muscle in a manner that is essentially irreversible, thereby preventing acetylcholine from interacting with its postsynaptic receptor. In addition to producing a powerful neurotoxin that is capable of paralyzing skeletal muscle, this snake also produces a larger protein toxin known as beta-bungarotoxin (Table 7.1), which inhibits the release of acetylcholine from the motor nerve terminal. The combination of these two toxins, which work together synergistically, can reduce the likelihood of neuromuscular transmission to zero. Elapid venoms typically contain phospholipase A and a peptide known as cardiotoxin, which is a cytolysin that has a tendency to attack cardiac myocardial cells. In addition to the postsynaptic alpha-neurotoxic peptides, their venoms also typically contain phospholipase A. Cardiotoxin causes the bilayer structure of membrane lipids to be disrupted, which in turn makes these lipids more accessible to the phospholipase A enzyme, which is responsible for their degradation.

In the new world, the only elapids that exist are coral snakes. Roughly fifty different species have been described. The United States of America is home to only two species, whereas the regions of Central America and the northern regions of South America are home to a considerably larger number of species. The amount of venom that is typically injected into a coral snake is typically quite low, which is one reason why coral snake bites are not nearly as dangerous as cobra bites. Because elapid snakes do not possess fangs like pit vipers do, they are forced to resort to a method of envenomation that involves chewing for a longer period of time, which is not nearly as effective as the previously mentioned method. The major danger for elapid snake envenomation victims is respiratory arrest due to neuromuscular arrest. It is common for there to be little or no localized edema shortly after the bite, as is the case with crotalid envenomations. This can sometimes lead to an incorrect initial perception that the victim's life is not in danger.

Despite the fact that antivenin therapy continues to be the most effective method for treating snake envenomations, there are many instances in which antivenin is not immediately available. As a result, a rational therapeutic approach that is based on knowledge of the actions of the toxic constituents is required.

There are only a few species of amphibians that pose a threat to human beings, but the majority of amphibians have skin toxins that serve as some kind of chemical defense against predators. Some of the brightly colored tropical South American frogs contain extremely potent toxins, and it is possible that simply touching these frogs is enough to cause intoxication. It would appear that some of these frogs are collected for the exotic pet market and kept in vivariums as pets. Fortunately for the owner, these frogs quickly lose their toxicity in captivity, which suggests that they produce their toxins from precursor molecules that are present in their natural diet. Because it is a lipophilic sodium channel activator, the component known as batrachotoxin, which originates from one of these frogs, is widely used by Indian hunters in the preparation of poison darts. Although human intoxication symptoms have not been reported, it is expected that they will be comparable to those that are brought on by the grayanotoxins or the veratrum alkaloids that are discovered in the false hellebore. Histrionicotoxin, which is another type of alkaloidal toxin found in frogs, is responsible for neuromuscular paralysis because it binds to the open channel of the nicotinic receptor found in skeletal muscle.

The parotid glands located behind the eyes of toads belonging to the genus Bufo contain a highly potent venom that is secreted through their skin. However, there are also biogenic amines, such as epinephrine and bufotenin, which is a methylated form of the neurotransmitter serotonin. The most toxic constituents are cardiac glycosides, which are referred to as bufotoxins. "Toad licking" is a practice that some enthusiasts have adopted due to the hallucinogenic properties of bufotenin. Getting high through this method is risky because the white milky venom contains a high concentration of bufotoxins (Lalloo & Theakston, 2003; Alirol et al., 2010; Bolt, 2021).

7.7.2. Fish Venoms and Toxins

Venomous fish are only found in a relatively small percentage of fish species, and the venoms that they produce are always used for defensive purposes, to ward off potential predators. Catfishes and sting rays are probably the two different types of venomous fish that are encountered the most frequently. Anglers with years of experience are aware of the painful stings that are caused by the venom of marine catfish, but novice anglers frequently learn this lesson the hard way. Despite the fact that a recent paper reports the smooth muscle stimulating and hemolytic activity of a large protein toxin, very little is known about the active constituents. Sting rays have a dorsal spine that is located near the base of their tail. When the ray is stepped on in shallow water, the tail is thrust upward so that the spine can penetrate the skin of the person who is stepping on it. As a result of the fact that the sting rays are almost always scared away when waders shuffle their feet along the surface of the bottom, this is the most effective method for avoiding this fish. On the other hand, the tropical Pacific stonefish, also known as *Synancega* sp., is not easily frightened and will simply raise its spine when it detects the presence of an intruder. Stonefish and sting ray spine venoms, similar to catfish venom, are likely to contain a number of protein toxins that cause smooth muscles to contract and cause inflammation. A large protein that stimulates the release of neurotransmitters from nerve terminals has been identified as the stonefish toxin, which was recently isolated and demonstrated to be a substance. Antihistamines and corticosteroids are two examples of anti-inflammatory medications that can typically be used to treat these stings, which, despite the fact that they are quite unpleasant, rarely pose a threat to the patient's life.

When it comes to fish toxins, tetrodotoxin is without a doubt one of the most powerful. As a result of the fact that pufferfish are regarded as a dangerous delicacy in Japan, chefs are required to undergo extensive training in the removal of poisonous viscera and skin before preparing "fugu" flesh for consumption. Even though pufferfish are not commonly consumed in the United States, there have been multiple reports of people becoming poisoned by them over the years. After ingesting pufferfish, a person who is intoxicated will typically experience tingling and numbness in the mouth region within an hour of the consumption of the pufferfish. There is muscular weakness and complete paralysis entailing removal of the consumed fish with symptomatic treatment. Further, slow passage of toxins like the cigua toxin is possible across the food chain.

An excellent illustration of this is ciguatoxin, which is responsible for activating voltage-gated sodium channels in nerve and muscle cells. There is a high degree of unpredictability associated with ciguatera poisoning; the highly predatory fish is typically edible in a specific location. Lethargy, tingling and numbness of the lips, weakness in the hands and/or feet, itching, joint pains, and gastrointestinal symptoms including diarrhea are some of the symptoms that are brought on by this condition. Due to the fact that this lipophilic toxin is eliminated very slowly, these problems may continue for a period of approximately several months. It is active in such minute concentrations that research on its structure was hampered for more than a decade because insufficient amounts were available for analysis.

This was due to the fact that that it is active. There have been reports of ciguatera infestations in both the Caribbean Sea and the tropical Pacific Ocean's waters. As a result of the fact that the symptoms are different in these locations, it is possible that the toxins are not identical. It would appear that the administration of hyperosmotic mannitol is an effective symptomatic therapy for controlling the Schwann cell edema that is brought on by this complex molecule.

7.7.3. Arthropod Toxins and Venoms

This animal phylum includes a wide variety of animals, including spiders, scorpions, and insects, among numerous others. A great number of arthropods employ neuroactive substances so that they can act as toxins, alarm pheromones, or repellents. Toxins appear to be present in only a small percentage of insect species, even though insects are the most diverse group in terms of biodiversity. On the other hand, almost all scorpions and spiders routinely use venomous secretions to capture their prey and to discourage predators from attacking them. To our great good fortune, the majority of arthropod toxins have developed in such a way that they are capable of immobilizing animals other than mammals. There is only a relatively small group of spider species that are known to be toxic to humans.

Scorpion venom is one of the most abundant sources of peptide toxins that are currently known; in terms of diversity, it is comparable to the cone shell venoms, which will be discussed in the following aforementioned section. Scorpions are able to quickly immobilize their prey, which is typically insects, by injecting a complex mixture of peptides that act on the voltage-gated sodium and potassium channels, which then produce action potentials. Within the sodium channel, there are two types of toxins, which are referred to as alpha and beta toxins, and they bind at sites 3 and 4, respectively, on the external surface of the channel. Both of these factors improve electrical excitability by modulating the probability that the sodium channel will remain open. This occurs even when the electrical potential of the membrane is nearly identical to what it was in the resting state (approximately 60–90 mV negative on the inside surface of the membrane). Specifically, the α-scorpion toxins can slow down a process known as inactivation, which is the process by which the open sodium channel becomes inactive when membrane depolarization is present. It is possible for an action potential that is normally short (with a duration of approximately one millisecond) to be transformed into an abnormally long signal with a duration that could be several hundred milliseconds. A significant amount of neurotransmitters are released at the peripheral nerve terminals of skeletal muscles and other muscles as a result of this happening. The victim is subjected to a series of disastrous consequences, including hyperexcitability, convulsions, paralysis, and even death in extraordinary cases.

By stimulating the nerves and muscles to generate trains of multiple action potentials in response to each depolarizing stimulus, the β-scorpion toxins also cause hyperexcitability in the peripheral nervous system. This occurs through a different mechanism than the one described above. The toxins derived from the β-scorpion are responsible for reducing the rate at which the sodium channel that has been opened returns to its resting state. This process is commonly known as "deactivation." In most cases, scorpions from the old world only contain sodium channel toxins of the alpha type, whereas scorpions from the new world frequently contain both α- and β-neurotoxins. It is possible to obtain antivenins for the most dangerous scorpions, which are also the most effective means of treatment.

Since the late 1980s, researchers have found that scorpion venom contains a different group of smaller peptide toxins that block a variety of potassium channels. In light of the fact that the electrical excitability of a nerve or muscle cell at any given moment is dependent on the relative permeability of the membrane to sodium and potassium ions, it is not surprising that a scorpion's venom would also contain toxins that block potassium channels. The calcium-activated potassium channels that are present in smooth and skeletal muscles are primarily blocked by charybdotoxin, which was the first of these toxins to be characterized. To prevent the cell from experiencing excessive membrane depolarization and calcium loading from within, this channel is present. In addition, charybdotoxin may inhibit the activity of certain voltage-activated potassium channels in the brain.

Because of this multiplicity of toxins in scorpion venom that enhance electrical excitability, an alternative approach for treating scorpion envenomation would be to reduce excitability, particularly in the peripheral nervous system (these peptides do not readily cross the blood–brain barrier). This could be at least partially achieved by reducing postsynaptic membrane responsiveness to Ach with nicotinic and muscarinic receptor antagonists. This potential method of treatment could supplement the use of antivenins.

Typically, spiders will use poison to kill their insect prey. Because the receptors in the nervous systems of vertebrates and insects are sufficiently distinct from one another from a pharmacological standpoint, the majority of spider toxins do not have a significant impact on human beings. The fact that we are so much larger than their typical prey and predators is also a factor that works in our favor. Nevertheless, there are a few spiders that pose significant harm to humans. Since black widow spiders, which belong to the genus Latrodectus, can be found all over the world, we will begin by focusing on them. Due to the presence of a potent protein toxin known as alpha-latrotoxin, their venom is classified as primarily neurotoxic (Table 7.1). This large protein not only increases the release of neurotransmitters from nerve terminals, but it also has the potential to cause the removal of secretory vesicles from nerve terminals. In addition to experiencing skeletal muscle spasms, victims also experience autonomic overstimulation, which can result in sweating, salivation, nausea, and elevated blood pressure symptoms. The administration of the antivenin Latrodectus is the primary component of the treatment, as stated previously. It is possible to alleviate some of these symptoms by taking centrally acting muscle relaxants such as diazepam. Additionally, autonomic overstimulation can be alleviated by taking muscarinic and/or adrenergic antagonists, depending on the symptoms.

Since its venom primarily contains an enzyme called sphingomyelinase, which is responsible for causing damage to tissue, the venom of the brown recluse spider (*Loxoceles* sp.) operates in an entirely different manner. It is possible for this venom to cause significant tissue necrosis at the site of the bite, even though it is less dangerous than the venom of the black widow.

The venoms of wasps, hornets, and bees are distinct from one another, even though they are all members of the order Hymenoptera. The most severe reactions to hymenopteran stings are what are known as immediate hypersensitivity reactions. These reactions are caused by an immune response that is mediated by immunoglobulin E and are a result of previous stings. It has been discovered that bee venom contains an extremely high concentration of enzymes and chemical substances. Phospholipase A is the most important enzyme because it works in conjunction with a peptide detergent known as mellitin, which is named after the common honeybee Apis mellifera. Together, these two enzymes work to break down phospholipids in the plasma membrane, which in turn releases prolytic fatty acids and lysolecithin. Although mellitin can disrupt the cell membrane on its own, the presence of these phospholipid breakdown products makes its performance significantly more efficient. For the same reason that many snake venoms do, bee venom also contains the enzyme hyaluronidase. This enzyme is responsible for breaking down connective tissue, which in turn makes it easier for the venom to spread from the site where it was injected. Apamin and mast cell degranulating peptide are two peptide toxins that are found in bee venom. These peptide toxins block calcium-activated potassium channels and voltage-activated potassium channels through their respective mechanisms.

Wasp and hornet venoms, in contrast to bee venom, primarily contain small peptides known as kinins. Kinins, which are similar to our own endogenous bradykinin, have a triple action, which includes the stimulation of sensory nerve endings, which leads to neurogenic inflammation, increased capillary permeability, and relaxation of vascular smooth muscle.

There are a great number of fire ants (Solenopsis) in the southeastern region of the United States, and each year, they sting a great number of people. The piperidine alkaloids that are found in the venom have been discovered to be capable of blocking the nicotinic receptor ion channel of the body. The painful sensation that is associated with the sting is thought to be caused, at least in part, by the constituents of proteins. At the site of the sting, it is possible that pustules that are irritated and some minor tissue necrosis will develop, which will cause the discomfort to last for several days. It is not entirely clear what part the alkaloids, which are known as solenopsins, play in the inflammatory responses that are associated with fire ant stings; however, it is known that solenopsins cause basophils to release histamine (Lalloo & Theakston, 2003; Alirol et al., 2010; Bolt, 2021).

7.7.4. Mollusk Venoms and Toxins

Although the exoskeleton of mollusks offers a significant degree of protection against predators, it also restricts the animals' mobility. In the case of predatory snails, this presents a challenge. On the other hand, a particular group of gastropods known as "cones" possesses a formidable venom apparatus that resembles a harpoon and is capable of paralyzing its prey. Conus venom was the subject of a significant amount of research in the 1990s. Each and every one of the Conus toxins is either a peptide or a small protein. There are several types of ion channel modulators that are present in the venom. These include nicotinic receptor antagonists (α-conotoxins), sodium channel blockers (μ-conotoxins), calcium channel blockers (ω-conotoxins), and glutamate channel blockers (conantokins). Only a relatively small fraction of the 300 known species of Conus are dangerous to humans, and these mainly occur in the tropical Pacific. Divers with little to no experience should steer clear of handling cone shells. A posterior salivary gland secretion is used by the octopus to envenomate its prey when it is hunting. The tiny Australian blue-ringed octopus, which was featured in the James Bond film "Octopussy," is the only species of octopus that, according to scientific research, is toxic to humans. People who go to the beach have been known to play with this adorable little animal, which can frequently be found among rocks on the beach, without being aware of how dangerous it is. While the venom of all other species of octopus contains protein toxins that are not harmful to humans, the venom of this species contains tetrodotoxin, which is the same toxin that pufferfish release into the environment. The capacity of bivalve mollusks to concentrate potentially lethal quantities of dinoflagellate toxins, such as saxitoxin and domoic acid, has already been covered in the preceding section.

7.7.5. Coelenterate (Cnidarian) Venoms

Cnidaria is a more recent name for this phylum, which indicates that all species contain something called cnidae, which are small stinging capsules. Nematocysts are another name for cnidae. Even within a single animal, there is a high degree of diversity in the cnidae family. It is not surprising that the majority of cnidarian human envenomations are caused by stings from jellyfish (Figure 7.4) or Portuguese man-o'-wars because the largest and most formidable cnidae, which are capable of discharging venom deep within the victim's skin, are found in the classes Scyphozoa (jellyfish) and Hydrozoa (man-o'-war, etc.). There are approximately 10,000 species that belong to this phylum, and all of them have the potential to be toxic or even venomous. The Chironex fleckeri, which is considered to be the most dangerous species of jellyfish in the world, can be found along the coast of Australia. There have been reports of swimmers collapsing within seconds of receiving multiple stings from this species, which makes it impossible for them to go swimming during certain occasions of the year. These jellyfish are kept out of swimming areas by means of barriers, and lifeguards are required to undergo extensive training to be able to assist those unfortunate individuals who have been affected by them. Stings from the majority of other types of jellyfish can also be extremely painful, but they are rarely considered to be life-threatening. Rather than being true corals, the fire corals that are found in tropical waters, such as the man-o'-war, are actually hydrozoans. It is likely that the presence of toxins that are comparable to those found in man-o'-war poison is the cause of their inflammatory sting.

Nematocysts are able to release their contents when the nematocyte cell in which they are housed is stimulated not only chemically but also mechanically. The tubule that is contained within the nematocyst undergoes an explosive evagination, which results in the injection of a protei-naceous venom into the skin of the victim. Due to the fact that jellyfish toxins are large, unstable proteins that are difficult to purify, only a few of the major jellyfish toxins have been isolated in recent times. According to the majority of the scant information available on these toxins, it appears that their primary function is that of pore-formers, which results in the depolarization of nerve, muscle, and inflammatory (basophil, etc.) cells.

Taking into account the massive release of numerous chemical mediators of inflammation and the transient stimulation of nerve terminals in various types of muscle, including cardiac and vascular muscle, it is possible to predict the majority of the symptoms that are observed in envenomated individuals and experimental animals during the experiment. Antihistamines, despite the fact that they offer a significant amount of relief for the symptoms that are solely associated with inflammation, are not adequate to counteract all of the actions that are carried out by the most potent venoms, such as Chironex. It has been suggested that alcohol, acetic acid, and protease mixtures like meat tenderizer are some of the treatments that could be used to limit the further discharge of nematocysts on the skin of the victim. It is likely that the most effective and common method of initial treatment is the application of vinegar (acetic acid) topically. The development of a therapy that is more rational for these envenomations is currently awaiting further investigations into the pharmacological actions of the various toxic components that are found in jellyfish venom.

Zoanthids, which are small colonial sea anemones that are found in tropical reefs, contain palytoxin, which is one of the most powerful contaminants found in marine environments. A marine bacterium that resides in the zoanthid is responsible for the production of this toxin, which exerts its effects by transforming the sodium-potassium pump into an ion channel rather than the other way around. Palytoxin, unlike ciguatoxin, has the potential to cause food-borne intoxications in humans. This is since it can also be transmitted up the food chain into fish that are edible.

Sea anemones have peptide toxins that interfere with signaling like those of scorpions. Some anemones also contain smaller peptide toxins that selectively block certain potassium channels. There are also powerful cytolytic proteins known as actinoporins that are found in the majority of sea anemones. These proteins permeabilize cell membranes, which ultimately leads to the death of cells. It is fortunate that only a small percentage of sea anemone species are capable of stinging humans when they are handled. This could be due to the fact that sea anemone nematocysts are typically too small to penetrate deep into the skin. On the other hand, it is best to avoid handling these organisms with your bare hands because there are some species that can cause quite a bit of pain!

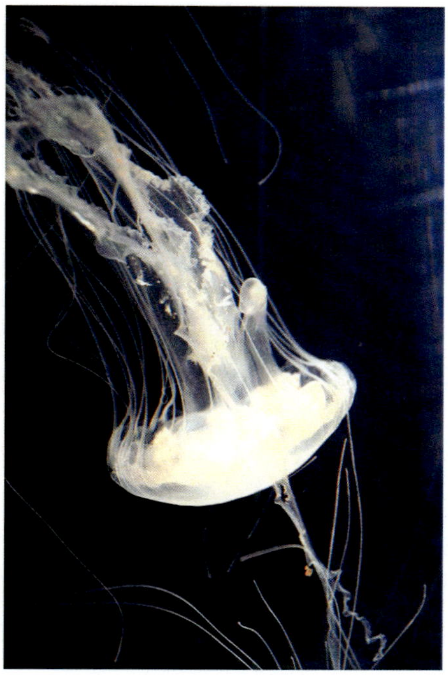

Figure 7.4. *The sea nettle jellyfish, Chrysaora quinquecirrha.*

7.7.6. Other Toxic Marine Invertebrates

The fact that only a relatively small number of species are harmful to humans is a fortunate circumstance, despite the fact that many invertebrates that are sedentary or slow-moving possess defensive toxins that are designed to discourage predators. Several species of sea urchins, primarily those found in the Indo-Pacific region, are equipped with either venomous spines or pedicellaria, which are venomous organs that resemble flowers and are known to rotate frequently around their base. These pedicellaria appear to protect the surface of the sea urchin from small predators or organisms that foul the surrounding environment. Recent research has led to the isolation of a number of inflammatory protein toxins that are responsible for contracting smooth muscle from the pedicellaria.

In addition to more immediate inflammatory action, certain sponges, such as the Caribbean fire sponge (*Tedania ignis*) and the nolitangere sponge (French for "do not touch!"), are known to cause chronic contact dermatitis. However, the active constituents of these sponges have not yet been identified.

There are some marine worms that are extremely poisonous. The phylum Annelida is home to a number of different species of segmented worms, which are included in this category. As a result of its ability to block nicotinic cholinergic receptors, the toxin extracted from a species that is found in Japanese waters, known as nereistoxin, has become an insecticide that is useful for agricultural purposes. In addition to the bothersome irritation caused by the fine bristles that are lodged in the skin, bristle worms, which are commonly found in coral reefs, are responsible for causing a sting that is quite irritating. This is likely due to the release of inflammatory substances. Another annelid that can cause stings and is used as bait for fishing in the New England region is the blood worm, also known as *Glycera dibranchiata*. The "fangs" of the proboscis of this relatively large worm inject a protein toxin that not only causes some tissue necrosis but also stimulates the release of neurotransmitters from nerve terminals.

7.8. Toxin and Venom Therapy

7.8.1. Identification of the Toxic Organism

It is typically essential to identify the toxic organism to select the appropriate treatment. This is due to the fact that the toxins of closely related species frequently have a different chemical structure and even a different mechanism of action. For the first time, an immunologic method that can identify the species of snake that is responsible for a bite is now available in Australia. There is a good chance that kits of this kind will become accessible in other regions of the world.

The readers who are interested in learning about the identification of poisonous plants and animals in the world have access to a number of excellent guides that provide information on the identification of these species. A significant number of intoxications that are caused by food occur when individuals sample natural or ornamental plants without proper identification, resulting in the consumption of the incorrect plant, which can sometimes have tragic consequences.

7.8.2. Immediate Therapeutic Procedures to Counteract Ingestion of Poisons

It is possible to induce vomiting with ipecac syrup, which is a mixture of plant alkaloids known as emetines. This is a highly effective initial response to the ingestion of a poisonous substance or plant. The only time it should be used is in the immediate aftermath of a poisoning that has already taken place. There are certain circumstances in which it should not be used, such as when the patient is extremely drowsy or unconscious. This is because the failure to vomit (which typically occurs 15–30 minutes later) could lead to additional difficulties due to the emetine alkaloids found in the medication. In the event that the patient does not throw up within a reasonable amount of time, an additional dose is ingested to finally cause vomiting and eliminate any poisons that have not been absorbed by the body.

Gastric lavage is a procedure that can be performed by trained medical personnel in the event that vomiting is unsuccessful or cannot be completed. This procedure involves inserting a tube into the stomach and applying suction to remove the harmful contents. This procedure is typically performed after the patient has been sedated. It is common practice to administer an oral dose of activated charcoal to the patient after this procedure. Activated charcoal is an effective method for removing many poisons from the gastrointestinal tract, and it is ultimately eliminated through the feces. It is common practice to administer a cathartic saline solution to hasten the elimination of the poisonous substance from the intestines, regardless of whether or not the charcoal has been adsorbed.

The sole purpose of this description is to bring the reader's attention to the various treatment options. As soon as possible, a medical professional who is trained to treat intoxications ought to be contacted to provide assistance to the patient!

7.8.3. Prospects for Improved Immunotherapy of Venoms and Toxins

It is common practice to use polyvalent antivenins to treat bites from related species of snakes. This is due to the fact that it is frequently difficult to differentiate between the bites of different snake species. The polyvalent serum that is used to treat crotalid bites is prepared by immunizing horses with a mixture of several species of Crotalus. This serum has been demonstrated to be effective in the treatment of bites caused by more than 65 different species of crotalids.

When it comes to immune therapy for venomous animal bites and stings, one of the traditional drawbacks is that the IgG antibody does not work effectively in neutralizing venom constituents once they have entered the interstitial fluid space. The preparation of truncated antibody molecules, such as the F(AB)2 fragments, has recently been discovered to be capable of enhancing the neutralization of tissue-bound toxins. This discovery was made relatively recently.

There is a high incidence of serum sickness, which is a human immune response to the intravenous administration of horse serum antivenin. This is one of the most significant issues that is associated with the use of antivenins. The antigenic mixture that is used to produce antivenin could be enriched with the major toxins or other proteins that are the most dangerous. This would be one method that could be used to reduce the problem. It is possible that this will allow for a reduction in the overall quantity of freeze-dried horse serum that is required for treatment. Monoclonal antibodies have not yet gained widespread acceptance for the immunotherapy of intoxications or envenomations. This is likely due to a combination of factors, including the following: (1) monoclonals are so specific that they would only work on single components of a venom; (2) they would be less likely to be of use against envenomation by a different species; and (3) they are significantly more expensive to produce. Due to the relatively small market for antivenins, the majority of pharmaceutical companies consider the production of antivenins to be more of a responsibility than a cost. As a result of the decreasing costs associated with the preparation of "humanized" monoclonal antibodies, it is highly probable that in the future, better antivenins will become freely available.

In Australia, it is customary to recommend that intramuscular epinephrine be administered before the injection of antivenin. This is done to lessen the severity of any immediate hypersensitivity reaction that may occur as a result of the antivenin. Following this, oral corticosteroids should be taken for several days after the antivenin injection to lessen the delayed hypersensitivity response that occurs because of the administration of antivenin. The incidence of serum sickness has been less than 10% thanks to these precautions, which is significantly lower than the nearly 30% that is estimated for victims in the United States (Lalloo & Theakston, 2003; Alirol et al., 2010; Bolt, 2021).

7.8.4. Towards a Rational Pharmacotherapy Based on Knowledge of the Toxic Constituents of Venom

There is a high probability that the majority of people who are envenomated do not receive antivenins promptly that allows them to fully respond to immunotherapy. This is especially true when the envenomation takes place outside of a geographical region that is prone to envenomations. Due to their extremely high levels of allergic sensitivity, some patients are unable to tolerate the antivenom. It would seem prudent to develop rational pharmacotherapies based on scientific knowledge of the chemistry and biological actions of the toxins involved, while at the same time acknowledging the therapeutic power of the immune approach. If the toxin in question is an agonist, then it is possible to use antagonists to counteract the effects of small toxins that act on receptors, and vice versa. By way of illustration, atropine can counteract the effects of the mushroom toxin muscarine. This phenomenon occurs most frequently when receptors for neurotransmitters are involved. In situations where a competitive antidote is not available, it may be possible to physiologically counteract the intoxication by utilizing knowledge of the system that is in opposition to the one being counteracted. It goes without saying that the biochemical and pharmacological understanding of the most active constituents is the very foundation upon which rational therapy is placed.

For a rational therapy to be successful, it must not only be founded on scientific knowledge of the individual actions of the constituents of venom, but it must also take into account the synergistic actions of a significant number of the constituents. Venom, after all, is typically the result of the evolution of a single toxic substance rather than a single venom. Therefore, to identify interactions between venom constituents, toxicological studies need to be conducted with both whole venoms and their purified constituents. This is necessary to avoid any potential contamination.

7.8.5. Toxins as Drugs

Certain naturally occurring toxins, in addition to serving as chemical defenses and offenses for the organisms that produce them, are also being utilized as chemical tools for the investigation of biomedical issues and as models for the development of novel new drugs. The utilization of toxins and venoms as therapeutic agents is not a recent phenomenon; rather, it is an activity that is likely to be as old as the most primitive humanoid species. Because of the development of organic chemistry in the nineteenth century, it became possible to create pharmaceuticals that were derived from natural constituents.

Recent years have seen the development of drug development processes. Several of the toxins that are discussed in this chapter are currently being utilized as molecular models for the purpose of developing drugs that have distinct mechanisms of action. One example is the modification of the worm toxin anabaseine, which has been altered to remove its peripheral nicotinic agonist activity. The resulting compound, DMXB-anabasine (also known as GTS-21), is currently being tested in human clinical trials as a potential treatment for Alzheimer's disease (Kem, 1995).

In the process of drug development, the objective is to disrupt the relationship between the toxicity and therapeutic activity of compounds that are intended to be used as drugs; however, this ideal is rarely completely attainable. By keeping in mind that the difference between a toxin and a drug is frequently a seemingly insignificant change in the chemical structure, or at the very least, the correct selection of dosage, it is helpful to keep this distinction in mind. When the physician and chemist Paracelsus, who lived in the sixteenth century, stated that drugs are also poisons, he demonstrated his understanding of the dual nature of Materia Medica. He also stated that it is frequently a matter of dose whether the therapeutic or toxic effect is more prevalent. Our collective capacity to use natural toxins and venoms as tools in biomedical research and drug design makes them valuable reagents in the field of medical research. This is even though natural toxins and venoms are responsible for many problems. In the end, these substances have the potential to be beneficial to human existence rather than harmful (Lalloo & Theakston, 2003; Alirol et al., 2010; Bolt, 2021).

A Closer Look

Toxicity of Tetrodotoxin

Tetrodotoxin (TTX) is a potent neurotoxin found in various marine and terrestrial species, notably pufferfish. Its toxicity primarily stems from its ability to inhibit voltage-gated sodium channels, which are crucial for the conduction of nerve impulses. When these channels are blocked, normal neuronal function is disrupted, leading to paralysis and potentially fatal respiratory failure. The lethal dose for humans is extremely low, with as little as 1-2 milligrams being sufficient to cause death. Symptoms of TTX poisoning include numbness, tingling, dizziness, and, in severe cases, complete paralysis and respiratory arrest. The onset of symptoms is rapid, often occurring within 30 minutes of ingestion. The toxin's mechanism involves binding to the sodium channels on nerve cell membranes, preventing sodium ions from entering the cells, which is necessary for action potential propagation. This blockade results in the cessation of electrical signaling in nerves and muscles, culminating in the clinical manifestations of toxicity. Despite its high toxicity, TTX has been the subject of medical research due to its potential applications in pain management and as a tool for studying ion channel function. However, there is no known antidote for TTX, and treatment primarily focuses on supportive care, including mechanical ventilation in cases of respiratory failure. The risk of TTX poisoning is particularly high in regions where pufferfish is considered a delicacy, such as Japan, where it is known as fugu. Strict regulations and meticulous preparation are crucial to minimize the risk of poisoning, as even trace amounts of TTX can be deadly. Overall, tetrodotoxin's extreme toxicity and rapid onset of action make it a significant concern in both clinical toxicology and food safety, while its unique properties continue to intrigue researchers exploring its potential therapeutic uses.

Summary

- In contrast to venom, which is a heterogeneous mixture of many substances, some of which are toxic, a toxin is a single substance that has a negative impact on a biological process or organism. Venom is a mixture of many substances. The term "poison" refers to either a single harmful substance or a combination of substances that can be the result of human creation (synthetic) or natural occurrence.
- When it comes to rational treatment of intoxication, having knowledge of the mechanism by which a toxin acts on a biological process is the ultimate basis for rational treatment. Although immunotherapy is effective in treating a significant number of protein intoxications, the treatment of smaller nonpeptide toxins must be based on pharmacologic antagonism in addition to symptomatic treatment. To choose the most appropriate treatment for an intoxication, it is of the utmost importance to determine the type of poison or venom that is involved.
- Initial treatments, such as inducing vomiting and gastric lavage, for toxins that have been ingested orally, as well as immobilization of individuals who have been bitten by poisonous snakes or other animals, can reduce the entry of the toxin(s) into the systemic circulation, which in turn delays the onset of the response and lessens its severity. An important factor in determining success is the training of personnel who are responsible for providing initial care to the victim.
- Even though only a small percentage of human intoxications caused by natural toxins or venoms are fatal when they are treated appropriately, the risk of death increases when treatment is delayed or is insufficient.
- Not only are toxins and venoms capable of causing harm to human health, but they also have the potential to be useful in the field of biomedical research by providing novel research tools and distinctive molecular models that can be used in the development of new medications.

References

1. Ainsworth, S., Slagboom, J., Alomran, N., Pla, D., Alhamdi, Y., King, S. I., Bolton, F. M., Gutiérrez, J. M., Vonk, F. J., & Toh, C. H. (2018). The Para specific neutralization of snake venom induced coagulopathy by antivenoms. *Communications Biology, 1*, 34.
2. Alirol, E., Sharma, S. K., Bawaskar, H. S., Kuch, U., & Chappuis, F. (2010). Snake bite in South Asia: A review. *PLoS Neglected Tropical Diseases, 4*(e603), e603.
3. Bergmeier, W., Bouvard, D., Eble, J. A., Mokhtarinejad, R., Schulte, V., Zirngibl, H., Brakebusch, C., Fässler, R., & Nieswandt, B. (2001). Rhodocytin (aggretin) activates platelets lacking $\alpha 2\beta 1$ integrin, GPVI, and the ligand binding domain of GPIbα. *Journal of Biological Chemistry, 276*(27), 25121–25126.
4. Bolt, H. M. (2021). New aspects in snake venom toxicology. *Archives of Toxicology, 95*(6), 1865–1866.

5. Cheng, C. L., Mao, Y. C., Liu, P. Y., Chiang, L. C., Liao, S. C., & Yang, C. C. (2017). Deinagkistrodon acutus envenomation: A report of three cases. *Journal of Venomous Animals and Toxins including Tropical Diseases, 23*, 20.

6. Deppermann, C., Kratofil, R. M., Peiseler, M., David, B. A., Zindel, J., Castanheira, F. V. E. S., van der Wal, F., Carestia, A., Jenne, C. N., & Marth, J. D. (2020). Macrophage galactose lectin is critical for Kupffer cells to clear aged platelets. *Journal of Experimental Medicine, 217*(e20190723), e20190723.

7. Dineshkumar, T., Dhanapriya, J., Sakthirajan, R., Thirumalvalavan, K., Kurien, A. A., Balasubramaniyan, T., & Gopalakrishnan, N. (2017). Thrombotic microangiopathy due to Viperidae bite: Two case reports. *Indian Journal of Nephrology, 27*(2), 161–164.

8. Fujita, M., Yamashita, S., Kawamura, Y., Tsuruta, R., Kasaoka, S., Okabayashi, K., & Maekawa, T. (2005). Viper (Agkistrodon halys blomhoffii "Mamushi") bite with remarkable thrombocytopenia. *Nihon Kyukyu Igakukai Zasshi, 16*(2), 126–130.

9. Gn, Y. M., Ponnusamy, A., & Thimma, V. (2017). Snakebite induced thrombotic microangiopathy leading to renal cortical necrosis. *Case Reports in Nephrology, 2017*, 1348749.

10. Gold, B. S., Barish, R. A., & Rudman, M. S. (2004). Refractory thrombocytopenia despite treatment for rattlesnake envenomation. *New England Journal of Medicine, 350*(19), 1912–1913; discussion 1912.

11. Gutierrez, J. M., Calvete, J. J., Habib, A. G., Harrison, R. A., Williams, D. J., & Warrell, D. A. (2017). Snakebite envenoming. *Nature Reviews Disease Primers, 3*, 17063.

12. Heemskerk, J., Mattheij, N., & Cosemans, J. (2013). Platelet-based coagulation: Different populations, different functions. *Journal of Thrombosis and Haemostasis, 11*(1), 2–16.

13. Hoffmeister, K. M., Josefsson, E. C., Isaac, N. A., Clausen, H., Hartwig, J. H., & Stossel, T. P. (2003). Glycosylation restores survival of chilled blood platelets. *Science, 301*(5632), 1531–1534.

14. Isbister, G. K. (2010). Snakebite doesn't cause disseminated intravascular coagulation: Coagulopathy and thrombotic microangiopathy in snake envenoming. *Seminars in Thrombosis and Hemostasis, 36*(4), 444–451.

15. Jansen, A., Josefsson, E. C., Rumjantseva, V., Liu, Q. P., Falet, H., Bergmeier, W., Cifuni, S. M., Sackstein, R., von Andrian, U. H., & Wagner, D. D. (2012). Desialylation accelerates platelet clearance after refrigeration and initiates GPIbα metalloproteinase-mediated cleavage in mice. *Blood, 119*(5), 1263–1273.

16. Josefsson, E. C., Gebhard, H. H., Stossel, T. P., Hartwig, J. H., & Hoffmeister, K. M. (2005). The macrophage αMβ2 integrin αM lectin domain mediates the phagocytosis of chilled platelets. *Journal of Biological Chemistry, 280*(18), 18025–18032.

17. Lalloo, D. G., & Theakston, R. D. G. (2003). Snake antivenoms: Antivenoms. *Journal of Toxicology: Clinical Toxicology, 41*(3), 277–290.

18. Lavonas, E. J., Schaeffer, T. H., Kokko, J., Mlynarchek, S. L., & Bogdan, G. M. (2009). Crotaline Fab antivenom appears to be effective in cases of severe North American pit viper envenomation: An integrative review. *BMC Emergency Medicine, 9*, 13.

19. Li, J., Callum, J. L., Lin, Y., Zhou, Y., Zhu, G., & Ni, H. (2014). Severe platelet desialylation in a patient with glycoprotein Ib/IX antibody-mediated immune thrombocytopenia and fatal pulmonary hemorrhage. *Haematologica, 99*(e61–e63), e61–e63.

20. Li, J., Van Der Wal, D. E., Zhu, G., Xu, M., Yougbare, I., Ma, L., Vadasz, B., Carrim, N., Grozovsky, R., & Ruan, M. (2015). Desialylation is a mechanism of Fc-independent platelet clearance and a therapeutic target in immune thrombocytopenia. *Nature Communications, 6*, 7737.

21. Li, M. F., Li, X. L., Fan, K. L., Yu, Y. Y., Gong, J., Geng, S. Y., Liang, Y. F., Huang, L., Qiu, J. H., Tian, X. H., et al. (2017). Platelet desialylation is a novel mechanism and a therapeutic target in thrombocytopenia during sepsis: An open-label, multicenter, randomized controlled trial. *Journal of Hematology & Oncology, 10*, 104.

22. Li, Y., Fu, J., Ling, Y., Yago, T., McDaniel, J. M., Song, J., Bai, X., Kondo, Y., Qin, Y., & Hoover, C. (2017). Sialylation on O-glycans protects platelets from clearance by liver Kupffer cells. *Proceedings of the National Academy of Sciences of the United States of America, 114*(31), 8360–8365.

23. Linglong, X., & Dijiong, W. (2018). Prolonged hemocoagulase Agkistrodon halys pallas administration induces hypofibrinogenemia in patients with hematological disorders: A clinical analysis of 11 patients. *Indian Journal of Hematology and Blood Transfusion, 34*(2), 322–327.

24. Liu, C. C., Lin, C. C., Hsiao, Y. C., Wang, P. J., & Yu, J. S. (2018). Proteomic characterization of six Taiwanese snake venoms: Identification of species-specific proteins and development of a SISCAPA-MRM assay for cobra venom factors. *Journal of Proteomics, 187*, 59–68.

25. Liu, M., Wang, G., Xu, R., Shen, C., Ni, H., & Lai, R. (2021). Soy isoflavones inhibit both GPIb-IX signaling and αIIbβ3 outside-in signaling via 14-3-3ζ in platelet. *Molecules, 26*, 4911.

26. Long, C., Liu, M., Tian, H., Li, Y., Wu, F., Mwangi, J., Lu, Q., Mohamed Abd El-Aziz, T., Lai, R., & Shen, C. (2020). Potential role of platelet-activating C-type lectin-like proteins in viper envenomation induced thrombotic microangiopathy symptom. *Toxins, 12*, 749.

27. Mackeigan, D. T., Ni, T., Shen, C., Stratton, T. W., & Ni, H. (2020). Updated understanding of platelets in thrombosis and hemostasis: The roles of integrin PSI domains and their potential as therapeutic targets. *Cardiovascular & Hematological Disorders Drug Targets, 20*(4), 260–273.

28. Maduwage, K., & Isbister, G. K. (2014). Current treatment for venom-induced consumption coagulopathy resulting from snakebite. *PLoS Neglected Tropical Diseases, 8*(10), e3220.

29. McNicholl, I. R., & McNicholl, J. J. (2001). Neuraminidase inhibitors: Zanamivir and oseltamivir. *Annals of Pharmacotherapy, 35*(1), 57–70.

30. Monzon Manzano, E., Alvarez Roman, M. T., Justo Sanz, R., Fernandez Bello, I., Hernandez, D., Martin Salces, M., Valor, L., Rivas Pollmar, I., Butta, N. V., & Jimenez Yuste, V. (2020). Platelet and immune characteristics of immune thrombocytopenia patients non-responsive to therapy reveal severe immune dysregulation. *British Journal of Haematology, 189*(5), 943–953.

31. Ni, H., & Freedman, J. (2003). Platelets in hemostasis and thrombosis: Role of integrins and their ligands. *Transfusion and Apheresis Science, 28*(3), 257–264.

32. Norris, P. A., Segel, G. B., Burack, W. R., Sachs, U. J., Lissenberg-Thunnissen, S. N., Vidarsson, G., Bayat, B., Cserti-Gazdewich, C. M., Callum, J., & Lin, Y. (2021). FcγRI and FcγRIII on splenic macrophages mediate phagocytosis of anti-glycoprotein IIb/IIIa autoantibody-opsonized platelets in immune thrombocytopenia. *Haematologica, 106*(2), 250–256.

33. Odeleye, A. A., Presley, A. E., Passwater, M. E., & Mintz, P. D. (2004). Rattlesnake venom-induced thrombocytopenia. *Annals of Clinical and Laboratory Science, 34*(4), 467–470.

34. Offerman, S. R., Barry, J. D., Schneir, A., & Clark, R. F. (2003). Biphasic rattlesnake venom-induced thrombocytopenia. *Journal of Emergency Medicine, 24*(3), 289–293.

35. Quach, M. E., Chen, W., & Li, R. (2018). Mechanisms of platelet clearance and translation to improve platelet storage. *Blood, 131*(14), 1512–1521.

36. Ravanat, C., Strassel, C., Hechler, B., Schuhler, S., Chicanne, G., Payrastre, B., Gachet, C., & Lanza, F. (2010). A central role of GPIb-IX in the procoagulant function of platelets that is independent of the 45-kDa GPIbα N-terminal extracellular domain. *Blood, 116*(7), 1157–1164.

37. Reheman, A., Yang, H., Zhu, G., Jin, W., He, F., Spring, C. M., Bai, X., Gross, P. L., Freedman, J., & Ni, H. (2009). Plasma fibronectin depletion enhances platelet aggregation and thrombus formation in mice lacking fibrinogen and von Willebrand factor. *Blood, 113*(8), 1809–1817.

38. Revilla, N., Corral, J., Miñano, A., Mingot-Castellano, M. E., Campos, R. M., Velasco, F., Gonzalez, N., Galvez, E., Berrueco, R., & Fuentes, I. (2018). Multirefractory primary immune thrombocytopenia; targeting the decreased sialic acid content. *Platelets, 30*(7), 743–751.

39. Seifert, S. A., & Cano, D. N. (2020). Late, new-onset thrombocytopenia following rattlesnake envenomation without early thrombocytopenia or post-antivenom platelet increase. *Clinical Toxicology, 58*(5), 424–425.

40. Seifert, S. A., Kirschner, R. I., & Martin, N. (2011). Recurrent, persistent, or late, new-onset hematologic abnormalities in crotaline snakebite. *Clinical Toxicology, 49*(4), 324–329.

41. Seifert, S., Mascarenas, D., Fullerton, L., Warrick, B., & Smolinske, S. (2020). Unpredicted late-, new-onset thrombocytopenia and hypofibrinogenemia in Fab antivenom-treated rattlesnake envenomation. *Toxicon, 184*, 55–56.

42. Shao, L., Wu, Y., Zhou, H., Qin, P., Ni, H., Peng, J., & Hou, M. (2015). Successful treatment with oseltamivir phosphate in a patient with chronic immune thrombocytopenia positive for anti-GPIb/IX autoantibody. *Platelets, 26*(5), 495–497.

43. Shen, C., Liu, M., Mackeigan, D. T., Chen, Z. Y., Chen, P., Karakas, D., Li, J., Norris, P. A., Li, J., & Deng, Y. (2021). Viper venoms drive the macrophages and hepatocytes to sequester and clear platelets: Novel mechanism and therapeutic strategy for venom-induced thrombocytopenia. *Archives of Toxicology, 95*(11), 3589–3599.

44. Shen, C., Liu, M., Tian, H., Li, J., Xu, R., Mwangi, J., Lu, Q., Hao, X., & Lai, R. (2020). Conformation-specific blockade of alphaIIbbeta3 by a non-RGD peptide to inhibit platelet activation without causing significant bleeding and thrombocytopenia. *Thrombosis and Haemostasis, 120*(8), 1432–1441.

45. Shen, C., Liu, M., Xu, R., Wang, G., Li, J., Chen, P., Ma, W., Mwangi, J., Lu, Q., Duan, Z., et al. (2020). The 14-3-3zeta-c-Src-integrin-beta3 complex is vital for platelet activation. *Blood, 136*(8), 974–988.

46. Su, H. Y., Huang, S. W., Mao, Y. C., Liu, M. W., Lee, K. H., Lai, P. F., & Tsai, M. J. (2019). Clinical and laboratory features distinguishing between *Deinagkistrodon acutus* and *Daboia siamensis* envenomation. *Journal of Venomous Animals and Toxins Including Tropical Diseases, 25*, e20190001.

47. Taniguchi, N. (2008). Toward cancer biomarker discovery using the glycomics approach. In *Wiley-VCH Verlag Weinheim* (Vol. 8, pp. 3205–3208).

48. Tao, L., Zeng, Q., Li, J., Xu, M., Wang, J., Pan, Y., Wang, H., Tao, Q., Chen, Y., & Peng, J. (2017). Platelet desialylation correlates with efficacy of first-line therapies for immune thrombocytopenia. *Journal of Hematology & Oncology, 10*(1), 46.

49. Than, T., Hutton, R., Lwin, M., Han, K. E., Soe, S., Swe, T. N., Phillips, R., & Warrell, D. (1988). Haemostatic disturbances in patients bitten by Russell's viper (*Vipera russelli siamensis*) in Burma. *British Journal of Haematology, 69*(4), 513–520.

50. Tian, H., Liu, M., Li, J., Xu, R., Long, C., Li, H., Mwangi, J., Lu, Q., Lai, R., & Shen, C. (2020). Snake C-type lectins potentially contribute to the prey immobilization in *Protobothrops mucrosquamatus* and *Trimeresurus stejnegeri* venoms. *Toxins, 12*(2), 105.

51. van Der Wal, D. E., Zhu, G., Li, J., Vadasz, B., Issaka, Y., Lang, S., Freedman, J., & Ni, H. (2012). Desialylation: A novel platelet clearance mechanism and a potential new therapeutic target in anti-GPIb antibody mediated thrombocytopenia. *Blood, 120*(7), 265.

52. Van Rooijen, N., & Sanders, A. (1994). Liposome mediated depletion of macrophages: Mechanism of action, preparation of liposomes and applications. *Journal of Immunological Methods, 174*(1–2), 83–93.

53. Wang, Y., Reheman, A., Spring, C. M., Kalantari, J., Marshall, A. H., Wolberg, A. S., Gross, P. L., Weitz, J. I., Rand, M. L., & Mosher, D. F. (2014). Plasma fibronectin supports hemostasis and regulates thrombosis. *Journal of Clinical Investigation, 124*(10), 4281–4293.

54. Warrell, D. A. (2010). Snake bite. *The Lancet, 375*(9708), 77–88.

55. Webster, M. L., Sayeh, E., Crow, M., Chen, P., Nieswandt, B., Freedman, J., & Ni, H. (2006). Relative efficacy of intravenous immunoglobulin G in ameliorating thrombocytopenia induced by antiplatelet GPIIbIIIa versus GPIbα antibodies. *Blood, 108*(3), 943–946.

56. Withana, M., Rodrigo, C., Gnanathasan, A., & Gooneratne, L. (2014). Presumptive thrombotic thrombocytopenic purpura following a hump-nosed viper (Hypnale hypnale) bite: A case report. *Journal of Venomous Animals and Toxins Including Tropical Diseases, 20*, 26.

57. Xu, M., Li, J., Neves, M. A. D., Zhu, G., Carrim, N., Yu, R., Gupta, S., Marshall, J., Rotstein, O., & Peng, J. (2018). GPIbα is required for platelet-mediated hepatic thrombopoietin generation. *Blood, 132*(6), 622–634.

58. Xu, X. R., Zhang, D., Oswald, B. E., Carrim, N., Wang, X., Hou, Y., Zhang, Q., Lavalle, C., McKeown, T., & Marshall, A. H. (2016). Platelets are versatile cells: New discoveries in hemostasis, thrombosis, immune responses, tumor metastasis and beyond. *Critical Reviews in Clinical Laboratory Sciences, 53*(6), 409–430.

59. Zeng, Q., Zhu, L., Tao, L., Bao, J., Yang, M., Simpson, E. K., Li, C., van der Wal, D. E., Chen, P., & Spring, C. M. (2012). Relative efficacy of steroid therapy in immune thrombocytopenia mediated by anti-platelet GPIIbIIIa versus GPIbα antibodies. *American Journal of Hematology, 87*(2), 206–208.

Chapter 8

TOXICOLOGY AND THEIR IMPACT ON HUMAN HEALTH

Contents

Introduction

Toxicology is the study of the adverse effects of chemicals on living organisms. It plays a crucial role in understanding how different substances can harm human health. By examining the toxicity of various compounds, toxicologists help assess risks and develop strategies to minimize exposure. Exposure to toxic substances can lead to a wide range of health effects, from mild irritation to severe illness or even death. Understanding the toxic properties of chemicals is essential for setting safety standards and regulations to protect public health.

Orientation and Directional Terms

Term	Definition	Illustration
Fatty Liver (Steatosis)	A condition characterized by the accumulation of excess fat in the liver cells, often associated with obesity, diabetes, and alcohol consumption.	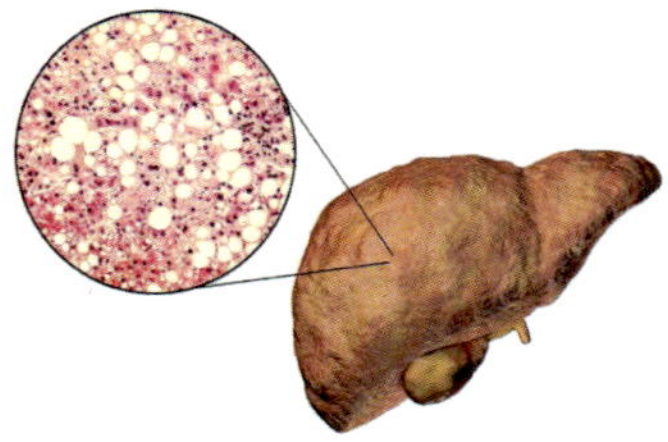
Liver Necrosis	The death of liver cells caused by various factors such as toxins, infections, or lack of blood supply, leading to liver dysfunction.	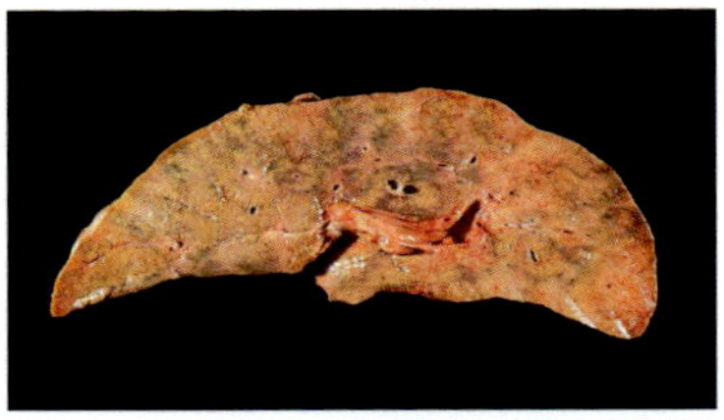
Cholestasis	A condition where bile flow from the liver is reduced or blocked, leading to the accumulation of bile in the liver and bloodstream.	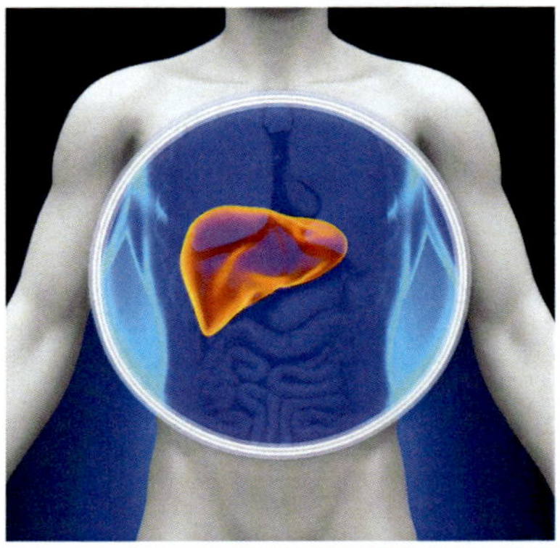
Immune System	The complex network of cells, tissues, and organs that work together to defend the body against harmful pathogens and foreign substances.	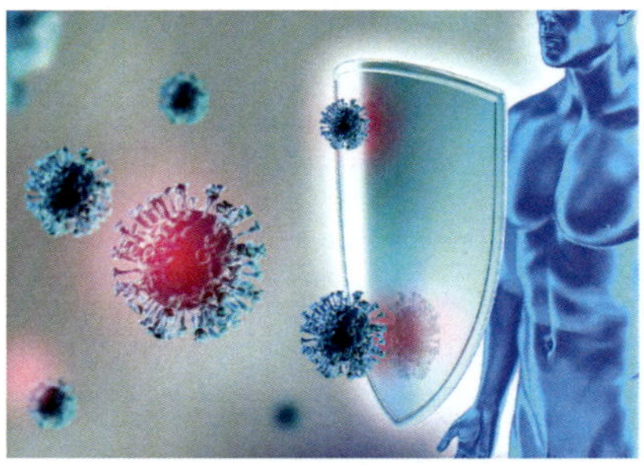
Neuronopathy	A disorder affecting neurons, the specialized cells of the nervous system, often resulting in neuronal degeneration and impaired function.	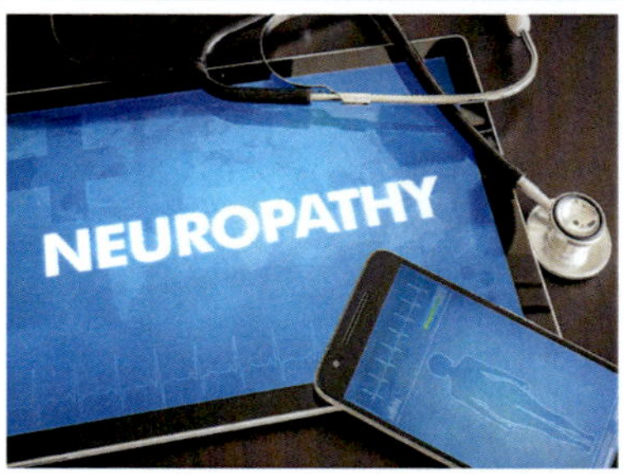

8.1. Toxicology of the Liver

For an adult, the liver weighs between 1.4 and 1.6 kilograms, making it the largest organ in the body. Although it is the most complicated organ in the body, the liver is also the largest organ. It is the organ that is responsible for the production of food, as well as the majority of medicines and toxins. The latter categories of drugs are typically the ones that undergo detoxification, even though the majority of these substances are capable of undergoing bioactivation and becoming more dangerous. It is the hepatocytes, also referred to as hepatic parenchymal cells, that make up the majority of the surface area of the liver. According to Adams et al. (1978), these cells play a role in the primary function of the liver, which is the metabolic process. All around the sinusoids that are filled with blood and the biliary passageways are where you will find them. Kupffer cells are an essential component of the reticuloendothelial system in the body. We can find them on the periphery of the hepatic sinusoids, where they are located. Specifically, the portal vein and the hepatic artery are the vessels that are accountable for the delivery of blood, and the vena cava, the portal vein, and the hepatic vein are the vessels that are accountable for the release of blood. It is the neighboring parenchymal cells that are responsible for the production of the minute bile canaliculi that make up the biliary pathways in the beginning. As depicted in Figure 8.1, these canaliculi will eventually converge into ductules, interlobular bile ducts, and larger hepatic vents later on. When the primary hepatic duct and the cystic duct of the gallbladder come together to form the pancreatic duct, Chen et al. (2013) state that this is the process that results in the formation of the pancreatic duct. After that, the duodenum is where this duct empties into.

The discovery of drug-induced liver damage (DILI) has resulted in the discontinuation of a significant number of newly developed active compounds (Watkins, 2011). It is because of the discovery of DILI that this has come about. The reason for this is that liver toxicity, which is also known as hepatotoxicity or hepatotoxicity, is frequently observed during the process of designing novel drugs. This is the reason why this is the case.

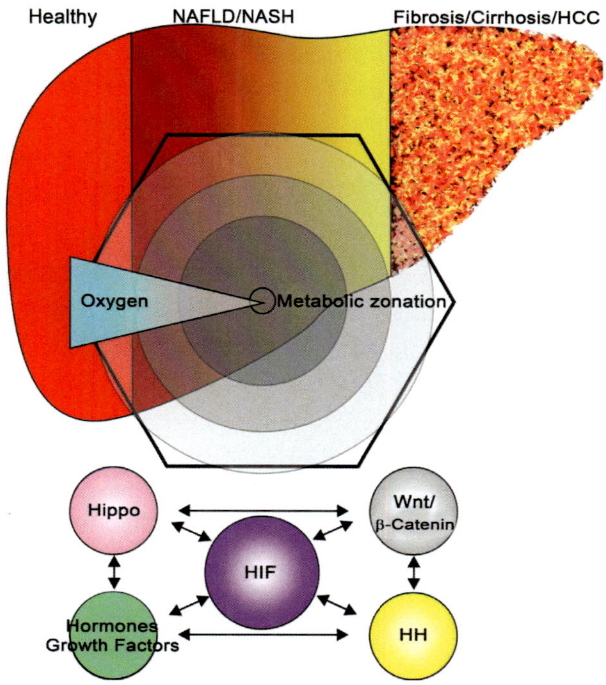

Figure 8.1. *A diagrammatic representation of the zonation and circulatory networks of the liver.*

Source: Kietzmann, T., (2019). Liver zonation in health and disease: Hypoxia and hypoxia-inducible transcription factors as concert masters. *International Journal of Molecular Sciences*, 20(9), 2347. https://doi.org/10.3390/ijms20092347.

Approximately 50% of the potential drugs have shown effects on the liver that are beyond what is considered therapeutic. These effects are superior to what is considered to be therapeutic. Overdoses of acetaminophen (APAP), a substance that is widely acknowledged to be hepatotoxic in the United States, were estimated to be responsible for the deaths of 458 people in the United States each year between the years 1990 and 1998 (Nourjah et al., 2006). This information was derived from a study that was conducted between the years 1990 and 1998. The findings of this study were obtained from a research project that was carried out by the National Institute of Health. One of the most dangerous adverse effects of medication is hepatotoxicity, which is a consequence of this. Hepatotoxicity is considered to be one of the most dangerous adverse conditions. It is possible for pharmaceuticals that are available without a prescription or over the counter, as well as herbal and nutritional products, to be the cause of a condition known as drug-induced liver injury (DILI) (LiverTox, 2016). The website LiverTox, which can be accessed at https://livertox.nih.gov/, provides information that is not only exhaustive but also up to date with regard to the disease. (Amacher Book, published in 1998).

8.1.1. Types of Liver Injury

Toxicants have a wide range of negative effects on the structures that are present in liver cells, which ultimately results in a variety of forms of tissue damage, which will be the subject of further discussion in the following paragraphs. According to Sanders et al. (1982), these liver damages are brought about by a variety of metabolic processes that are distinct from one another. Oxidative and covalent binding, suppression of protein formation, biliary formation and/or circulation perturbation, immune disease, and disruption of calcium homeostasis are some of the processes that are involved in this process.

8.1.2. Fatty Liver (Steatosis)

It is a condition that is characterized by a fatty liver that contains more than 5% lipid by mass. This condition is known as fatty liver disease (FLD) or hepatic steatosis. It is possible to observe, from a histochemical standpoint, the presence of additional fat in this liver that is resistant to staining. There is a possibility that you will develop acute lesions, similar to those that are brought on by tetracycline, phosphorus, or ethionine. In addition to the potential to cause persistent lesions, methotrexate, and ethanol both have the capability of causing acute lesions simultaneously. As stated by Agostinis et al. (2011), there are a number of distinct types of FLD, which can be broken down into the following categories:

1. **Microvascular Fatty Liver Disease:** It is a subtype of fatty liver disease that affects the liver's blood vessels. Several toxic substances, including tetracycline and valproic acid, are responsible for the production of a large number of microvascular fat globules within a cell, which ultimately results in a high mortality rate.
2. **Macrovascular Fat Droplets:** Both ethanol and malnutrition have the potential to cause large fat droplets to form inside of a cell. These droplets are referred to as macrovascular fat droplets. There is a possibility that these droplets will cause the nucleus to shift, which may even result in a lower mortality rate. Additionally, there is a connection between metabolic syndrome (which includes conditions such as diabetes, high blood pressure, and obesity, among others) and FLD.
3. **Non-Alcoholic Fatty Liver Disease (NAFLD) and Alcoholic Fatty Liver Disease (AFLD):** According to Youssef & McCullough (2002), non-alcoholic fatty liver disease (NAFLD)

is the most common type of liver disease and the primary cause of chronic liver disease. Alcoholic fatty liver disease (AFLD) involves the accumulation of fat in the liver.

8.1.3. Liver Necrosis

The death of hepatocytes is a consequence of necrosis of the liver. The necrosis could be localized (middle, semi, and peripheral) or widespread (central, mid-zonal, and peripheral). Any of these three scenarios is possible. The majority of the time, it is a severe injury. According to Aitken et al. (1993), a number of different compounds have been demonstrated or asserted to be capable of inducing liver necrosis. This is a significant adverse effect, but it does not necessarily result in death due to the astounding capacity of the liver to regenerate itself.

The destruction of the cell membrane is what ultimately leads to the death of the cell. There were no ultrastructural changes discovered in the envelope prior to the break. As a matter of fact, Ali et al. (2014) found that there are numerous variations that occur prior to cell damage. In the early stages of the disease, morphologic changes include cytoplasmic edema, endoplasmic reticulum dilatation, and polysome disaggregation. Triglycerides are developing into fat droplets within the cells of the body. Late changes include cellular membrane disruption, cytoplasmic swelling, organelle, and nucleus breakup, and mitochondrial enlargement with cristae breakdown (Bridges et al., 1983). Other late changes include cytoplasmic swelling. The liver is known to be negatively affected by microcystins, which are produced by blooms of cyanobacteria. Several significant deformations in the cell membrane have been associated with microcystins. These deformations include the production of blebs and the removal of microvilli. Microcystins, in addition, are responsible for severe hypoglycemia because they disrupt the process of hepatic gluconeogenesis (Zurawell et al., 2005).

8.1.4. Cholestasis

Cholestasis is a liver disorder in which regular bile circulation and/or production in the liver cells is reduced or impaired, resulting in intrahepatic bile acid accumulation. With the probable exception of steroids, this form of liver injury, which is generally rapid, is less common than liver fibrosis and necrosis and is also more difficult to produce in animals (Manchon et al., 1964). Cholestatic agents appear to act in several ways. Cholestasis, hyperbilirubinemia, and inhibition of mixed-function microsomal oxygenases are all caused by naphthyl isocyanate (ANIT). Cholestasis appears to be caused by a decrease in the biliary excretory function of the duct wall. ANIT also appears to alter the accessibility of ductular cells. According to Bailie et al. (1994), platelets appear to play a role in ANIT-induced liver injury. In addition, cholestasis is associated with complicated transcriptional and post-transcriptional changes in hepatobiliary transporters (e.g., ATP-binding cassette transporters) and bile-forming enzymes (Wagner et al., 2009).

8.2. Toxicology of Kidney

The kidneys are a pair of organelles arranged in the direction of the lower spine on both sides of the spinal column. The kidney purifies the blood and excretes numerous toxins from the body through the urine, with the majority of toxins being excreted (Auger et al., 1995). The kidney is the second most common organ responsible for drug-induced damage. The kidneys perform about 25% of cardiac function, resulting in an enormous amount of blood circulation and intense toxins that are transported through the renal tubules and bioactivated or detoxified, depending on the toxins. Since the kidneys are among the major excretory organs, they are associated with a greater percentage of flowing drugs and toxins (Amaro et al., 2014). Consequently, it is the main target organ for adverse effects. The characteristics and composition of the kidneys are briefly described to help explain these effects. One of the most common kidney problems is nephrotoxicity, which occurs whenever our body is exposed to drugs or toxins that damage the tissues. When kidney damage occurs, the kidney is no longer able to excrete extra urine and toxins. As a result, blood electrolytes (such as potassium and magnesium) increase (Amacher, 1998).

8.2.1. The Structure

On average, there are approximately 1.3×106 nephrons in the kidney, making them the most prominent organelles in the organ. Nephrons in two normal kidneys are capable of filtering between 150 and 180 liters of plasma on a daily basis, processing the filtrate to maintain the equilibrium of liquids, electrolytes, and acid-bases, and removing waste products. The glomerulus and a pair of glomeruli are the components that make up each nephron (Figure 8.2). The glomerulus receives its nourishment from a capillary system that operates at high pressure, and it is responsible for producing various filters from the plasma (Axelsson, 1969).

The filtrate that is deposited in Bowman's capsule travels through the proximal tubule, the Henle loop, and the distal tubule before draining into the renal pelvis and being excreted as urine through a gathering tubule. S_1, S_2, and S_3 are the three sections that make up the proximal tubule itself. The direct section and the major sections of the convoluted tubule are the components that make up S_1 and S_3, respectively. The conclusion of the convoluted section and the beginning of the straight section are the components that make up S_2 (Bailie et al., 1994). Figure 8.3 illustrates this process.

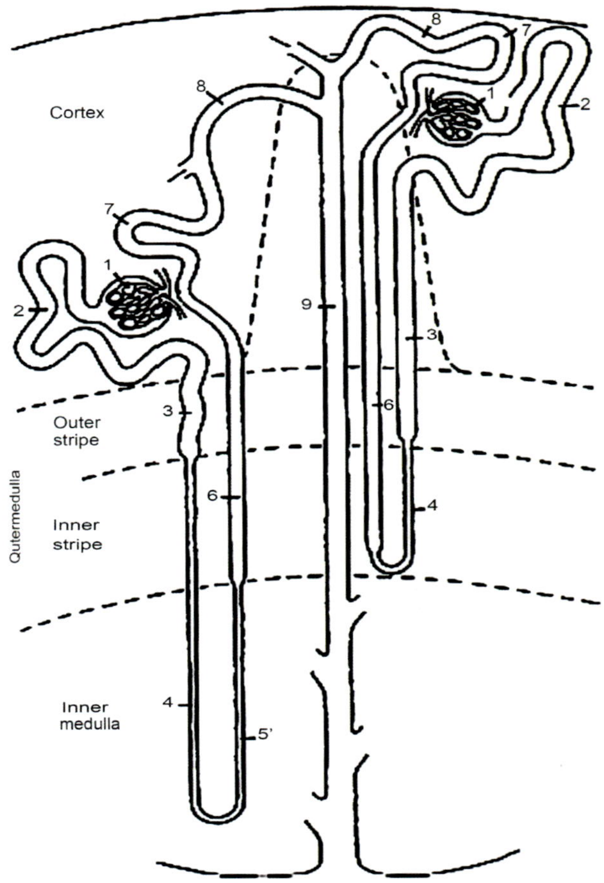

Figure 8.2. *Cortical and a juxtamedullary (long-looped) nephron, as well as the collecting network, are shown schematically. (1) Glomerulus with Bowman's capsule; (2) proximal tubule (convoluted section); (3) proximal tubule (straight portion); (4) descent narrow limb (loop of Henle); (5) ascend limb (loop of Henle); (6) wide moving up limb; (7) distal convoluted tubule; (8) linking tubule; and (9) gathering tubule.*

Source: https://pubmed.ncbi.nlm.nih.gov/3352156/.

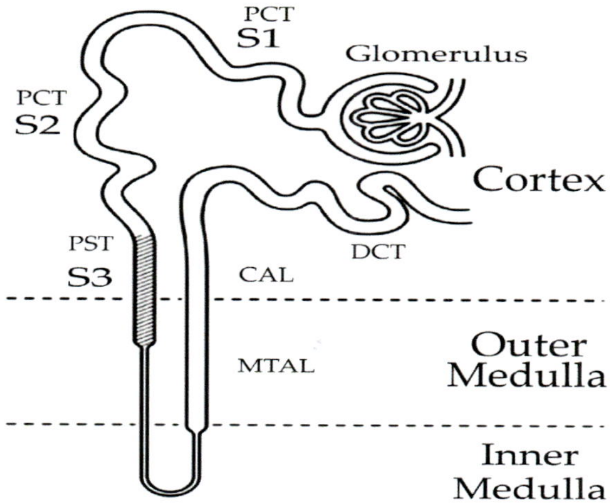

Figure 8.3. *The tubule is made up of a proximal convoluted tubule (PCT), which is made up of an S_1, S_2, and S_3 section, as well as a proximal straight tubule (PST), the loop of Henle, the medullary ascending limb (MTAL), the cortical ascending limb (CAL), and a distal convoluted tubule (DCT).*

Source: https://www.ncbi.nlm.nih.gov/pmc/articles/PMC6629462/.

8.2.2. The Production of Urine

Urine synthesis is a complicated procedure that starts with glomerular filtration. Each day, roughly 180 liters of filtrate are produced by individuals. Since only 500–2,500 ml of urination is discharged, 99% of purified water is absorbed into the body (Bardin et al., 1978). Water is first recycled back by diffusion in the renal tubular, whereby Na+ is rapidly absorbed by the body. Just at the descending limb of the Henle loop, water diffusion continues into the hyperosmolar interstitium. The hyperosmolarity is caused by the rapid absorption of nutrients of Cl–(in addition to Na+) just at the ascending limb. The design and layout of the rings and vasa recta create an efficient countercurrent multiplier mechanism (Baillie-Hamilton, 2002).

As Na+ is rapidly absorbed by the body, more water is eliminated from the filtration in the proximal as well as collecting ducts. The degree of water loss from such tubules is determined by the action of antidiuretic hormone (ADH). ADH decreases urinary excretion by raising such structures' permeability (Balazs & Ferrans, 1978).

8.2.3. Tubular Resorption and Secretion

Molecules with a molecular mass that is less than 60,000 Da can enter Bowman's capsules because the glomerular capillaries have quite large holes (70 nm). The ducts are responsible for absorbing a few of the filtering molecules that are necessary for the organism. These molecules include sugars and proteins. In contrast, ammonia (NH_3), which is a waste product of amino acids, travels through the cells to the filtration process, where it combines with hydrogen ions to produce NH+4, which is nondiffusible and is therefore expelled (Bates et al., 2001).

Almost all of the electrolytes that are used in glomerular filtration are recycled back into the system. This helps to ensure that the inert water is reabsorbed and that the body remains healthy. Mineralocorticoids are responsible for calcium reabsorption in both the proximal and distal tubules, while parathyroid hormone (PAH) is responsible for phosphorus reabsorption, and acid-base balance is responsible for bicarbonate (HCO_3) reabsorption. Furthermore, the ducts are responsible for the release of both K+ and H+ (Kauffmann et al., 1982).

8.3. Toxicology of the Immune System

The immune system is responsible for protecting the body from different types of foreign organisms, such as cancer cells, viruses, bacteria, and fungi, as well as other foreign particles, such as xenobiotics. Infections and cancers are more likely to occur in individuals who suffer from immunodeficiency, which is a condition that demonstrates the significance of the immune response. Both congenital and acquired immunodeficiency syndrome (AIDS) are common names for immunodeficiency illnesses (Bennett et al., 2008). Immunodeficiency can be either congenital or acquired. There are a number of organs, cell types, and noncellular components that make up the immune system. In general, the functions of the various components are dependent upon one another by a certain degree. A cascade of interactions involving a variety of cellular and humoral components frequently takes place as a result of the encounter with a foreign material. According to Beringer et al. (2009), these responses consist of identification, memory, and responses to foreign chemicals. The purpose of these responses is to eliminate or regulate the foreign chemicals (Figure 8.4).

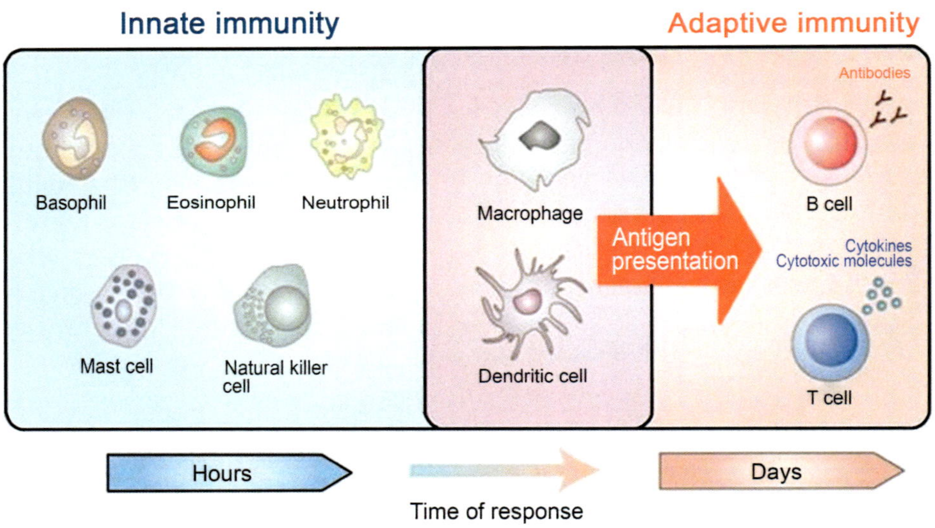

Figure 8.4. *Depicts the fundamentals of the immune system in mammals.*

Source: Yamauchi, T., & Moroishi, T., (2019). Hippo pathway in mammalian adaptive immune system. Cells, 8(5), 398. https://doi.org/10.3390/cells8050398.

Numerous toxicants are known to inhibit immunological activities. This action reduces the host's resistance to the bacterial, parasite, or viral infections, as well as the ability to inhibit the formation of cancer cells. In addition, some toxicants may induce heightened immune responses that result in local or systemic reactions. Moreover, toxicants may sometimes cause "autoimmune responses." Immune system toxicity is thus indicated not only by immunosuppression but also by immunoenhancement, in which the immune function is inappropriately activated or accelerated (Berti-Mattera et al., 1990). Numerous drugs have been shown to negatively impact the immune system. Based on amount, duration, and method of administration, the influence of foreign chemicals inhibits or stimulates immune reaction (Kreitinger et al., 2016). Many parent substances might profoundly change immune processes or need metabolism. The substances may be classified as follows (Birchenough et al., 2002):

1. Amongst them, the antineoplastic medications cyclophosphamide, nitrogen mustards, 6-mercaptopurine, azathioprine, methotrexate, 5-fluorouracil, actinomycin, doxorubicin, and diazepam are implicated more often.

2. Heavy metals and organometals: beryllium, nickel, chromium, lead, gold, methylmercury, platinum, organic tin compounds, sodium arsenite and arsenate, and arsenic trioxide.
3. Pyrethroids, chlordane, DDT, dieldrin, methyl parathion, carbofuran, maneb, hexachlorobenzene, carbaryl, 2,4-D, paraquat, and diquat are examples of pesticides.
4. Halogenated hydrocarbons: 2,3,7,8-tetrachlorodibenzo-p-dioxin (TCDD), polybrominated biphenyls, trichloroethylene, chloroform, carbon tetrachloride, pentachlorophenol, perfluorooctanoic acid, and perfluorooctane sulfonate
5. Aflatoxins, benzo(a)pyrene, methylcholanthrene, diethylstilbestrol, 2-methoxyethyl, benzene, corticosteroids, deoxynivalenol, and other chemicals. Toluene diisocyanates, 12-O-tetradecanoylphorbol-13-O-acetate, ochratoxin, penicillin, sulfites, subtilisin, formaldehyde, and drugs of abuse, such as cocaine, are toxic (Song et al., 2008).

8.4. Toxicology of Respiratory System

Through the process of inhalation, humans are directly exposed to air toxins such as cigarette smoke, small particles, toxic substances, fumes from modern automobiles, volatile organic compounds (VOCs), and microbes. What is meant by the term "inhalation toxicity" is the toxic reactions that are brought about in the respiratory system as a consequence of toxicants. According to Blake et al. (1997), the Meuse Valley air pollution episode (which occurred in Belgium in 1930), the Donora air pollution event, and the Donora episode (which occurred in Pennsylvania in 1948) were all responsible for the deaths of human beings.

8.4.1. Respiratory Defense System

The respiratory system is a complex structure, both in terms of its structure and its function. The nasopharynx, the tracheal and bronchial tracts, and the pulmonary acini, which are composed of respiratory bronchioles, alveolar ducts, and alveoli, are the components that make up this structure (Figure 8.5).

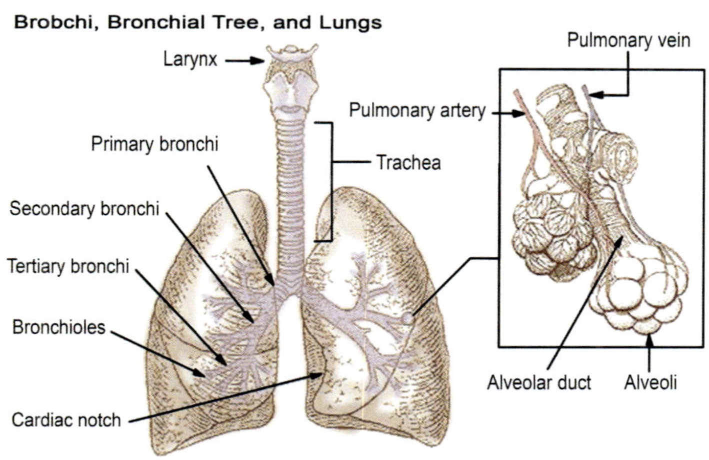

Figure 8.5. *Lung framework: Trachea, bronchi, bronchioles, respiratory terminal bronchioles, alveolar channel, and alveoli.*

Source: Public Domain; https://commons.wikimedia.org/w/index.php?curid=789698.

The nasopharynx is responsible for regulating body temperature, supplying moisture, and filtering large particulates from the air that breathes in. According to McClellan & Henderson (2009), the tracheal and bronchial tubes serve as the ventilation pathways that lead to the alveoli.

8.4.2. Toxicants and Their Effects

Studies have shown that a number of toxic substances can cause damage to the circulatory system in both humans and animals. As examples of inhalation exposure toxicants, vapors, gases, water vapor, and solid particle debris are all examples of these types of substances. It is possible to absorb gases and vapors in a short amount of time. In addition to particles, vapors can also be consumed; however, the size of the particles varies, which has a significant influence on the amount of uptake that occurs. Granules more than ten millimeters in size do not typically penetrate the respiratory system. An inhalation of very granules (0.01 m) is possible. In terms of retention, the optimal particle size range is between one and three meters (Boor et al., 1995).

Effects on the entirety of the system: As a result of the influence, the air may collect a wide variety of gases. After they have been absorbed, they are transported to various parts of the body by the bloodstream, where they exert their effects, which may include anesthesia. As well as other parts of the respiratory system, the nasopharynx is a potential entry point for potentially hazardous fumes. The alveoli, on the other hand, are the primary region that absorbs substance, and the primary route of absorption is through the process of simple diffusion. Further, according to Boro & Bromberg (2006), there are a number of different ways in which liquid aerosols, solid particulate matter, and solid particulates can be taken in.

Complications affecting the lungs: There has been a wide variety of documented pulmonary effects. The two are separated into five distinct groups, each of which is described in a brief manner (Bouldin et al., 1981; Gordon & Amdur, 1994 have provided additional information and references).

Many gases, such as ammonia and chlorine, are known to be irritating to the human body. The bronchial constriction and edema that they cause ultimately lead to dyspnea, although the long-term consequences of these conditions are relatively uncommon. Arsenicals are irritating when present for a short period of time; however, if they are present for an extended period of time, they have the potential to cause lung cancer. In a similar vein, smoking tobacco for an extended period of time causes inflammation in the lungs, which ultimately results in the development of lung cancer. It has been demonstrated that living in highly developed areas or in close proximity to transportation can cause lung malfunctions, including the development of conditions such as asthma, as a result of environmental particulate matter and diesel fumes particulates. Dust that is produced during storms has been associated with discomfort in the lungs as well as an increase in the number of instances in which breathing difficulties occur (Brain, 1980).

8.5. Toxicology of the Skin

For the most part, the skin covers the entirety of the living organism as well as the skin of other species. As a consequence, it is confronted with a variety of substances, comprising cosmetics components, home items, topical treatments, and environmental toxins like toxic substances as well as chemical contaminants, particularly in specific jobs (Castello et al., 2007). Chemical contact with the skin has the potential to result in a wide range of disorders. Ultraviolet light is another common form of stimulation that can lead to direct skin problems. Compounds that come into contact with the skin have the potential to be photoactivated by UV irradiation, which can lead to chemical phototoxicity. Additionally, skin conditions may manifest themselves as a consequence of environmental contamination that is systemic and the subsequent chemical dispersion that occurs through the dermal microcirculation tissue. The epidermis and the dermis, which are responsible for covering the subcutaneous tissue, are the components that comprise the skin (Figure 8.6). On average, the epidermis is only 0.1–0.2 millimeters thick, whereas the dermis is approximately 2 millimeters thick. Bridges et al. (1983) found that a foundation membrane was responsible for separating these two levels.

Basal cells, also known as stratum germinativum, are the cells that make up the living layer of the epidermis. These cells are responsible for supplying new cells to the other layers. This type of new cell eventually transforms into prickle neurons, also known as stratum spinosum, and then granular cells, also known as stratum granulosum, with nuclei that have disintegrated. In addition, these cells produce keratohyalin, which is then converted into keratin on the outer surface of the stratum corneum, which is the horny layer that is gradually removed. Approximately four weeks are required to make this procedure a success. It is also possible to find lymphocytes, macrophage-like Langerhans cells, and pigment-producing melanocytes within the epidermis. It is the other two types of cells that are responsible for mediating immune responses. As a consequence of this, the epidermis performs the function of an essential outside covering for the body (Cao et al., 2003).

Collagen and elastin, which appear to be extremely important components for the stability of the skin, make up the majority of the dermis. According to Carlsen et al. (1992), the most numerous cells in this region are fibroblasts. Additionally, fibroblasts play a significant role in the production of fibrous proteins and ground compounds such as hyaluronic acid, chondroitin sulfates, and mucopolysaccharides.

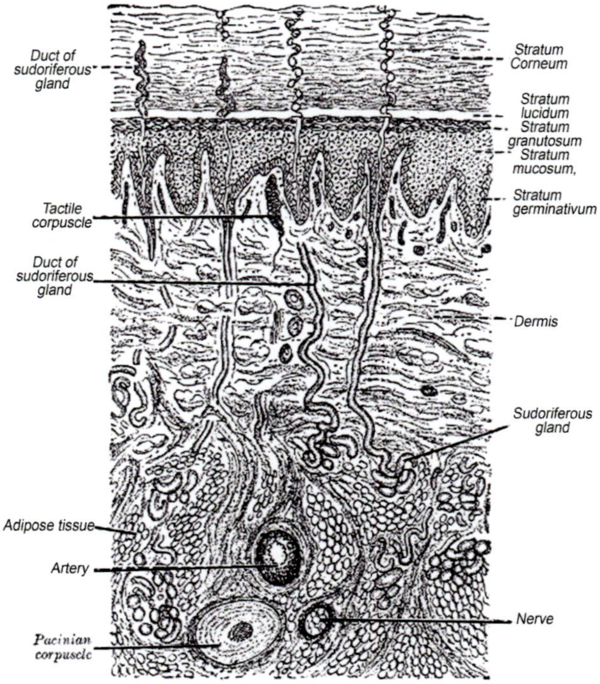

Figure 8.6. *Structure of the skin. The two principal sections of the epidermis and dermis, as well as the different structures in the dermis, are shown in these cross-sections of the skin.*

Source: By Henry Vandyke Carter – Henry Gray (1918). Anatomy of the Human Body (see "Book" section below) Bartleby.com: Gray's Anatomy, Plate 940, Public Domain; https://commons.wikimedia.org/w/index.php?curid=566886.

Other types of cells include mast cells, fat cells, macrophages, and histiocytes. Mast cells are specific to the immune system. It is located beneath the dermis and is known as the subcutaneous tissue. Systemic administration of toxicants, in particular, has the potential to result in cutaneous responses (Chapin et al., 1999). When the skin reacts to substances such as strong alkalis, acids, solvents, and detergents, it can cause irritation. There is a wide range of severity of irritation, which can include hyperemia, edema, and vesiculation, all the way up to ulceration (corrosion). When first encountered, initial irritations typically occur at the point of contact and, more often than not, during the first encounter. The difference between irritation and sensitization lies in this particular aspect (Choi & Lee, 2004).

The response to sensitization: After being subjected to a chemical for the very first time, the skin may not react very strongly to the substance present. On the other hand, a response or a more severe reaction will occur after a single subsequent exposure to the chemical. It is possible that the injection phase could last anywhere from a few days to a big number of years. Repeated exposure to the same toxicant causes a response after a delay of from twelve to forty-eight hours. The condition is known as "delayed type IV hypersensitivity" as a consequence of this characteristic. Complex immunological mechanisms are responsible for eliciting this response. The toxicant, as it enters the skin, binds to the top of certain cells, which are known as antigen-presenting cells. Once it reaches the skin, it is processed by T lymphocytes, which are responsible for the immune response. Whenever hypersensitive T cells are subjected to a similar toxicant for a second time, they have the potential to produce a multitude of chemicals, which can lead to hyperemia as well as edema (Chen et al., 2013).

8.6. Toxicology of the Eye

On the other hand, despite their diminutive size, the eyes are extremely important to one's health and possess a complex anatomy (Cheon et al., 2016).

The sclera, the choroids, and the retina are the three layers of tissue that cover the eye, which is a sphere-shaped body. The components that comprise such coatings include neural impulses, cells, and specific receptors, in addition to fibrous tissues, pigments, and blood vessels. They do not go through the cracks. Light, on the other hand, enters the eye from the front, in which the three layers are substituted by a multitude of issues, most prominently the cornea and lens (Figure 8.7) (Chen et al., 1993).

The cornea is composed of a relatively thick stroma that is covered in the front by an epithelium that is composed of several layers of cells as well as Bowman's membranes. In the back, the cornea is covered by Descemet's membrane and endothelium. The cornea, the front region of the sclera, and the inside of the eyelids are all typically covered by a thin layer of conjunctiva (Christofk et al., 2008; Katz et al., 1977).

One of the components of the lens is a lens capsule, which contains fibers that are translucent. A ciliary zonule is responsible for its attachment to the ciliary body, and the constriction of the ciliary muscle is responsible for controlling the curvature of the ciliary body. Moreover, the aqueous humor is responsible for filling the space between the cornea and the lens. Moreover, the iris can be found in this region, which is situated just beyond the lens. In addition to having a lot of blood vessels, it has a dense coloration. The iris contains a central aperture that is known as the pupil. Choi et al. (2004); and Christofk et al. (2008) found that the vitreous humor is responsible for filling the space that exists between the lens and the retina.

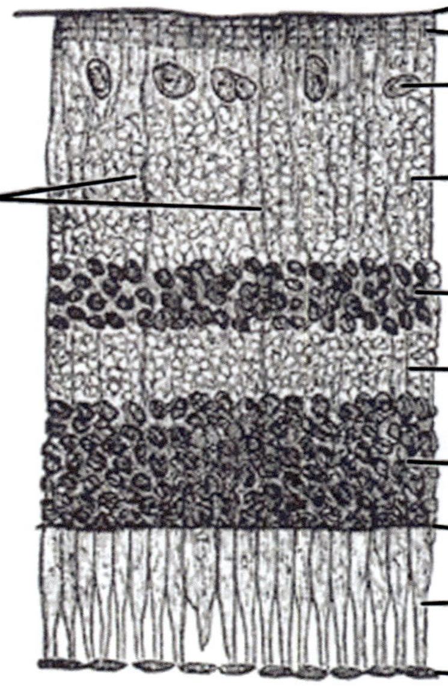

Figure 8.7. *The retina structure in cross-section.*

Source: By Henry Vandyke Carter – Henry Gray (1918). Anatomy of the Human Body, p. 1,016 (see "Book" section below) Bartleby.com: Gray's Anatomy, Plate 881, Public Domain; https://commons.wikimedia.org/w/index.php?curid=566820.

Cornea: The cornea is a delicate structure that is vulnerable to the toxic effects of external factors, particularly those that are chemical in nature. The cornea is susceptible to damage from a variety of substances, including but not limited to acids, alkalis, detergents, volatile compounds, and fog. According to Chang et al. (2005), the cornea is susceptible to damage from both acids and alkalis. The severity of the injury can range from just a slight degradation of the surface tissue that heals properly to corneal opacity or even piercing of the membranes of the eye. Having a low pH and the anion's affinity for ocular tissue are both factors that contribute to the development of acid wounds. Alkali's effects typically take longer to become apparent than those of either acid, and the majority of them are dependent on the pH of the environment. According to Potts (1996); and Phalen et al. (2010), the ammonium ion, which is present in a number of common household items, is able to enter the cornea more rapidly and, as a consequence, can alter the appearance of the iris.

In the home and in commercial settings, cleaning products are common items that have the potential to cause corneal damage. Cationic cleansers are more harmful than anionic detergents, according to Draize and Kelley's research from 1952. Nonionic detergents, on the other hand, are generally less problematic than ionic chemicals. Organic solvents such as acetone, hexane, and toluene have the potential to enter the eye as a result of accidents that occur in the workplace or in the laboratory. In addition to causing damage to corneal epithelial cells, these chemicals degrade fat. In addition to fog, smog is a mixture of smoke from industrial sources. Nevertheless, it is currently more commonly used to describe the photochemical byproducts of automotive emissions that accumulate to a certain degree under specific climatic conditions (Commandeur & Vermeulen, 1990). The respiratory system is the primary organ that they affect; however, even at low doses, they have the potential to disrupt the sensory nerve endings in the eyes and cause reflex lacrimation. When administered through the systemic route, other substances have an effect on the cornea. There are a few of them, including quinocrine, chloroquine, and chlorpromazine. Potts (1996) investigated the effects that these medications and other substances had on the cornea from a scientific perspective. One of the potential causes of corneal damage is the flow of tears through the blood-aqueous barrier. According to Colnot & Perret (2011), humans, on the other hand, are only experiencing adverse effects in extremely rare instances and only after receiving extremely high dosages.

8.7. Toxicology of the Nervous System

Both the blood-brain barrier (BBB) and the blood-nerve barrier (BNB) protect the nervous system, which is an essential component of the body, from the harmful effects of toxins that are present in the blood. In spite of this, it is susceptible to a number of different toxins. For instance, methylmercury (MeHg) has a significant impact on the nervous system, despite the fact that the concentration of MeHg in the brain is comparable to that in other tissues, and the fact that it is significantly lower than the concentration in the kidneys and liver (Dean et al., 1982).

It is possible that the increased susceptibility is at least partially attributable to the rapid metabolic rate of neurons and their limited capacity for anaerobic metabolism. Excitable neurons are also more likely to degrade the permeability of the cell membrane. This is because excitable neurons are more likely to be excitable. The extensive duration of the axons is a contributing factor to the vulnerability of the nervous system. This is because the cell is required to provide both structural and functional support to the axon. According to Boni et al. (1976), the various components of the nervous system are defined below to facilitate the explanation of the numerous types of harmful effects as well as the testing procedures for them.

8.7.1. Neurotoxic Effects and Neurotoxicants

Depending on the location of the impacts, it is possible to classify them into different categories. Neurons, axons, glial cells, and the vascular system are the components that encompass these components. On the other hand, a toxin may cause damage in more than one location. According to Dhouib et al. (2016), the following is a concise summary of specific neurotoxicity and the presumptive mechanism of action associated with it, organized according to the site of action.

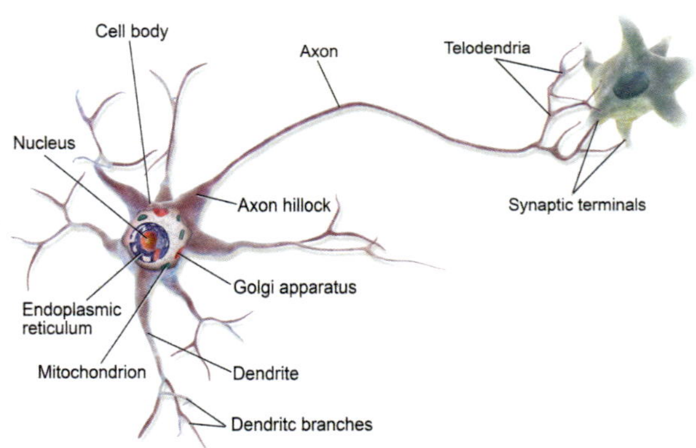

Figure 8.8. *A neuron.*

Source: By BruceBlaus - Own work, CC BY 3.0; https://commons.wikimedia.org/w/index.php?curid=28761830.

Figure 8.8 depicts the destruction of neurons, axons, and the myelin sheath that surrounds them. According to Donehower et al. (1979), neuropathy is characterized by the destruction of a second-order sensory nerve (4), which stimulates corpuscle A, as well as a neuron in the dorsal root (3), which stimulates corpuscle B.

The injured central axonal procedure of a sensory neuron, which innervates corpuscle C, and the axons of the lower motor neurons (2), that innervate muscle fibers D and E, are representative of axonopathy. Myelinopathy is seen along the axons of the upper (1) and lower (2) motor neurons that innervate muscle fiber F.

8.7.2. Neuronopathy

The fact that neurons are dependent on glucose as a source of energy makes them particularly vulnerable to hypoxia and hypoglycemia effects. The anoxygenic physiological effects of a number of substances are the subject of widespread recognition. Barbiturates play a role in the development of anoxia in the brain, particularly in the hippocampus and the cerebellum. Jacobs et al. (1977); and Diamond et al. (2003) found that even after a barbiturate-induced coma, persistent central nervous system injury is uncommon. This is likely due to a decrease in cell metabolism. Continuous exposure to carbon monoxide, on the other hand, may result in long-term changes to the brain as a consequence of the development of white matter diffuse sclerosis, also known as leukoencephalopathy. Both cyanide and azide inhibit cytochrome oxidase, which results in the production of cytotoxic anoxia. There is evidence that tricresyl phosphate contamination of food items can lead to chronic neuropathy by inhibiting the activity of "neuropathy target esterase." This activity is responsible for causing damage to neurons, the spinal cord, the brain, and other tissues (Craig & Barth, 1999). Also linked to organophosphorus (OP) pesticide exposure is this particular form of neuropathy (Pope, 1999; see below for further explanation).

There is a possibility that toxicants will have an effect on the neuronal cell body. Beginning with the induction of localized ribosome loss, methylmercury then proceeds to cause the breakdown and removal of Nissl substances, particularly in very small cells. The nucleus and perinuclear alterations come next, and then the loss of the entire neuron in its entirety, including the axon, comes after that. According to Yang & Tiffany-Castiglioni (2008), the pesticide paraquat causes oxidative stress, which ultimately results in the death of dopaminergic neurons. The neuronal effects that you get from paraquat are very similar to those that you get from Parkinson's disease.

8.8. Toxicology of the Cardiovascular System

These two components make up the cardiovascular system: the heart and the blood vessels. Due to the fact that it supplies each organ in the body with vital energy supplies, the heart is an essential organ in the body. Despite the fact that the heart is not typically a target organ for xenobiotic-associated toxicity, it is susceptible to damage from a wide variety of substances (Draize & Kelley, 1952). It is possible for these substances to exert their influence on the myocardium either directly or indirectly by way of the nervous system or the blood vessels. According to Pope (1999); and Kirmaz et al. (2004), smooth muscle cells and endothelial cells may be the primary target cells for chemically-mediated damage in blood vessels. This is due to the fact that these cells are constantly exposed to xenobiotics that are absorbed by the systemic circulation circulating throughout the body.

Toxic effects on the heart Myocardial cells, which measure approximately 15 to 80 millimeters in length, make up the majority of the heart. When compared to the cells that make up skeletal muscle, which are all innervated, only a subset of the cells that make up heart muscle are nerve-connected. On the other hand, these cells are linked together at their extremities by a low-resistance nexus, which makes it possible for electrical stimuli to be transferred from one cell to the next in a very short amount of time (Driscoll et al., 1993). To properly sequence the contractions that occur in the different chambers of the heart, these characteristics are absolutely necessary. A difference between the myocardium and skeletal muscle is that the myocardium contains less contractile material (50% versus 80%) and more mitochondrial material (35% versus 2%). Accordingly, mitochondria are a frequent subcellular target of cardiotoxicity (Ebino et al., 2001). This is because mitochondria play a significant role in the rate at which the heart contracts.

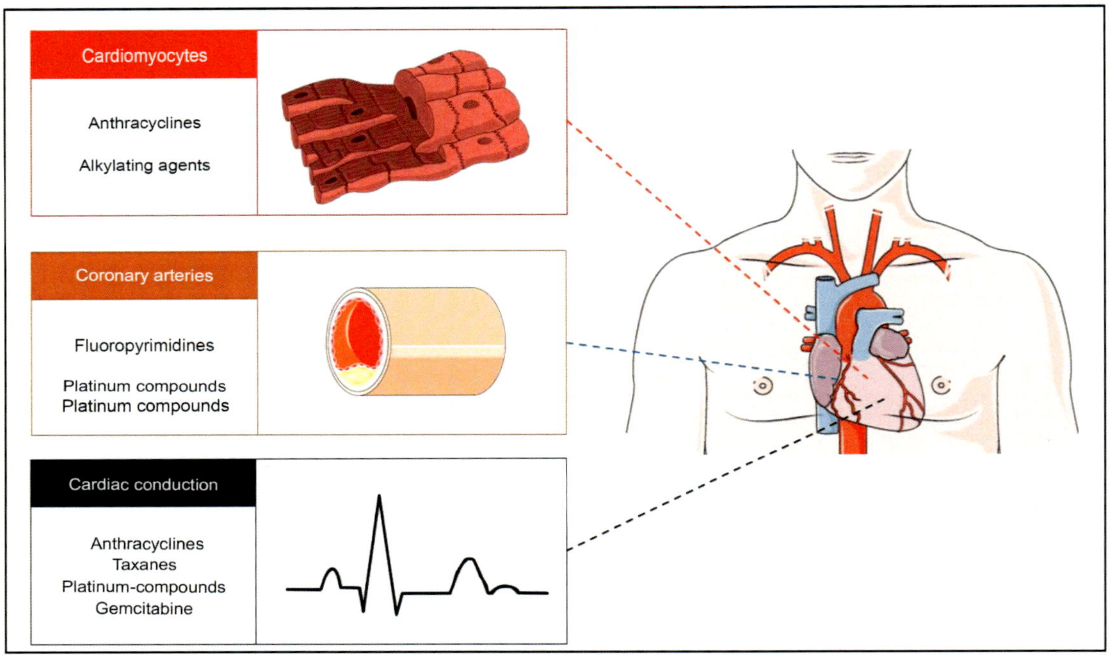

Figure 8.9. *The cardiotoxicity of chemotherapy.*

Source: Trapani, D., Zagami, P., Nicolò, E., Pravettoni, G., & Curigliano, G., (2020). Management of cardiac toxicity induced by chemotherapy. *Journal of Clinical Medicine*, 9(9), 2885. https://doi.org/10.3390/jcm9092885.

The release of energy from oxidative metabolism, the conservation of energy by adenosine triphosphate and creatine phosphate, and the uptake of energy by contractile proteins are all necessary for myocardial contraction. The processes that are the most sensitive are the utilization of energy and the movement of calcium ions within the cell (Eyler & Mueller, 2011). These processes are involved in the contractility of the myocardium, the regulation of enzyme activities, and the translation of hormonal information. Considering that the contraction of cardiac cells and the function of the systolic chamber are both controlled by intricate signaling networks at both the cellular and organ levels, alterations to these pathways can lead to cardiotoxicity (Ellinsworth, 2015).

Chemotherapy-related cardiac dysfunction (Figure 8.9) demonstrates that there is a growing concern about drug-induced cardiotoxicity. As a result, there is a need for more in-depth monitoring and knowledge of the mechanism of action to prevent chemical-associated cardiotoxicity (Ghare et al., 2011).

8.9. Toxicology of the Reproductive System

Reproduction begins with the process known as gametogenesis. In the process of oogenesis, which takes place in females, mitosis takes place during the formation of initial oocytes from precursor cells (oogonia). This progression takes place throughout the entirety of the fetal stage and reaches its zenith at the time of delivery. Before ovulation, primary oocytes go through the process of meiosis, which results in the formation of secondary oocytes (Gold & Austin, 1991).

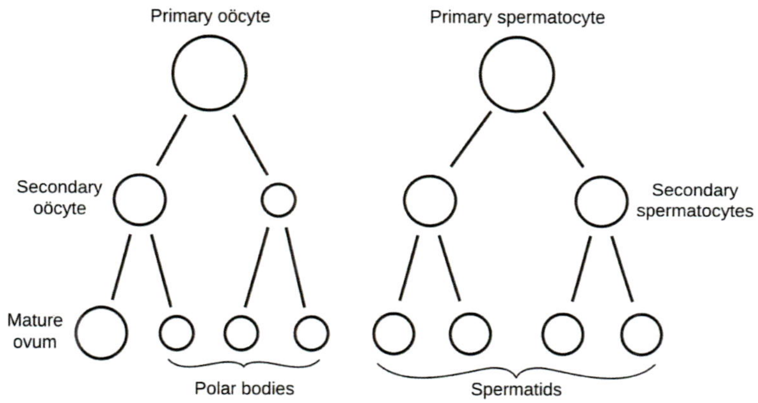

Figure 8.10. *Gametogenesis.*

Source: By Fred the Oyster – Own work, Public Domain; https://commons.wikimedia.org/w/index.php?curid=35184498.

During the process of spermatogenesis, gonocytes undergo a transformation into spermatogonia, which marks the beginning of the process among males. Spermatogonia do not begin to proliferate until puberty, at which point they emerge from their dormant state. According to Meier-Ruge (1969); and Wilkie (2013), a significant number of spermatogonia undergo a process of division, resulting in the formation of new spermatogonia. There are three distinct stages that occur during the process of spermatogenesis. First, spermatogonia go through the process of mitosis, which results in the production of primary spermatocytes. These spermatocytes then divide through the process of meiosis, which results in the production of secondary spermatocytes. Finally, spermatids undergo metamorphosis, which results in the formation of spermatozoa. It takes approximately sixty days for spermatogonia to transform into spermatozoa, which is a process that occurs continuously (Figure 8.10) (Fu et al., 2010; Jacobs et al., 1977).

The term "reproductive toxicity" refers to the detrimental effects that a toxin has on the reproductive capacity of an organism as well as the development of its offspring within that organism. The Globally Harmonized Framework defines reproductive toxicity as the adverse effects of air pollution on erectile function as well as reproduction in both males and females.

This is in addition to the effect that air pollution has on the development of children. According to Whitehead & Rice (2006); and Francis & Kimmel (1988), a wide range of toxins have the potential to hinder the reproductive processes of both sexes. This is because of the impact that these toxins have on the reproductive tracts of both sexes. There is a possibility that males will experience difficulties in the generation, maturation, storage, and transit of spermatozoa. Similarly, the oocytes of females are susceptible to the effects of certain poisons. It is also possible that the implantation of fertilized eggs, the growth of the fetus, and the development of the fetus will be compromised.

According to Thayer et al. (2012), many potentially harmful effects are mediated by mechanisms that are associated with the neurological or hormonal systems in both sexes. For example, exposure to TCDD alters the process of folliculogenesis in the ovary and reduces the number of antral follicles without causing an increase in atresia. According to Karman et al. (2012), these findings indicate that TCDD was able to inhibit the growth of ovarian cells in rats. Although there is evidence that TCDD is associated with changes in hormone levels and ovarian function in animals, the effects of this substance on humans have not been investigated. Residents of Seveso, Italy encountered the highest levels of TCDD in their blood as a result of an explosion that occurred on July 10, 1976. Twenty years later, Turner et al. (2006); and Gordon & Amdur (1991) launched the Seveso Women's Health Study with the purpose of investigating reproductive health.

8.10. Toxicology of Endocrine-Disrupting Chemicals

The study of endocrine-disrupting chemicals, also known as EDCs, is considered to be extremely important in the field of toxicology because of the significant impact that these chemicals have on both public health and the environment. According to DeRosa et al. (1998); and Grice & Carlson (1972), the endocrine process is a complicated organ that controls a number of different functions and physiological changes in the body. In addition to the hypothalamus, the pituitary gland (which produces luteinizing hormones as well as follicle-stimulating hormones), the pineal gland (which produces melatonin), the pancreas (which produces insulin), and sex organs such as the ovaries (which produce estrogens and progestins) and testes (which produce androgens), the thyroid, the parathyroid gland, and the adrenal glands all contribute to the endocrine system (which produces corticosteroids) (Grant, 1980). Specialized cells that are responsible for the production of hormones make up endocrine glands. Arachidonic acid and cholesterol, proteins, and amino acids are the components that make up these hormones. They are categorized as lipid derivatives (for example, eicosanoids and steroids), peptides, and amines, in that order (for example, tyrosine and tryptophan) (Seegal, 1999).

When it comes to the organization of metabolic processes, the endocrine system is absolutely necessary. According to Choi et al. (2004); and Harber & Baer (1972), excessive or insufficient levels of hormones are the root cause of reproductive and developmental toxicity, as well as carcinogenicity, mutagenicity, neurotoxicity, and immunotoxicity. It is also the cause of carcinogenicity. According to Baillie-Hamilton (2002), numerous chemicals have been linked to a variety of diseases and conditions, including cancer, cardiovascular disease, obesity, diabetes, and behavioral and learning disorders such as attention deficit hyperactivity disorder (ADHD). These chemicals function as endogenous estrogens on their own. One of Rachel Carson's books, published in 1962 and titled Silent Spring, was about EDCs. The last fifty years have seen an increase in the level of concern regarding EDCs. It is not going to be possible to cover the entire endocrine system in this chapter; rather, it is going to concentrate on the most important endocrine systems that are affected by EDCs. Taking this viewpoint into consideration, the danger that is posed by EDCs that have endocrine effects, whether they are agonistic or antagonistic, has become an increasingly important concern, not only for people but also for ecosystems (Birnbaum, 2013).

8.10.1. Endocrine-Disrupting Chemicals

EDCs, which are also referred to as endocrine-disrupting chemicals or endocrine-disruptors, are exogenous chemicals that are physically identical to one another and interact with the production, release, transportation, digestion, and binding task of normal endogenous hormones (Green, 2019; Griffith et al., 1980). It is possible for endocrine drugs to mimic or inhibit the activity of all endocrine hormones, including, androgens, thyroid hormones, adrenal hormones, and pituitary hormones. EDCs canimitate or interact with the effects of all endocrine hormones, including, androgens, thyroid hormones, adrenal hormones, and pituitary hormones. In the beginning, the focus was on substances that possessed estrogen-like characteristics (Colborn et al., 1993). In addition, an EDC may have additional hormonal effects, such as estrogenic and antiestrogenic effects, androgenic, and antiandrogenic effects, and thyroid and antithyroid effects (McKinney & Waller, 1998). According to Carlsen et al. (1992), environmental and food sources of EDCs include all of the following: pesticides, combustion products, plasticizers, detergents, and heavy metals of various types.

8.10.2. Effect on Humans

Even though there is a high probability that EDCs will cause harm to humans, there is not much evidence to back up this assertion. Taiwanese children whose mothers used cooking oil that was contaminated with PCBs were found to have developmental delays, attention deficit hyperactivity disorder (ADHD), and very small penises when they reached puberty (Yu et al., 2000). A girl who had been exposed to synthetic estrogen was found to have a rare form of vaginal cancer, and her son was found to have a malformed penis (Mericskay et al., 2005). The woman had been exposed to synthetic estrogen previously. There was a relatively high incidence of children with developmental disorders among mothers whose diets included fish from the Great Lakes when the children were young. Sperm counts among Danish men dropped from 113 million/ml to 66 million/ml over the course of the study. During the year 1976, the number of male sperm in France decreased from 89 million per milliliter to 60 million per milliliter, and the motility of sperm also decreased (Halliwell & Cross, 1994; Auger et al., 1995). In Japan, a man in his twenties who lived in the suburbs of Tokyo used to have a sperm production of 46 million per milliliter, which was significantly lower than the 84 million per milliliter that a man in his forties had. There has been some speculation among researchers that estrogen could be the cause. Women who were exposed to DDT or PCBs in the United States were found to have a higher risk of developing breast cancer. This was determined through empirical research. According to Wolff & Toniolo (1995), exposure to EDC may very well be associated with a decrease in the number of sperm, an increase in the severity of cancers (breast, prostate, and testicular), an increase in sterility, malformations, attention deficit hyperactivity disorder (ADHD), and learning impairments in children.

A Closer Look

Toxicity of Neuronopathy

Neuronopathy is a condition marked by the degeneration of nerve cells that can arise from various toxic exposures. Toxicity-induced neuronopathy typically results from substances that disrupt neuronal function or lead to cell death through several mechanisms. Heavy metals, such as lead and mercury, are well-known culprits; they can interfere with neuronal ion channels, disrupt neurotransmitter release, and induce oxidative stress, ultimately leading to neurodegeneration. Pesticides, particularly organophosphates, also contribute to neuronopathy by inhibiting acetylcholinesterase, leading to overstimulation of neurons and subsequent neuronal damage. Certain medications and recreational drugs can further exacerbate this condition, either through direct neurotoxicity or by triggering secondary effects like oxidative stress or excitotoxicity.

The clinical presentation of toxic neuronopathy can vary depending on the toxin involved and the affected neural pathways. Common symptoms include sensory disturbances, motor dysfunction, and cognitive impairment. For instance, lead poisoning often presents with peripheral neuropathy and cognitive deficits, while mercury exposure may cause a range of neurological symptoms from tremors to memory loss.

Preventive measures and early detection are crucial in managing toxin-induced neuronopathy. Regular screening for toxic exposures, especially in at-risk populations, and prompt intervention when symptoms arise can mitigate long-term damage. Treatment typically involves removing or reducing exposure to the offending toxin, alongside supportive therapies to manage symptoms and promote neuronal recovery.

Summary

- Toxicology is the scientific study of the adverse effects of chemicals or physical agents on living organisms. It encompasses understanding how substances interact with biological systems, the mechanisms by which toxicity occurs, and the implications for human health. Toxicologists evaluate the toxicity of substances through various tests and experiments, aiming to assess risks and establish safe exposure levels.
- The impact of toxicology on human health is profound. It informs regulatory decisions, healthcare policies, and environmental protection measures. By identifying toxic substances and their effects, toxicology contributes to the development of safer products, environmental remediation strategies, and medical treatments. It plays a crucial role in addressing public health concerns related to pollution, occupational hazards, food safety, and pharmaceuticals. Ultimately, toxicology strives to minimize human exposure to harmful substances and mitigate their adverse health effects through rigorous research, risk assessment, and the dissemination of evidence-based recommendations.

References

1. Agency for Toxic Substances and Disease Registry Division of Toxicology and Environmental Medicine. (2005). *Toxicological Profile for Zinc*. Atlanta, GA, USA.
2. Agren, M. S. (1990). Percutaneous absorption of zinc from zinc oxide applied topically to intact skin in man. *Dermatologica, 180*(1), 36–39.
3. Agren, M. S., Franzen, L., & Chvapil, M. (1993). Effects on wound healing of zinc oxide in a hydrocolloid dressing. *Journal of the American Academy of Dermatology, 29*(2), 221–227.
4. Agren, M. S., Krusell, M., & Franzen, L. (1991). Release and absorption of zinc from zinc oxide and zinc sulfate in open wounds. *Acta Dermato-Venereologica, 71*(4), 330–333.
5. Bentley, P. J., & Grubb, B. R. (1991). Experimental dietary hyperzincemia tissue disposition of excess zinc in rabbits. *Trace Elements in Medicine, 8*(4), 202–207.
6. Blanc, P., Wong, H., Bernstein, M. S., & Boushey, H. A. (1991). An experimental human model of metal fume fever. *Annals of Internal Medicine, 114*(11), 930–936.
7. Brown, J. J. (1988). Zinc fume fever. *British Journal of Radiology, 61*(726), 327–329.
8. Brown, M. A., Thom, J. V., Orth, G. L., Cova, P., & Juarez, J. (1964). Food poisoning involving zinc contamination. *Archives of Environmental Health, 8*(6), 657–660.
9. Callender, G. R., & Gentzkow, C. J. (1937). Acute poisoning by the zinc and antimony content of limeade prepared in a galvanized iron can. *Military Surgeon, 80*(1), 67–71.
10. Chimienti, F., Aouffen, M., Favier, A., & Seve, M. (2003). Zinc homeostasis-regulating proteins: New drug targets for triggering cell fate. *Current Drug Targets, 4*(4), 323–338.
11. Drinker, P., Thompson, R. M., & Finn, J. L. (1927). Metal fume fever: IV. Threshold doses of zinc oxide, preventive measures, and the chronic effects of repeated exposures. *Journal of Industrial Hygiene, 9*(4), 331–345.
12. Fox, M. R. S. (1989). Zinc excess. In C. F. Mills (Ed.), *Zinc in Human Biology* (pp. 366–368). Springer Verlag.

13. Freitag, A., & Caduff, B. (1996). ARDS caused by military zinc fumes exposure. *Schweizerische Medizinische Wochenschrift, 126*(20), 1006–1010.

14. Haase, H., & Maret, W. (2003). Intracellular zinc fluctuations modulate protein tyrosine phosphatase activity in insulin/insulin-like growth factor-1 signaling. *Experimental Cell Research, 291*(2), 289–298.

15. Haase, H., Overbeck, S., & Rink, L. (2008). Zinc supplementation for the treatment or prevention of disease: Current status and future perspectives. *Experimental Gerontology, 43*(5), 394–408.

16. Hammond, J. W. (1944). Metal fume fever in crushed stone industry. *Journal of Industrial Hygiene, 26*(3), 117–119.

17. He, L. S., Yan, X. S., & Wu, D. C. (1991). Age-dependent variation of zinc-65 metabolism in LACA mice. *International Journal of Radiation Biology, 60*(6), 907–916.

18. Homma, S., Jones, R., Qvist, J., Zapol, W. M., & Reid, L. (1992). Pulmonary vascular lesions in the adult respiratory distress syndrome caused by inhalation of zinc chloride smoke: A morphometric study. *Human Pathology, 23*(1), 45–50.

19. Igic, P. G., Lee, E., Harper, W., & Roach, K. W. (2002). Toxic effects associated with consumption of zinc. *Mayo Clinic Proceedings, 77*(7), 713–716.

20. Johnson, F. A., & Stonehill, R. B. (1961). Chemical pneumonitis from inhalation of zinc chloride. *Diseases of the Chest, 40*(6), 619–626.

21. Jones, M. M., Schoenheit, J. E., & Weaver, A. D. (1979). Pretreatment and heavy metal LD50 values. *Toxicology and Applied Pharmacology, 49*(1), 41–44.

22. Krezel, A., & Maret, W. (2007). Dual nanomolar and picomolar Zn(II) binding properties of metallothionein. *Journal of the American Chemical Society, 129*(35), 10911–10921.

23. Laity, J. H., & Andrews, G. K. (2007). Understanding the mechanisms of zinc-sensing by metal-response element binding transcription factor-1 (MTF-1). *Archives of Biochemistry and Biophysics, 463*(2), 201–210.

24. Lansdown, A. B. (1991). Interspecies variations in response to topical application of selected zinc compounds. *Food and Chemical Toxicology, 29*(1), 57–64.

25. Lansdown, A. B. (1993). Influence of zinc oxide in the closure of open skin wounds. *International Journal of Cosmetic Science, 15*(2), 83–85.

26. Lewis, M. R., & Kokan, L. (1998). Zinc gluconate: Acute ingestion. *Journal of Toxicology: Clinical Toxicology, 36*(1–2), 99–101.

27. Lichten, L. A., & Cousins, R. J. (2009). Mammalian zinc transporters: Nutritional and physiologic regulation. *Annual Review of Nutrition, 29*(1), 153–176.

28. Liu, C. H., Lee, C. T., Tsai, F. C., Hsu, S. J., & Yang, P. M. (2006). Gastroduodenal corrosive injury after oral zinc oxide. *Annals of Emergency Medicine, 47*(3), 296.

29. Llobet, J. M., Domingo, J. L., Colomina, M. T., Mayayo, E., & Corbella, J. (1988). Subchronic oral toxicity of zinc in rats. *Bulletin of Environmental Contamination and Toxicology, 41*(1), 36–43.

30. Magee, A. C., & Matrone, G. (1960). Studies on growth, copper metabolism of rats fed high levels of zinc. *Journal of Nutrition, 72*(2), 233–242.

31. Maret, W. (2006). Zinc coordination environments in proteins as redox sensors and signal transducers. *Antioxidants and Redox Signaling, 8*(9–10), 1419–1441.

32. Marquart, H., Smid, T., Heederik, D., & Visschers, M. (1989). Lung function of welders of zinc-coated mild steel: Cross-sectional analysis and changes over five consecutive work shifts. *American Journal of Industrial Medicine, 16*(3), 289–296.

33. Martin, C. J., Le, X. C., Guidotti, T. L., Yalcin, S., Chum, E., Audette, R. J., Liang, C., Yuan, B., Zhang, X., & Wu, J. (1999). Zinc exposure in Chinese foundry workers. *American Journal of Industrial Medicine, 35*(6), 574–580.

34. Oestreicher, P., & Cousins, R. J. (1985). Copper and zinc absorption in the rat: Mechanism of mutual antagonism. *Journal of Nutrition, 115*(2), 159–166.

35. Ogiso, T., Moriyama, K., Sasaki, S., Ishimura, Y., & Minato, A. (1974). Inhibitory effect of high dietary zinc on copper absorption in rats. *Chemical and Pharmaceutical Bulletin (Tokyo), 22*(1), 55–60.

36. Ogiso, T., Ogawa, N., & Miura, T. (1979). Inhibitory effect of high dietary zinc on copper absorption in rats. II. Binding of copper and zinc to cytosol proteins in the intestinal mucosa. *Chemical and Pharmaceutical Bulletin, 27*(2), 515–521.

37. OSHA. (2003). Occupational safety and health standards; Occupational Safety and Health Administration: Washington, DC, USA, 2003; Volume 29, CFR 1910.1000, pp. Table Z-1.

38. Porea, T. J., Belmont, J. W., & MahoneyJr., D. H. (2000). Zinc-induced anemia and neutropenia in an adolescent. *Journal of Pediatrics, 136*(5), 688–690.

39. Rohrs, L. C. (1957). Metal-fume fever from inhaling zinc oxide. *AMA Archives of Industrial Health, 16*(1), 42–47.

40. Samman, S., & Roberts, D. C. (1987). The effect of zinc supplements on plasma zinc and copper levels and the reported symptoms in healthy volunteers. *Medical Journal of Australia, 146*(6), 246–249.

41. Scott, B. J., & Bradwell, A. R. (1983). Identification of the serum binding proteins for iron, zinc, cadmium, nickel, and calcium. *Clinical Chemistry, 29*(4), 629–633.

42. Stromberg, H. E., & Agren, M. S. (1984). Topical zinc oxide treatment improves arterial and venous leg ulcers. *British Journal of Dermatology, 111*(4), 461–468.

43. Sturgis, C. C., Drinker, P., & Thompson, R. M. (1927). Metal fume fever: I. Clinical observations on the effect of the experimental inhalation of zinc oxide by two apparently normal persons. *Journal of Industrial Hygiene, 9*(2), 88–97.

44. Tapiero, H., & Tew, K. D. (2003). Trace elements in human physiology and pathology: Zinc and metallothioneins. *Biomedicine & Pharmacotherapy, 57*(9–10), 399–411.

45. Taylor, K. M., Vichova, P., Jordan, N., Hiscox, S., Hendley, R., & Nicholson, R. I. (2008). ZIP7-mediated intracellular zinc transport contributes to aberrant growth factor signaling in antihormone-resistant breast cancer cells. *Endocrinology, 149*(10), 4912–4920.

46. Trumbo, P., Yates, A. A., Schlicker, S., & Poos, M. (2001). Dietary reference intakes: Vitamin A, Vitamin K, arsenic, boron, chromium, copper, iodine, iron, manganese, molybdenum, nickel, silicon, vanadium, and zinc. *Journal of the American Dietetic Association, 101*(3), 294–301.

47. Vallee, B. L., & Falchuk, K. H. (1993). The biochemical basis of zinc physiology. *Physiological Reviews, 73*(1), 79–118.

48. Van Campen, D. R. (1969). Copper interference with the intestinal absorption of zinc-65 by rats. *Journal of Nutrition, 97*(1), 104–108.

49. Vogelmeier, C., Konig, G., Bencze, K., & Fruhmann, G. (1987). Pulmonary involvement in zinc fume fever. *Chest, 92*(5), 946–948.

50. Wastney, M. E., Aamodt, R. L., Rumble, W. F., & Henkin, R. I. (1986). Kinetic analysis of zinc metabolism and its regulation in normal humans. *American Journal of Physiology, 251*(2 Pt 2), R398–R408.

51. Zerahn, B., Kofoed-Enevoldsen, A., Jensen, B. V., Molvig, J., Ebbehoj, N., Johansen, J. S., & Kanstrup, I. L. (1999). Pulmonary damage after modest exposure to zinc chloride smoke. *Respiratory Medicine, 93*(12), 885–890.

Chapter 9

PREVENTION AND MITIGATION OF TOXIC EFFECTS

Contents

Introduction

Prevention and mitigation of toxic effects are critical components in safeguarding human health and the environment from harmful substances. These strategies encompass a broad range of practices, techniques, and regulations aimed at reducing exposure to toxic chemicals and pollutants. Effective implementation of these measures is essential in various sectors including industrial, agricultural, healthcare, and residential settings.

Prevention of toxic effects starts with identifying and understanding the hazardous properties of chemicals. This involves thorough research and testing to ascertain toxicity levels, potential health impacts, and environmental persistence. Once identified, the use of such chemicals can be minimized or substituted with safer alternatives in industrial processes and products. This proactive approach is fundamental in chemical safety and is often guided by principles of green chemistry, which promotes the design of chemical products and processes that reduce or eliminate the use and generation of hazardous substances.

On the regulatory front, strict guidelines and standards are established to control the release of toxins into the environment. These regulations are enforced by agencies such as the Environmental Protection Agency (EPA) in the United States, which mandates compliance with laws like the Toxic Substances Control Act (TSCA). These laws ensure that chemicals are properly managed throughout their life cycle, from manufacturing to disposal, to prevent environmental contamination and protect public health.

Mitigation, on the other hand, involves steps taken to reduce the severity of toxic effects after exposure has occurred. This includes emergency response measures such as decontamination, medical interventions like antidotes for poisonings, and long-term strategies such as environmental cleanup projects and remediation of polluted sites. Education and training also play a crucial role in mitigation by informing the public and workers about the risks associated with toxic substances and the best practices for handling them safely.

Both prevention and mitigation require collaboration among government bodies, industries, scientists, and the public to be effective. Through comprehensive policies, continued scientific research, and community awareness, it is possible to significantly reduce the risks associated with toxic substances and create a safer and healthier environment for all.

Orientation and Directional Terms

Term	Definition	Illustration
Exposure Guidelines	Recommendations or regulations that limit the amount and duration of exposure to hazardous substances to ensure safety and health.	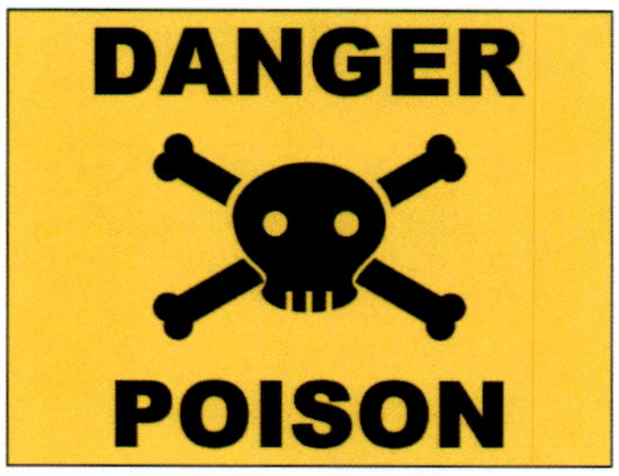
Time-Weighted Average (TWA)	The average exposure to a hazardous substance over a specified period, usually an 8-hour workday or 40-hour workweek.	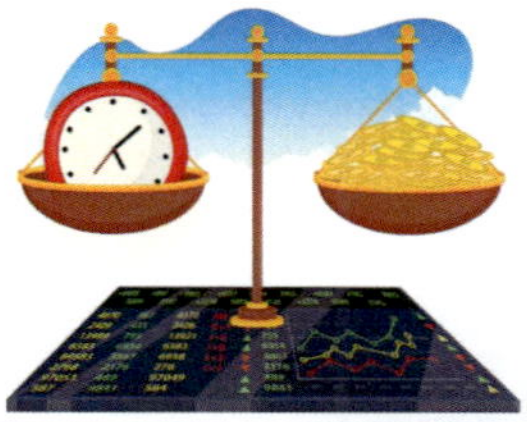
Short-Term Exposure Limit (STEL)	The maximum concentration of a hazardous substance to which workers can be exposed for a short period, typically 15 minutes, without suffering adverse health effects.	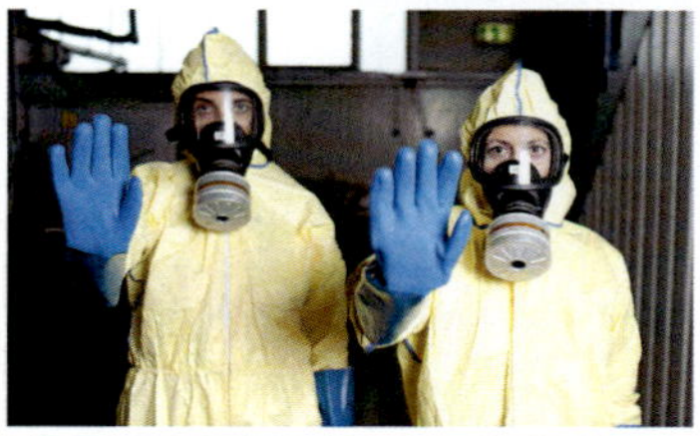
Ceiling (C)	The maximum concentration of a hazardous substance that should not be exceeded at any time during exposure.	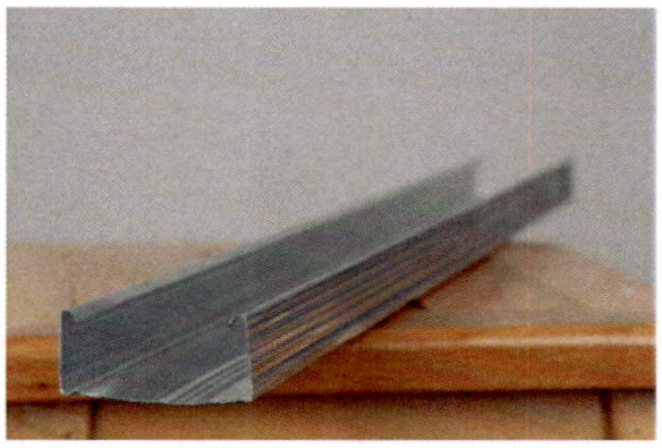

9.1. Toxicity

Toxicity is always the result of exposure, and consequently, there is no toxic impact without exposure, regardless of the conclusions that risk assessments come to, it is self-evident but sometimes overlooked. With the confirmation of both the danger and the exposures, as well as the fact that the risk appears to be high, there appear to be several different options for lowering the risk. From outright bans on both the manufacturing and the use of the chemical in question to exposure restrictions and impact restrictions, these actions range from the former to the latter (Blakley et al., 2002; Landrigan et al., 1999). To reduce exposure, it may be helpful to take preventative measures such as preventing production, controlling usage patterns, managing application methods, modifying the environment, and offering education. By utilizing preventative and therapeutic measures, as well as by educating people, it is possible to lessen the impact of the circumstances. There are several different pieces of legislation that govern or at least partially govern a good number of these methods. When all these things are taken into consideration together, they constitute the material that will be discussed in this chapter (Farooqui et al., 2001) (Figure 9.1).

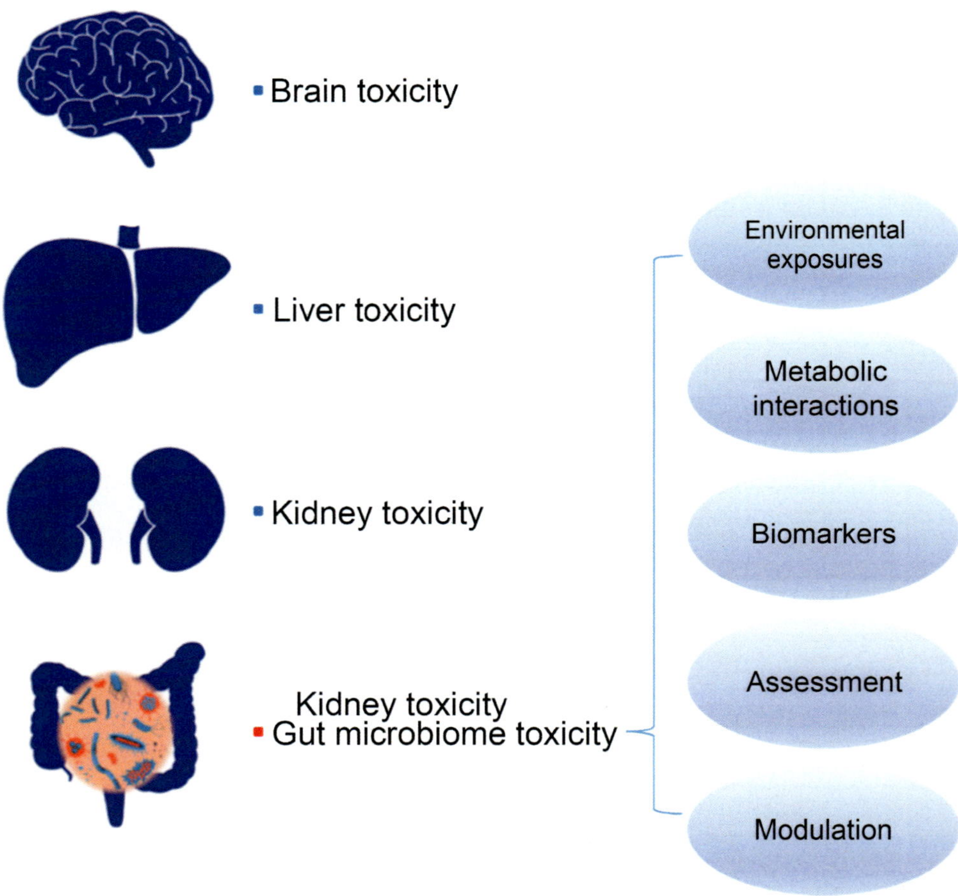

Figure 9.1. *An illustration of toxicity.*

Source: Tu, P., Chi, L., Bodnar, W., Zhang, Z., Gao, B., Bian, X., Stewart, J., Fry, R., & Lu, K., (2020). Gut microbiome toxicity: Connecting the environment and gut microbiome-associated diseases. *Toxics*, 8(1), 19. https://doi.org/10.3390/toxics8010019.

To prevent individuals who lack social consciousness from knowingly exposing their fellow citizens to toxic threats, it is necessary to have consequences in place. Rules and regulations provide us with the foundation for coordinated efforts to avoid toxicity. The rules, on the other hand, will never be successfully implemented if there is no requirement for a population that is informed about hazardous risks or how to avoid them. Furthermore, actions that are not always specified by law are often prescribed by wisdom in a variety of situations, particularly those that occur within the home. The most important factors in preventing exposure to toxic substances are education and information, while the law, regulations, and sanctions provide the highest level of protection. According to Akira et al. (1990), the likelihood of being required to comply with regulations decreases in proportion to the degree to which the general public is well-informed and educated.

9.2. Exposure Guidelines for Prevention of Toxicity

There are multiple organizations that work together to develop recommendations regarding exposure. On the other hand, the kinds of instructions that they generate are comparable (Bellinger et al., 2017).

9.2.1. Time-Weighted Average (TWA)

This exposure is obtained by taking the average of the concentrations of all the exposures, with each concentration being weighted based solely on the amount of time that the exposure was exposed. For instance, Ahmed & Siddiqui (2007) found that an exposure to acetone at all the following concentrations and for the following amount of time:

1,000 ppm for 3 hours 500 ppm for 2 hours

200 ppm for 3 hours would have an 8-hour,

TWA exposure of:

[(3 hrs)(1000 ppm) + (2 hrs)(500 ppm) + (3 hrs)(200 ppm)] / 8 hrs

= [3000 ppm + 1000 ppm + 600 ppm] / 8

= 575 ppm

That exposure would've been contrasted to a TWA limit of 8 hours.

A TWA is the average concentration that is above a particular time. Most TWAs, on the other hand, are the average concentration of the chemical that most workers may be exposed to over the course of a typical eight-hour workday or a forty-hour work week without experiencing any adverse effects. On the other hand, the NIOSH TWA guidelines may be dependent on exposures that last for up to ten hours. The moment average allows for exposure to concentrations that are higher than the limit (Fanni et al., 2014; Figure 9.2). This occurs when exposure at a concentration that is just above the limit is balanced by equivalent exposure to concentrations that are below the limit.

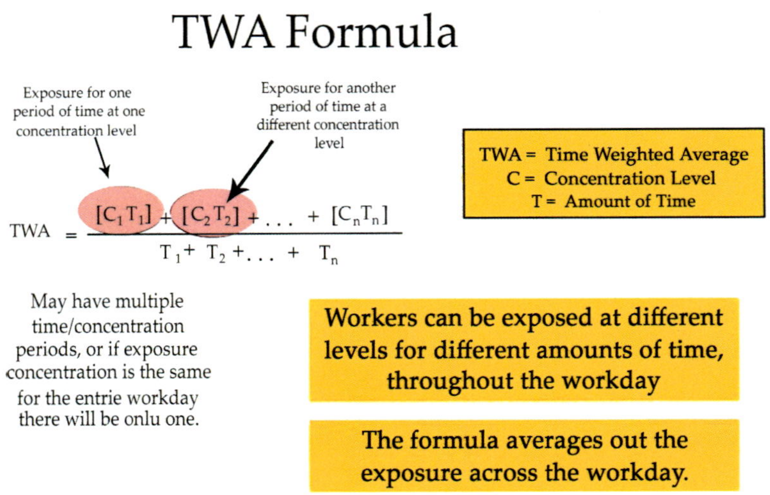

Figure 9.2. *TWA formula.*

Source: https://ehs.unl.edu/documents/tox_exposure_guidelines.pdf.

9.2.2. Short-Term Exposure Limit (STEL)

The TWA permits deviations that may involve extremely high concentrations and have a detrimental impact while still falling within the acceptable range of the average. Several organizations are of the opinion that the number of these trips ought to be restricted. The inclusion of STELs in ACGIH's TLVs occurred in the year 1976 (Bassett et al., 2004).

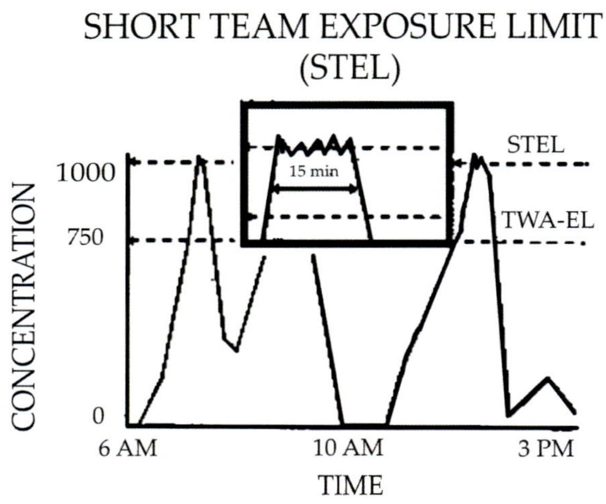

Figure 9.3. *Short-term exposure limit.*

Source: https://ehs.unl.edu/documents/tox_exposure_guidelines.pdf.

The TWA exposure that is known as the STEL lasts for fifteen minutes. A minimum of sixty minutes must pass between each outing to a STEL, there must be a duration of fifteen minutes or more, and there must be at least four outings per day. Since the excursions are incorporated into the 8-hour TWA, the exposure should always be controlled to prevent exceeding the TWA. Figure 9.3 illustrates a dosage that is higher than the 15-minute limit for a STEL of 1,000 ppm (Guidotti & Ragain, 2007).

9.2.3. Ceiling (C)

Chemicals that can cause a rapid and kind of reaction have certain maximum levels that they can reach. It is utilized in situations where a TWA, with its permitted excursions, is not capable of being conducted. An ACGIH and OSHA recommendation states that a maximum value should not be exceeded, even for a short period of time. An ACT that comes before the exposure limit is a representation of a ceiling, which they represent. NIOSH takes into consideration ceiling values as well. On the other hand, their ceiling values are more comparable to a STEL measurement. There are many exposures that have time limits, which can range anywhere from five to sixty minutes. According to Damalas & Koutroubas (2016), Figure 9.4 depicts an exposure that does not go beyond a ceiling limit of 5 parts per million.

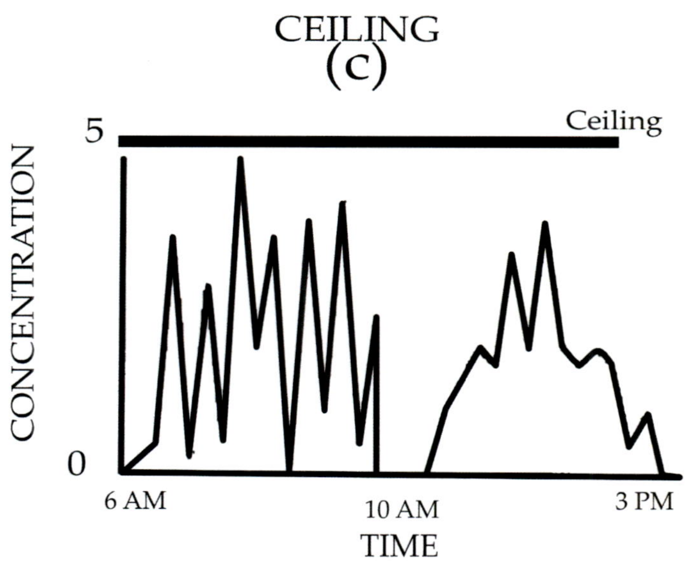

Figure 9.4. *The exposure that does not exceed a ceiling value of 5 ppm.*

Source: https://ehs.unl.edu/sop/tox_exposure_guidelines.pdf.

9.2.4. Peaks

The American National Standards Institute (ANSI), the Occupational Safety and Health Administration (OSHA), and ANSI had previously utilized a maximum exposure limit. This maximum exposure represents the maximum conceivable departure from their ceiling values. This maximum value places limitations on both the duration of exposures and the number of exposures. The American National Standards Institute (ANSI) claims that the benzene limit value of 25 parts per million (ppm) could be exceeded to 50 ppm for ten minutes within eight hours. It was in 1982 when the American National Regulations Institute (ANSI) decided to abandon its occupational exposure compliance standards. During the revision of the PELs in 1989, most OSHA's peaks were removed (Sutton et al., 2012).

9.2.5. Immediately Dangerous to Life or Health (IDLH)

According to the National Institute of Occupational Safety and Health's Respirator Decision Logic report from May 1987, an IDLH is defined as a state that "provides a danger of exposure to airborne pollutants when such exposure is likely to cause death or instant or delayed persistent ill-health consequences or the prohibition of escape from such an environment." A worker should be able to leave a hazardous workplace if their respiratory protection fails (Silbergeld, 1990). This is the objective of determining an IDLH exposure threshold.

IDLH has been defined in the same manner by the Mine Safety and Health Administration (MSHA), the American National Standards Institute (ANSI), and the Occupational Safety and Health Administration (OSHA). Each of these organizations agrees that IDLH circumstances include not only dangerous levels of pollutants but also oxygen-deficient environments, explosive, and near-explosive situations (beyond, at, or around the lowest detection limits) (Watson et al., 2003). There is also a lack of oxygen in the environment.

9.3. Application of Exposure Guidelines

According to the rule known as "Harmful Waste Operations and Urgent Response" (29 CFR 1910.120), the utilization of specific exposure limits is required. The declared exposure limits are the permissible and "published exposure levels" exposure limits (PLEs) made by the Occupational Safety and Health Administration (OSHA). In situations where a PEL is not available, the "published exposure limits" are utilized as an alternative. It is defined as "the exposure limits specified in 'NIOSH Guidelines for Employee Health Guidelines' dated 1986 incorporated by reference." This is the definition of the "published exposure limit." Even though there are no exposure limits specified, the exposure limits that are found in the book Threshold Value Values and Biological Sensitivity Indices published by the American Council of Governmental Industrial Hygienists will be utilized (Watson et al., 2006).

9.3.1. Engineered Controls and Work Practices

"Engineering controls, as well as working conditions, shall be implemented to decrease and retain workers' exposure to below the allowable limits for materials regulated by 29 CFR Part 1910, to the extent necessary by Subpart Z, other than to the large extent that kind control systems and procedures aren't feasible," according to 29 CFR 1910. Workers' exposure must be kept below the allowable limits for materials regulated by 29 CFR Part 1910.120 grams) (1) I (Italics added) It is necessary to make use of personal protective equipment (PPE) to reduce and maintain exposures in situations where control activities and working conditions are not feasible (Woskie, 2010).

If there is no PEL for a drug or hazard, the documented exposure levels, established literature, and material safety data sheets (MSDS) will be utilized to evaluate it. It is necessary to implement a combination of engineering controls, work practices, and personal protective equipment (PPE) to reduce and maintain exposures (Gerberding, 1993).

9.3.2. Personal Protective Equipment

This exposure limit is being used to evaluate the

effectiveness of personal protective equipment (PPE) because it is necessary to select it based on the dangers that are present at the location. Depending on the results of a comparison between the actual or projected exposure and a PEL or even other exposure limits, the wearer may decide which personal protective equipment (PPE) to use (Schulte et al., 2008).

9.3.3. Medical Surveillance

The 29 CFR 1910.120(f)(2)(i) mandates the implementation of a medical monitoring program for all personnel who are exposed to chemicals or dangers that exceed the PEL for a period of thirty days or more than once per year. For the purpose of assessing the situation, the published exposure values are utilized if there is no PEL. Even in situations where a mask was only worn during the time of exposure, exposure is still taken into consideration (Leso et al., 2019).

9.4. Limitations/Restrictions of Exposure Guideline Use

A combination of industry experience, experimental human research, and animal experimental studies served as the foundation for the exposure recommendations that are presented in this section. Members of the workforce working in the industrial environment were the intended recipients of the recommendations. As a consequence of this, they should not be useful for any other purpose. According to the ACGIH's Thresholds Permissible Limits and Biological Exposure Indexes for 1992–1993 (Daniell et al., 2002), these limits have been destined to be used in the exercise of occupational health as guidance or suggestions inside the regulation of potential health risks for no other purpose, such as evaluating or controlling community poor air quality nuisances, predicting the potential toxicity of continuous, undisrupted exposures or other working extended periods, as evidence or refutation of an associated disease or physical state, or implementation by states whose workplace environments vary from the United States. These limits are not precise lines between acceptable and harmful concentrations, nor are they a relative measure of toxicity, and they should not be utilized by anyone who is not skilled in occupational safety (Iavicoli et al., 2019). Rather, they are a relative measure of toxicity.

Any application of the exposure guidelines as a relative indicator of toxicity falls under the category of having certain limitations. This is because the exposure limits for different substances are based on the effects of particular substances. To prevent irritation of the eyesight and respiratory problems, for instance, the TLV-TWA of acetone was chosen as the appropriate concentration. To reduce the likelihood of developing cancer, the TLV-TWA for acrylonitrile was chosen. The exposure of these substances to higher concentrations may result in additional consequences. Consequently, when determining the level of risk associated with chemical exposure, it is necessary to take into account all of the toxicological information (Baker et al., 1994).

9.5. Legislation and Regulation

In its most fundamental form, the legislation functions as an act that has been passed, defining the segments of the economy that are to be protected by law and the general way they are controlled. Additionally, it designates an executive agency with the responsibility of developing and implementing specific rules that are in line with the objective of the governmental body. For instance, the Toxic Substances Control Act (TSCA) was enacted by Congress to regulate the introduction of chemicals into the market, assess the risks that these chemicals pose to both people and the environment, and either restrict or outright ban those chemicals that are deemed to be harmful. It was the responsibility of the Environmental Protection Agency (EPA) to formulate and carry out the implementation of specific regulations. It is not uncommon for legislators to be unsuccessful in their efforts to enshrine restrictions in legislation. They lacked versatility and rarely dealt with the issues in a rigorous scientific manner (Methner et al., 2010). This was since solicitors, rather than toxicologists, were responsible for the design of the laws.

Remember that the law is the result of a combination of research, political pressure, and pressure from both the government and non-government organizations. This is an important point to keep in mind. Within the context of the public interest, this is an evaluation of the risks that it is willing to accept to prevent them, as well as the costs that it is willing to pay at that moment in time. Such decisions should be based on more than just scientific evidence. It is the responsibility of the toxicologist to ensure that the scientific information is accurate and clearly understood. This is, in many respects, a complicated jumble of overlapping rules and jurisdictions that places an unnecessary burden on the legal industry and causes it to exert unnecessary effort. At the same time, there are very few, if any, hazardous dangers that are not addressed within the home, industry, or environment (Cristini et al., 2003).

9.6. Prevention of Toxicity at Home

Young students are responsible for nearly half of all deaths that occur because of accidental poisoning in the United States. (Eastlake et al., 2012) (Figure 9.5) As a consequence of this, toxicity avoidance is of utmost importance in households that contain minors.

1. It is imperative that you always store prescription medications in their original packaging. In the United States of America and a few other countries, it is now mandatory for the packaging to have safety closures. These should be used by the individual for the medication that they were prescribed, and any medications that are left over after the disease has been completely eradicated should be disposed of in a careful manner. When children are present, prescription medications should be kept in a cabinet that is locked; there are some cabinets that are impossible for a child to open, even if they are determined to do so. It is common practice to flavor nonprescription medications in an appealing manner, even though these medications are typically less hazardous. Because of this, it is necessary to adhere to the same guidelines that are applicable to the use of prescription medications (Amyotte et al., 2009).
2. Chemicals that are used in the home, such as lye, polish, and gasoline, should be kept in closed storage if possible; if this is not possible, then these chemicals should be kept in a secure location that is as far away from children as is possible. When it comes to storing substances of this nature, we should only use the appropriate container. It is completely unacceptable to store them in glass bottles, kitchen containers, or any other containers of a similar nature. Items that have not been used should be disposed of

in a careful manner at facilities that are designated for disposal (Hackman, 1978).

3. It is important to ensure that adequate ventilation is present when performing several tasks around the house, such as decorating the interior. Insecticide treatment must be carried out in a manner that is fully consistent with the instructions provided on the label.

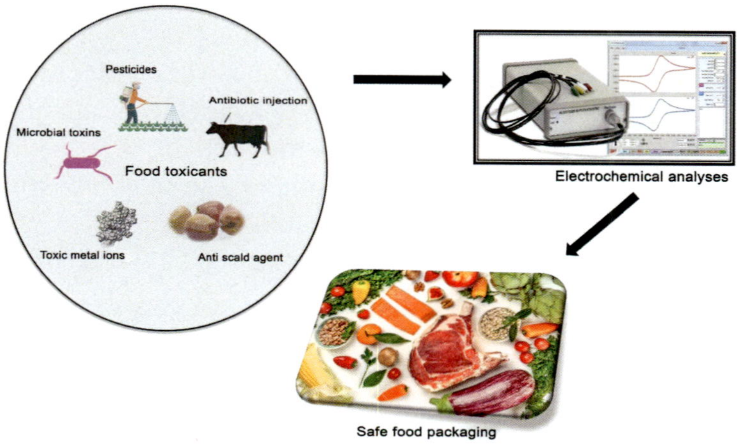

Figure 9.5. *Methods for reducing toxicity at home.*

Source: Raja, I. S., Vedhanayagam, M., Preeth, D. R., Kim, C., Lee, J. H., & Han, D. W., (2021). Development of two-dimensional nanomaterials based electrochemical biosensors on enhancing the analysis of food toxicants. *International Journal of Molecular Sciences*, 22(6), 3277. https://doi.org/10.3390/ijms22063277.

The rise in the cost of fuel has led to a number of changes in lifestyle, some of which may be associated with the risk of some adverse consequences. The use of more firewood and coal for combustion, as well as the construction of homes that are well-insulated and have less ventilation, are several of these factors. In the latter scenario, furnaces that are burned improperly may produce large quantities of carbon monoxide (CO) or aromatic hydrocarbons. On the other hand, furnaces that are burned correctly can produce oxides of nitrogen (NOx) at levels that are high enough to irritate the respiratory tracts of individuals who are sensitive to such chemical substances. For the purpose of preventing these impacts, it is imperative that all thermal equipment, including heaters, wood-burning stoves, and heaters, be properly vented, maintained, and inspected on a regular basis. Furthermore, it is imperative that the building always has adequate ventilation. However, when the temperature is in the middle range, the homeowner should never attempt to produce a sealed home (Thompson, 2017). This is because the amount of ventilation that is required decreases when the temperature is too high or too low, and increases when the temperature is too low.

9.7. Prevention at the Workplace

Workplaces are required to comply with OSHA's exposure limit levels for hazardous substances that are present in the air. NIOSH is the organization that is responsible for conducting the necessary research to determine these levels. On the other hand, the American Conference of Governmental Industrial Hygienists (ACGH) is responsible for keeping a more exhaustive list of well-known threshold permissible limits (TLVs). In spite of the fact that they are not legally binding, TLVs provide employers with valuable guidance. However, in practice, OSHA frequently employs them as exposure limit values. These are the weighted concentrations that are generally considered to be safe for an exposure that occurs for eight hours per day, five days per week. Absolute higher bounds, also known as excursion values, are another option that can be considered. According to Salin (2008), Table 9.1 illustrates a number of exposure limits. It is common practice to implement environmental control measures to maintain concentrations at or below those of regular or occupational exposures whenever possible. Large-scale operations that generate a significant amount of dust or fumes are carried out in enclosed facilities that are equipped with vents or that are located beneath hoods. There is adequate ventilation in other areas, and humidity and temperature controls are installed in accordance with the requirements (Loomis et al., 2002).

Table 9.1. *Threshold Limit Values in a Few Cases*

Chemical	TLV-TWA (ppm)	TLV-STEL[b] (ppm)	TLV-C[c] (ppm)
Acetaldehyde	100	150	–
Boron trifluoride	–	–	1
o-Dichlorobenzene	–	–	50
p-Dichlorobenzene	75	110	–
N-Ethylmorpholine	5	20	–
Fluorine	1	2	–
Phosgene	0.1	–	–
Trichloroethylene	50	200	–

Source: (Marras & Karwowski, 2006)

To prevent concentrations from increasing by accident or on a consistent basis, additional strategies are required. The material must be transported in containers that are "safe," any spilled material must be cleaned up as soon as possible, and the materials used for the floor and walls should be selected to prevent contamination and make cleaning easier (Bryan Jr., 1990).

The use of personal safety equipment, the most important of which are protective gear, gloves, and goggles, is yet another method for preventing the presence of toxic substances in the workplace. It is possible that jobs that are extremely hazardous will require the use of closed-circuit air masks, respirators, and other types of protective equipment (Johnson, 2015).

Pre-employment training and physical examinations are required for most job assignments that involve the handling of hazardous materials. The earlier should make it abundantly clear what the risks are, why it is necessary to minimize exposure in regular working situations, and what the measures are for limiting exposure. It is also important for workers to be aware of when to manage spills, as well as when and how to evacuate the area where the spill occurred. It is important to provide the location and procedures for emergency supplies, showers, eye washes, and other processes, with the procedures that are most pertinent to the workspace being highlighted (Berry & Mirabito, 2011; Hills & Joyce, 2013).

9.8. Prevention from Pollution of Air, Water, and Land

There is a possibility that environmental contamination could be toxicologically significant as a result of employment, such as in the form of agricultural laborers, or as a result of the environments that people encounter in their day-to-day lives. Toxicology is something that agricultural laborers should avoid experiencing at all costs. For example:

1. When storing insecticides and other agrochemicals, make sure to keep them in their original containers and label them with the information that is required by either the EPA or the FIFRA.
2. Waste containers and surplus chemicals are required to be disposed of in an appropriate manner in special locations designated for the management of hazardous waste, burned if it is possible, or decontaminated in certain circumstances.
3. Before returning to the treatment area, workers are required to wait until after a reasonable amount of time has passed.
4. Certain employees, such as those who apply the substance and those who prepare the mixture for the tank, are required to wear protective clothing, gloves, and masks, among other protective gear. The development of closed solutions for combining pesticides as a means of protecting pesticide mixing and loader from exposure is currently underway.
5. Activities involving spraying should be carried out in a way that reduces the risk of drift, water pollution, and other kinds of problems.

Over the course of history, pesticides have been the cause of a significant number of fatalities. According to Artiola et al. (2019), the current practice in several countries of restricting the use of the most hazardous chemicals to only authorized operators should result in a significant reduction in the exposure of these regions to the toxic effects of pesticides.

It is possible for individuals to take no action to protect themselves from chemical exposure in the water and air, unless they demand that toxicants be discharged into the air in the least amount possible. In comparison to the levels of exposure that are present in situations of acute toxicity, the levels of exposure are relatively low, and the consequences may be indirect, such as an increase in the inflammation that is already present in the airways when smog is present. Because of this, the only way to assess these effects is through an epidemiologic perspective. Some people believe that environmental pollution is unimportant because many people are not harmed by it, or because they may not have been affected by it for hundreds of years.

In the context of the entire population, a relatively small percentage increase might be indicative of a significant number of people. However, chronic toxicity is not always reversible in its effects. As a result of the fact that most developed nations already have regulations in place to address emission issues, the occurrence of such issues in such countries is primarily due to a lack of enforcement (Hilson, 2000).

When it comes to preventing the toxicity that is caused by pollution, one of the most important areas to focus on is the dumping of waste. Historical practices in many developed nations have resulted in many waste sites, where garbage is frequently misidentified, inadequately kept, and leaches into the environment. This is made abundantly clear by the fact that the situation has become so widespread. It is only now that efforts are being made to address the enormous challenge of rectifying errors that have been made in the past (Rondinelli & Berry, 2000).

The ideal situation for both existing practices and those that will be implemented in the future is to reduce harmful byproducts to the absolute minimum and then protect the ones that remain. It is possible to reduce waste in several different ways (De Koning, 1981).

1. Improve the operating procedures of the factory to produce less waste. You can turn waste into valuable goods through recycling.
2. Collect and sort different types of garbage.
3. Cause to burn. Present-day technology allows for the incineration of virtually all waste, resulting in the production of artificial slag. It is unfortunate that the technology is both cutting-edge and expensive. Inappropriate incineration poses a threat to the environment because it has the potential to release dioxins and other toxic substances into the atmosphere for the first time. They need to be less complicated and easier to maintain if incinerators are going to play a significant role in the reduction of trash.

9.9. Education

Education is likely the most effective method for avoiding toxicity because chemicals, the majority of which are hazardous, are an unavoidable component of life in developed nations. There is no way to avoid exposure to chemicals. To our great regret, it is one of the things that is least appreciated. The primary protagonists in a typical public debate about the possibility of a chemical threat fell into two distinct camps regarding their positions. The main characters who have the belief that "everything will be okay" and those who have the belief that "ban it entirely." According to Geake (2008), the press does not appear to educate the audience very often, but rather it seems to be fueling the fire. It is the responsibility of the toxicologist to serve as a voice of reason, providing a fair evaluation of the advantages and disadvantages of the substance in question and, whenever possible, describing alternative courses of action. According to Peters (2010), it is essential for all parties involved to have a fundamental understanding of the fact that science deals with levels of certainty rather than absolute certainty. In every level of education—middle school, high school, university, continuing education, and multimedia education—there should be opportunities for students to participate in continuing education programs. When conditions are ideal, there are a variety of approaches that can be utilized to educate the community (Dewey, 1986):

A Closer Look

Toxicity of (NOx)

Nitrogen oxides (NOx), primarily comprising nitrogen dioxide (NO_2) and nitric oxide (NO), are significant environmental pollutants with considerable implications for both human health and ecosystems. These gases are produced through combustion processes, such as those occurring in vehicles and industrial activities. NO_2, in particular, is known for its toxic effects, as it can irritate the respiratory system, leading to conditions such as asthma, bronchitis, and reduced lung function. Chronic exposure to NOx can exacerbate pre-existing respiratory diseases and compromise overall lung health. In addition to its direct health impacts, NOx contributes to the formation of ground-level ozone and fine particulate matter (PM2.5), which further aggravate respiratory conditions and cardiovascular diseases. Beyond human health, NOx emissions play a role in environmental degradation by contributing to acid rain, which can damage forests, soil, and water bodies. Acid rain results from the interaction of NOx with atmospheric moisture, leading to the formation of nitric acid, which can leach nutrients from the soil and harm aquatic life. Additionally, NOx can contribute to the formation of smog, reducing air quality and visibility. Mitigating NOx emissions is crucial for protecting public health and the environment. Strategies include adopting cleaner technologies, improving fuel efficiency, and implementing stricter emission standards for industrial and transportation sources. Addressing NOx pollution requires a comprehensive approach that considers both emission reductions and the promotion of sustainable practices to minimize its harmful effects.

Summary

- Prevention and mitigation of toxicity are essential strategies to protect public health and the environment from the adverse effects of toxic substances. These approaches encompass a wide range of actions, policies, and technologies aimed at minimizing exposure and reducing the impact of toxic agents.
- Prevention focuses on avoiding the introduction of toxic substances into the environment and reducing human exposure. This proactive approach involves the identification of hazardous chemicals and their potential health risks. Key prevention strategies include the use of safer alternatives through green chemistry, which aims to design products and processes that reduce or eliminate the use and generation of hazardous substances. Regulatory measures also play a crucial role in prevention, with agencies such as the EPA enforcing strict guidelines to control chemical use and manage waste. Additionally, public and occupational health initiatives promote best practices in handling chemicals, enhancing safety in workplaces and communities.
- Mitigation, on the other hand, deals with reducing the severity of toxic effects after exposure has occurred. This includes emergency responses like decontamination and medical treatments such as antidotes. Long-term mitigation may involve environmental cleanup and remediation efforts to restore contaminated sites, thereby reducing ongoing exposure risks. Educational programs are also vital, providing training and information to the public and professionals on how to respond to and manage toxicity effectively.
- Both strategies require integrated efforts across multiple sectors, including government, industry, academia, and the community. By implementing stringent regulations, encouraging safer chemical practices, and fostering a culture of safety and awareness, it is possible to significantly diminish the risks posed by toxic substances. These efforts not only protect individual health but also preserve environmental integrity for future generations.

References

1. Abdelfattah, A., Ali, S. S., Ramadan, H., El-Aswar, E. I., Eltawab, R., Ho, S. H., Elsamahy, T., Li, S., El-Sheekh, M. M., Schagerl, M., et al. (2022). Microalgae-based wastewater treatment: Mechanisms, challenges, recent advances, and future prospects. *Environmental Science and Ecotechnology, 13*, 100205. https://doi.org/10.1016/j.ese.2021.100205.
2. Al Hossain, M. M. A., Yajima, I., Tazaki, A., Xu, H., Saheduzzaman, M., Ohgami, N., Ahsan, N., Akhand, A. A., & Kato, M. (2019). Chromium-mediated hyperpigmentation of skin in male tannery workers in Bangladesh. *Chemosphere, 229*, 611–617. https://doi.org/10.1016/j.chemosphere.2019.04.187.
3. Al-Tohamy, R., Ali, S. S., Li, F., Okasha, K. M., Mahmoud, Y. A. G., Elsamahy, T., Jiao, H., Fu, Y., & Sun, J. (2022). A critical review on the treatment of dye-containing wastewater: Ecotoxicological and health concerns of textile dyes and possible remediation approaches for environmental safety. *Ecotoxicology and Environmental Safety, 231*, 113160. https://doi.org/10.1016/j.ecoenv.2021.113160.
4. Ali, H., Khan, E., & Ilahi, I. (2019). Environmental chemistry and ecotoxicology of hazardous heavy metals: Environmental persistence, toxicity, and bioaccumulation. *Journal of Chemistry, 2019*, 1–14. https://doi.org/10.1155/2019/6730305.
5. Ali, S. S., Abdelkarim, E. A., Elsamahy, T., Al-Tohamy, R., Li, F., Kornaros, M., Zuorro, A., Zhu, D., & Sun, J. (2023). Bioplastic production in terms of life cycle assessment: A state-of-the-art review. *Environmental Science and Ecotechnology, 15*, 100254. https://doi.org/10.1016/j.ese.2022.100254.
6. Ali, S. S., El-Sheekh, M., Manni, A., Ruiz, H. A., Elsamahy, T., Sun, J., & Schagerl, M. (2022). Microalgae-mediated wastewater treatment for biofuels production: A comprehensive review. *Microbiological Research, 265*, 127187. https://doi.org/10.1016/j.micres.2022.127187.
7. Ali, S. S., Elsamahy, T., Abdelkarim, E. A., Al-Tohamy, R., Kornaros, M., Ruiz, H. A., Zhao, T., Li, F., & Sun, J. (2022). Biowastes for biodegradable bioplastics production and end-of-life scenarios in circular bioeconomy and biorefinery concept. *Bioresource Technology, 363*, 127869. https://doi.org/10.1016/j.biortech.2022.127869.
8. Amadou, A., Praud, D., Coudon, T., Danjou, A. M. N., Faure, E., Deygas, F., Grassot, L., Leffondré, K., Severi, G., Salizzoni, P., et al. (2021). Exposure to airborne cadmium and breast cancer stage, grade and histology at diagnosis: Findings from the E3N cohort study. *Scientific Reports, 11*, 23088. https://doi.org/10.1038/s41598-021-02621-7.
9. Anyanwu, B., Ezejiofor, A., Igweze, Z., & Orisakwe, O. (2018). Heavy metal mixture exposure and effects in developing nations: An update. *Toxics, 6*(4), 65. https://doi.org/10.3390/toxics6040065.
10. Baszuk, P., Janasik, B., Pietrzak, S., Marciniak, W., Reszka, E., Białkowska, K., Jabłońska, E., Muszyńska, M., Lesicka, M., Derkacz, R., et al. (2021). Lung cancer occurrence-correlation with serum chromium levels and genotypes. *Biological Trace Element Research, 199*(4), 1228–1236. https://doi.org/10.1007/s12011-020-02299-7.
11. Büyüköztürk, S., Gelincik, A., Ünal, D., Demirtürk, M., Çelik, D. D., Erden, S., Çolakoğlu, B., & Kuruca, S. E. (2015). Oral nickel exposure may induce type I hypersensitivity reaction in

nickel-sensitized subjects. *International Immunopharmacology, 26*(1), 92–96. https://doi.org/10.1016/j.intimp.2015.02.016.

12. Chakraborty, R., Renu, K., Eladl, M. A., El-Sherbiny, M., Elsherbini, D. M. A., Mirza, A. K., Vellingiri, B., Iyer, M., Dey, A., & Valsala Gopalakrishnan, A. (2022). Mechanism of chromium-induced toxicity in lungs, liver, and kidney and their ameliorative agents. *Biomedicine and Pharmacotherapy, 151*, 113119. https://doi.org/10.1016/j.biopha.2022.113119.
13. Charkiewicz, A. E., & Backstrand, J. R. (2020). Lead toxicity and pollution in Poland. *International Journal of Environmental Research and Public Health, 17*(12), 4385. https://doi.org/10.3390/ijerph17124385.
14. Chen, S. Y., Wu, J. Q., & Sung, S. (2022). Effects of sulfur dosage on continuous bioleaching of heavy metals from contaminated sediment. *Journal of Hazardous Materials, 424*, 127257. https://doi.org/10.1016/j.jhazmat.2021.127257.
15. Chen, X., Li, Y., Zhang, B., Zhou, A., Zheng, T., Huang, Z., Pan, X., Liu, W., Liu, H., Jiang, Y., et al. (2018). Maternal exposure to nickel in relation to preterm delivery. *Chemosphere, 193*, 1157–1163. https://doi.org/10.1016/j.chemosphere.2017.11.121.
16. Dehghan, S. F., Mehrifar, Y., & Ardalan, A. (2019). The relationship between exposure to lead-containing welding fumes and the levels of reproductive hormones. *Annals of Global Health, 85*(1), 125. https://doi.org/10.5334/aogh.2594.
17. Deng, Y., Wang, M., Tian, T., Lin, S., Xu, P., Zhou, L., Dai, C., Hao, Q., Wu, Y., Zhai, Z., et al. (2019). The effect of hexavalent chromium on the incidence and mortality of human cancers: A meta-analysis based on published epidemiological cohort studies. *Frontiers in Oncology, 9*, 24. https://doi.org/10.3389/fonc.2019.00024.
18. Duffus, J. H. (2002). “Heavy metals” a meaningless term? (IUPAC technical report). *Pure and Applied Chemistry, 74*(5), 793–807. https://doi.org/10.1351/pac200274050793.
19. Farzan, S. F., Howe, C. G., Chen, Y., Gilbert-Diamond, D., Korrick, S., Jackson, B. P., Weinstein, A. R., & Karagas, M. R. (2021). Prenatal and postnatal mercury exposure and blood pressure in childhood. *Environment International, 146*, 106201. https://doi.org/10.1016/j.envint.2020.106201.
20. Fergusson, J. E. (1990). *The Heavy Elements: Chemistry, Environmental Impact and Health Effects* (Vol. 614). Pergamon Press.
21. Genchi, G., Carocci, A., Lauria, G., Sinicropi, M. S., & Catalano, A. (2020). Nickel: Human health and environmental toxicology. *International Journal of Environmental Research and Public Health, 17*(3), 679. https://doi.org/10.3390/ijerph17030679.
22. Jacob, J. M., Karthik, C., Saratale, R. G., Kumar, S. S., Prabakar, D., Kadirvelu, K., & Pugazhendhi, A. (2018). Biological approaches to tackle heavy metal pollution: A survey of literature. *Journal of Environmental Management, 217*, 56–70. https://doi.org/10.1016/j.jenvman.2018.03.078.
23. Joseph, S. J., Arunachalam, K. D., Murthy, P. B., Ramalingam, R., & Musthafa, M. S. (2021). Uranium induces genomic instability and slows cell cycle progression in human lymphocytes in acute toxicity study. *Toxicology in Vitro, 73*, 105149. https://doi.org/10.1016/j.tiv.2021.105149.
24. Kahlson, M. A., & Dixon, S. J. (2022). Copper-induced cell death. *Science, 375*, 1231–1232. https://doi.org/10.1126/science.abm6561.
25. Kang, P., Shin, H. Y., & Kim, K. Y. (2021). Association between dyslipidemia and mercury

exposure in adults. *International Journal of Environmental Research and Public Health, 18*, 775. https://doi.org/10.3390/ijerph18020775.

26. Koutra, E., Mastropetros, S. G., Ali, S. S., Tsigkou, K., & Kornaros, M. (2021). Assessing the potential of *Chlorella vulgaris* for valorization of liquid digestates from agro-industrial and municipal organic wastes in a biorefinery approach. *Journal of Cleaner Production, 280*, 124352. https://doi.org/10.1016/j.jclepro.2020.124352.
27. Kumar, L., & Bharadvaja, N. (2020). Microbial remediation of heavy metals. In *Microbial Bioremediation & Biodegradation* (pp. 139–165). Springer. https://doi.org/10.1007/978-981-15-4106-3_7.
28. Kumar, V., & Dwivedi, S. K. (2021). Bioremediation mechanism and potential of copper by actively growing fungus *Trichoderma lixii* CR700 isolated from electroplating wastewater. *Journal of Environmental Management, 277*, 111370. https://doi.org/10.1016/j.jenvman.2020.111370.
29. Lee, S., Cho, S. R., Jeong, I., Park, J. B., Shin, M. Y., Kim, S., & Kim, J. H. (2020). Mercury exposure and associations with hyperlipidemia and elevated liver enzymes: A nationwide cross-sectional survey. *Toxics, 8*(3), 47. https://doi.org/10.3390/toxics8030047.
30. Li, R., Wu, H., Ding, J., Fu, W., Gan, L., & Li, Y. (2017). Mercury pollution in vegetables, grains and soils from areas surrounding coal-fired power plants. *Scientific Reports, 7*, 46545. https://doi.org/10.1038/srep46545.
31. Mitra, S., Chakraborty, A. J., Tareq, A. M., Emran, T. B., Nainu, F., Khusro, A., Idris, A. M., Khandaker, M. U., Osman, H., Alhumaydhi, F. A., et al. (2022). Impact of heavy metals on the environment and human health: Novel therapeutic insights to counter the toxicity. *Journal of King Saud University–Science, 34*, 101865. https://doi.org/10.1016/j.jksus.2021.101865.
32. Nakhaee, S., Amirabadizadeh, A., Brent, J., & Mehrpour, O. (2018). Impact of chronic lead exposure on liver and kidney function and hematologic parameters. *Basic & Clinical Pharmacology & Toxicology, 124*(6), 621–628. https://doi.org/10.1111/bcpt.13078.
33. Negahdari, S., Sabaghan, M., Pirhadi, M., Alikord, M., Sadighara, P., Darvishi, M., & Nazer, M. (2021). Potential harmful effects of heavy metals as a toxic and carcinogenic agent in marine food-an overview. *Egyptian Journal of Veterinary Science, 52*(3), 379–385. https://doi.org/10.21608/ejvs.2021.208689.
34. Niu, Y., Zhang, Y., Zhu, Z., Zhang, X., Liu, X., Zhu, S., Song, Y., Jin, X., Lindholm, B., & Yu, C. (2020). Elevated intracellular copper contributes a unique role to kidney fibrosis by lysyl oxidase mediated matrix crosslinking. *Cell Death & Disease, 11*, 211. https://doi.org/10.1038/s41419-020-2396-6.
35. Obeng-Gyasi, E., Ferguson, A. C., Stamatakis, K. A., & Province, M. A. (2021). Combined effect of lead exposure and allostatic load on cardiovascular disease mortality—A preliminary study. *International Journal of Environmental Research and Public Health, 18*, 6879. https://doi.org/10.3390/ijerph18136879.
36. Papadopoulou, E., Botton, J., Caspersen, I. H., Alexander, J., Eggesbø, M., Haugen, M., Iszatt, N., Jacobsson, B., Knutsen, H. K., Meltzer, H. M., et al. (2021). Maternal seafood intake during pregnancy, prenatal mercury exposure and child body mass index trajectories up to 8 years. *International Journal of Epidemiology, 50*(4), 1134–1146. https://doi.org/10.1093/ije/dyaa259.
37. Peng, Y., Hu, J., Li, Y., Zhang, B., Liu, W., Li, H., Zhang, H., Hu, C., Chen, X., Xia, W., et al.

(2018). Exposure to chromium during pregnancy and longitudinally assessed fetal growth: Findings from a prospective cohort. *Environment International, 121*, 375–382. https://doi.org/10.1016/j.envint.2018.09.054.

38. Redvers, N., Chischilly, A. M., Warne, D., Pino, M., & Lyon-Colbert, A. (2021). Uranium exposure in American Indian communities: Health, policy, and the way forward. *Environmental Health Perspectives, 129*(8), 085002. https://doi.org/10.1289/EHP8142.
39. Rehman, A. U., Nazir, S., Irshad, R., Tahir, K., ur Rehman, K., Islam, R. U., & Wahab, Z. (2021). Toxicity of heavy metals in plants and animals and their uptake by magnetic iron oxide nanoparticles. *Journal of Molecular Liquids, 321*, 114455. https://doi.org/10.1016/j.molliq.2020.114455.
40. Sarker, A., Al Masud, M. A., Deepo, D. M., Das, K., Nandi, R., Ansary, M. W. R., Islam, A. R. M. T., & Islam, T. (2023). Biological and green remediation of heavy metal contaminated water and soils: A state-of-the-art review. *Chemosphere, 332*, 138861. https://doi.org/10.1016/j.chemosphere.2023.138861.
41. Sears, C. G., Poulsen, A. H., Eliot, M., Howe, C. J., James, K. A., Harrington, J. M., Roswall, N., Overvad, K., Tjønneland, A., Raaschou-Nielsen, O., et al. (2021). Urine cadmium and acute myocardial infarction among never smokers in the Danish diet, cancer and health cohort. *Environment International, 150*, 106428. https://doi.org/10.1016/j.envint.2021.106428.
42. Sundseth, K., Pacyna, J., Pacyna, E., Pirrone, N., & Thorne, R. (2017). Global sources and pathways of mercury in the context of human health. *International Journal of Environmental Research and Public Health, 14*(1), 105. https://doi.org/10.3390/ijerph14010105.
43. Surdyk, S., Itani, M., Al-Lobaidy, M., Kahale, L. A., Farha, A., Dewachi, O., Akl, E. A., & Habib, R. R. (2021). Weaponized uranium and adverse health outcomes in Iraq: A systematic review. *BMJ Global Health, 6*, e004166. https://doi.org/10.1136/bmjgh-2020-004166.
44. Tchounwou, P. B., Yedjou, C. G., Patlolla, A. K., & Sutton, D. J. (2012). Heavy metal toxicity and the environment. *Experientia Supplementum, 101*, 133–164. https://doi.org/10.1007/978-3-7643-8340-4_6.
45. Teixeira, F. B., de Oliveira, A. C. A., Leão, L. K. R., Fagundes, N. C. F., Fernandes, R. M., Fernandes, L. M. P., da Silva, M. C. F., Amado, L. L., Sagica, F. E. S., de Oliveira, E. H. C., et al. (2018). Exposure to inorganic mercury causes oxidative stress, cell death, and functional deficits in the motor cortex. *Frontiers in Molecular Neuroscience, 11*, 125. https://doi.org/10.3389/fnmol.2018.00125.
46. Titcomb, T. J., Liu, B., Lehmler, H., Snetselaar, L. G., & Bao, W. (2021). Environmental nickel exposure and diabetes in a nationally representative sample of US adults. *Exposure and Health, 13*(4), 697–704. https://doi.org/10.1007/s12403-020-00367-7.
47. Tvrda, E., Peer, R., Sikka, S. C., & Agarwal, A. (2015). Iron and copper in male reproduction: A double-edged sword. *Journal of Assisted Reproduction and Genetics, 32*(1), 3–16. https://doi.org/10.1007/s10815-014-0380-2.
48. Verma, S., Bhatt, P., Verma, A., Mudila, H., Prasher, P., & Rene, E. R. (2021). Microbial technologies for heavy metal remediation: Effect of process conditions and current practices. *Clean Technologies and Environmental Policy, 25*(38), 1–23. https://doi.org/10.1007/s10098-021-02029-8.

49. Vijayakumar, V., Abern, M. R., Jagai, J. S., & Kajdacsy-Balla, A. (2021). Observational study of the association between air cadmium exposure and prostate cancer aggressiveness at diagnosis among a nationwide retrospective cohort of 230,540 patients in the United States. *International Journal of Environmental Research and Public Health, 18*(16), 8333. https://doi.org/10.3390/ijerph18168333.

50. Wang, T., Zhang, J., & Xu, Y. (2020). Epigenetic basis of lead-induced neurological disorders. *International Journal of Environmental Research and Public Health, 17*(13), 4878. https://doi.org/10.3390/ijerph17134878.

51. Wang, X., Dai, X., Shi, C., Wan, J., Silver, M. A., Zhang, L., Chen, L., Yi, X., Chen, B., Zhang, D., et al. (2019). A 3,2-hydroxypyridinone-based decorporation agent that removes uranium from bones in vivo. *Nature Communications, 10*, 2570. https://doi.org/10.1038/s41467-019-10452-3.

52. Wang, X., Wu, Y., Sun, X., Guo, Q., Xia, W., Wu, Y., Li, J., Xu, S., & Li, Y. (2021). Arsenic exposure and metabolism in relation to blood pressure changes in pregnant women. *Ecotoxicology and Environmental Safety, 222*, 112527. https://doi.org/10.1016/j.ecoenv.2021.112527.

53. Witt, B., Stiboller, M., Raschke, S., Friese, S., Ebert, F., & Schwerdtle, T. (2021). Characterizing effects of excess copper levels in a human astrocytic cell line with focus on oxidative stress markers. *Journal of Trace Elements in Medicine and Biology, 65*, 126711. https://doi.org/10.1016/j.jtemb.2021.126711.

54. Wu, C., Li, F., Yi, S., & Ge, F. (2021). Genetically engineered microbial remediation of soils co-contaminated by heavy metals and polycyclic aromatic hydrocarbons: Advances and ecological risk assessment. *Journal of Environmental Management, 296*, 113185. https://doi.org/10.1016/j.jenvman.2021.113185.

55. Xia, B., Yuan, J., Pang, L., & He, K. (2022). Chromium [Cr (VI)] exposure causes cytotoxicity of human bronchial epithelial cells (16-HBE) and proteomic alterations. *International Journal of Toxicology, 41*(3), 225–233. https://doi.org/10.1177/10915818221104094.

56. Yan, L. J., & Allen, D. C. (2021). Cadmium-induced kidney injury: Oxidative damage as a unifying mechanism. *Biomolecules, 11*(11), 1575. https://doi.org/10.3390/biom11111575.

57. Yang, H., Liu, C. N., Wolf, R. M., Ralle, M., Dev, S., Pierson, H., Askin, F., Steele, K. E., Magnuson, T. H., Schweitzer, M. A., et al. (2019). Obesity is associated with copper elevation in serum and tissues. *Metallomics, 11*(8), 1363–1371. https://doi.org/10.1039/c9mt00122j.

58. Yu, M., & Zhang, J. (2017). Serum and hair nickel levels and breast cancer: Systematic review and meta-analysis. *Biological Trace Element Research, 179*(1), 32–37. https://doi.org/10.1007/s12011-017-0962-y.

59. Zhou, C. C., He, Y. Q., Gao, Z. Y., Wu, M. Q., & Yan, C. H. (2020). Sex differences in the effects of lead exposure on growth and development in young children. *Chemosphere, 250*, 126294. https://doi.org/10.1016/j.chemosphere.2020.126294.

INDEX

MIX
Papier | Fördert gute Waldnutzung
FSC® C083411

Kolibri 360 GmbH
Ferdinand-Jühlke-Straße 7
99095 Erfurt, Deutschland
produktsicherheit@kolibri360.de